Hepatitis C Infection as a Systemic Disease: Extra-Hepatic Manifestation of Hepatitis C

Editor

ZOBAIR M. YOUNOSSI

CLINICS IN LIVER DISEASE

www.liver.theclinics.com

Consulting Editor
NORMAN GITLIN

August 2017 • Volume 21 • Number 3

ELSEVIER

1600 John F. Kennedy Boulevard • Suite 1800 • Philadelphia, Pennsylvania, 19103-2899

http://www.theclinics.com

CLINICS IN LIVER DISEASE Volume 21, Number 3
August 2017 ISSN 1089-3261, ISBN-13: 978-0-323-53239-6

Editor: Kerry Holland
Developmental Editor: Meredith Madeira

Clinics in Liver Disease (ISSN 1089-3261) is published quarterly by Elsevier Inc., 360 Park Avenue South, New York, NY 10010-1710. Months of issue are February, May, August, and November. Business and Editorial Offices: 1600 John F. Kennedy Blvd., Ste. 1800, Philadelphia, PA 19103-2899. Customer Service Office: 3251 Riverport Lane, Maryland Heights, MO 63043. Periodicals postage paid at New York, NY and additional mailing offices. Subscription prices are $281.00 per year (U.S. individuals), $100.00 per year (U.S. student/resident), $476.00 per year (U.S. institutions), $403.00 per year (international individuals), $200.00 per year (international student/resident), $590.00 per year (international instituitions), $347.00 per year (Canadian individuals), $200.00 per year (Canadian student/resident), and $590.00 per year (Canadian institutions). Foreign air speed delivery is included in all *Clinics* subscription prices. All prices are subject to change without notice. **POSTMASTER:** Send address changes to *Clinics in Liver Disease*, Elsevier Health Sciences Division, Subscription Customer Service, 3251 Riverport Lane, Maryland Heights, MO 63043. **Customer Service: Telephone: 1-800-654-2452 (U.S. and Canada); 314-447-8871 (outside U.S. and Canada). Fax: 314-447-8029. E-mail: journalscustomer service-usa@elsevier.com (for print support); journalsonlinesupport-usa@elsevier.com (for online support).**

Reprints. For copies of 100 or more of articles in this publication, please contact the Commercial Reprints Department, Elsevier Inc., 360 Park Avenue South, New York, NY 10010-1710. Tel.: 212-633-3874; Fax: 212-633-3820; E-mail: reprints@elsevier.com.

Clinics in Liver Disease is covered in *MEDLINE/PubMed (Index Medicus)*, Science Citation Index Expanded, Journal Citation Reports/Science Edition, and Current Contents/Clinical Medicine.

Contributors

CONSULTING EDITOR

NORMAN GITLIN, MD, FRCP (LONDON), FRCPE (EDINBURGH), FAASLD, FACP, FACG
Formerly, Professor of Medicine, Chief of Hepatology, Emory University, Currently, Consultant, Atlanta Gastroenterology Associates, Atlanta, Georgia

EDITOR

ZOBAIR M. YOUNOSSI, MD, MPH, FACG, FACP, AGAF, FAASLD
Chairman, Department of Medicine and Center for Liver Diseases, Inova Fairfax Hospital Vice President for Research, Inova Health System Professor of Medicine, Inova Campus Betty and Guy Beatty Center for Integrated Research, Falls Church, Virginia

AUTHORS

LUIGI ELIO ADINOLFI, MD
Department of Medicine, Surgery, Neurology, Metabolism, and Aging Sciences, University of Study of Campania "Luigi Vanvitelli", Naples, Italy

NEZAM H. AFDHAL, MD, DSc
Division of Gastroenterology and Hepatology, Beth Israel Deaconess Medical Center, Boston, Massachusetts

ALESSIO AGHEMO, MD, PhD
A.M. and A. Migliavacca Center for Liver Disease, Division of Gastroenterology and Hepatology, Fondazione IRCCS CA' Granda Ospedale Maggiore Policlinico, Università degli Studi di Milano, Milan, Italy

AIJAZ AHMED, MD
Division of Gastroenterology and Hepatology, Stanford University School of Medicine, Palo Alto, California

MAYA BALAKRISHNAN, MD, MPH
Section of Gastroenterology and Hepatology, Department of Medicine, Baylor College of Medicine, Houston, Texas

HALEY BUSH, MSPH
Betty and Guy Beatty Center for Integrated Research, Inova Health System, Inova Fairfax Hospital, Falls Church, Virginia

PATRICE CACOUB, MD
Inflammation-Immunopathology-Biotherapy Department, Sorbonne Universités, INSERM, CNRS, Department of Internal Medicine and Clinical Immunology, AP-HP, Groupe Hospitalier Pitié-Salpêtrière, Paris, France

MICHELE COLACI, MD
Assistant Professor, Rheumatology Unit, University of Modena and Reggio Emilia, Azienda Ospedaliero-Universitaria Policlinico di Modena, Modena, Italy

MASSIMO COLOMBO, MD
Professor, Humanitas Clinical and Research Center, Rozzano, Italy

CLOÉ COMARMOND, MD, PhD
Inflammation-Immunopathology-Biotherapy Department, Sorbonne Universités, INSERM, CNRS, Department of Internal Medicine and Clinical Immunology, AP-HP, Groupe Hospitalier Pitié-Salpêtrière, Paris, France

MICHAEL P. CURRY, MD
Division of Gastroenterology and Hepatology, Beth Israel Deaconess Medical Center, Boston, Massachusetts

ELISABETTA DEGASPERI, MD
A.M. and A. Migliavacca Center for Liver Disease, Division of Gastroenterology and Hepatology, Fondazione IRCCS CA' Granda Ospedale Maggiore Policlinico, Università degli Studi di Milano, Milan, Italy

ANNE CLAIRE DESBOIS, MD
Inflammation-Immunopathology-Biotherapy Department, Sorbonne Universités, INSERM, CNRS, Department of Internal Medicine and Clinical Immunology, AP-HP, Groupe Hospitalier Pitié-Salpêtrière, Paris, France

JEAN-FRANÇOIS DUFOUR, MD
Professor, Division of Hepatology, Department of Visceral Surgery and Medicine, Bern University Hospital, Bern, Switzerland

FREBA FARHAT, MD
Department of Medicine, Center for Liver Disease, Inova Fairfax Hospital, Falls Church, Virginia

CLODOVEO FERRI, MD
Professor and Chair, Rheumatology Unit, University of Modena and Reggio Emilia, Azienda Ospedaliero-Universitaria Policlinico di Modena, Modena, Italy

VALTER GATTEI, MD
Chief of the Clinical and Experimental Onco-Hematology Unit, Centro di Riferimento Oncologico, I.R.C.C.S., Aviano, Italy

LYNN H. GERBER, MD
Betty and Guy Beatty Center for Integrated Research, Inova Health System, Department of Medicine, Center for Liver Disease, Inova Fairfax Hospital, Falls Church, Virginia

MAURO GIORDANO, MD
Department of Medicine, Surgery, Neurology, Metabolism, and Aging Sciences, University of Study of Campania "Luigi Vanvitelli", Naples, Italy

DILIA GIUGGIOLI, MD
Assistant Professor, Rheumatology Unit, University of Modena and Reggio Emilia, Azienda Ospedaliero-Universitaria Policlinico di Modena, Modena, Italy

MATTHEW T. GLOVER, MD
Section of Gastroenterology and Hepatology, Department of Medicine, Baylor College of Medicine, Houston, Texas

PEGAH GOLABI, MD
Betty and Guy Beatty Center for Integrated Research, Inova Health System, Inova Fairfax Hospital, Falls Church, Virginia

NICOLAS GOOSSENS, MD, MSc
Division of Gastroenterology and Hepatology, Geneva University Hospitals, Geneva, Switzerland

SENTIA IRIANA, MD
Division of Gastroenterology and Hepatology, Beth Israel Deaconess Medical Center, Boston, Massachusetts

FASIHA KANWAL, MD
Section of Gastroenterology and Hepatology, Department of Medicine, Baylor College of Medicine, Department of Medicine, Houston Veterans Affairs Health Services Research and Development Center for Innovations in Quality, Effectiveness and Safety, Michael E. DeBakey Veterans Affairs Medical Center, Houston, Texas

CESARE MAZZARO, MD
Clinical and Experimental Onco-Hematology Unit, Centro di Riferimento Oncologico, I.R.C.C.S., Aviano, Italy

FRANCESCO NEGRO, MD
Divisions of Gastroenterology and Hepatology and Clinical Pathology, Geneva University Hospitals, Geneva, Switzerland

RICCARDO NEVOLA, MD
Department of Medicine, Surgery, Neurology, Metabolism, and Aging Sciences, University of Study of Campania "Luigi Vanvitelli", Naples, Italy

GABRIELE POZZATO, MD
Associate Professor of Blood Diseases, Department of Medicine, Surgery and Health Sciences, University of Trieste, Trieste, Italy

LUCA RINALDI, MD
Department of Medicine, Surgery, Neurology, Metabolism, and Aging Sciences, University of Study of Campania "Luigi Vanvitelli", Naples, Italy

CIRO ROMANO, MD
Department of Medicine, Surgery, Neurology, Metabolism, and Aging Sciences, University of Study of Campania "Luigi Vanvitelli", Naples, Italy

SAMMY SAAB, MD, MPH
Departments of Medicine and Surgery, David Geffen School of Medicine, University of California at Los Angeles, Los Angeles, California

DAVID SAADOUN, MD, PhD
Inflammation-Immunopathology-Biotherapy Department, Sorbonne Universités, INSERM, CNRS, Department of Internal Medicine and Clinical Immunology, AP-HP, Groupe Hospitalier Pitié-Salpêtrière, Paris, France

MEHMET SAYINER, MD
Betty and Guy Beatty Center for Integrated Research, Inova Health System, Department of Medicine, Center For Liver Disease, Inova Fairfax Hospital, Falls Church, Virginia

DANIEL SEGNA, MD
Department of General Internal Medicine, Bern University Hospital, Bern, Switzerland

LAWRENCE SERFATY, MD
Hepatology Department, INSERM, APHP, Saint-Antoine Hospital, Paris, France

MARIA STEPANOVA, PhD
Center for Outcomes Research in Liver Diseases, Washington, DC; Betty and Guy Beatty Center for Integrated Research, Inova Health System, Inova Fairfax Hospital, Falls Church, Virginia

, MD, MS
Clinical Professor of Medicine, Director of Research and Education, Division of Gastroenterology and Hepatology, Alameda Health System–Highland Hospital, Oakland, California

ZOBAIR M. YOUNOSSI, MD, MPH, FACG, FACP, AGAF, FAASLD
Chairman, Department of Medicine and Center for Liver Diseases, Inova Fairfax Hospital Vice President for Research, Inova Health System Professor of Medicine, Inova Campus Betty and Guy Beatty Center for Integrated Research, Falls Church, Virginia

Contents

It is critical to recognize that hepatitis C virus (HCV) infection is, in fact, a multifaceted systemic disease with both hepatic and extrahepatic complications. It is also important to recognize that the comprehensive burden of HCV should include not only its clinical burden but also its burden on th economic and patient-reported outcomes. It is only through this compr hensive approach to HCV infection that we can fully appreciate its tru burden and understand the full benefit of curing HCV for the patient and the society.

Hepatitis C virus (HCV) infection is associated with a morbidity and mortality due to liver complications. HCV infection is also frequently associated with rheumatic disorders, such as arthralgia, myalgia, cryoglobulinemia vasculitis, and sicca syndrome, as well as the production of autoantibodies. The treatment of HCV infection with interferon alpha (IFN) has been contraindicated for a long time in many rheumatologic autoimmune/inflammatory disorders. New oral IFN-free combinations offer an opportunity for HCV-infected patients with extrahepatic manifestations, including rheumatologic autoimmune/inflammatory disorders, to be cured with a short treatment duration and a low risk of side effects.

Hepatitis C virus (HCV) infection is a prevalent condition associated with numerous extrahepatic manifestations. Epidemiologic studies have found that HCV is associated with increased cardiovascular morbidity and mortality, in particular with carotid atherosclerosis, cerebrovascular events, and coronary heart disease. The mechanisms involved encompass a chronic systemic inflammatory state, insulin resistance, and a potential, direct infection of the vascular endothelium. Sustained virologic response with interferon-based regimens is associated with reduced cardiovascular events, although this must be validated with newer direct-acting antivirals. This clear association between HCV and cardiovascular events may have significant economical and public health implications.

Metabolic disorders are common in patients with chronic hepatitis C virus (HCV) infection. Epidemiologic and clinical data indicate an overprevalence of lipids abnormalites, steatosis, insuline resistance (IR) and diabetes mellitus in HCV patients, suggesting that HCV itself may interact with glucido-lipidic metabolism. HCV interacts with the host lipid metabolism by several mechanisms leading to hepatic steatosis and hypolipidemia which are reversible after viral eradication. Liver and peripheral IR are HCV genotype/viral load dependent and improved after viral eradication. This article examines the relationship between HCV, lipid abnormalities, steatosis, IR, and diabetes and the pathogenic mechanisms accounting for these events in HCV-infected patients.

Hepatitis C virus (HCV) is a hepatotropic and lymphotropic virus responsible for hepatic and extrahepatic autoimmune and neoplastic disorders, including renal involvement, which is the consequence of immune-mediated organ damage due to glomerular deposition of immune-complex and/or anti-HCV IgG antibodies and complement. It can appear at any time during the natural history of HCV infection, more often as membranoproliferative glomerulonephritis, alone or in association with other HCV-related disorders. The presence of renal involvement should be investigated in HCV-infected individuals at the first referral and during clinical follow-up.

Eradication of hepatitis C virus (HCV) in indolent non-Hodgkin lymphomas (NHLs), especially in marginal zone lymphomas, determines the regression of the hematologic disorder in a significant fraction of cases. Because direct antiviral agents show an excellent profile in terms of efficacy, safety, and rapid onset of action, these drugs can be used in any clinical situation and in the presence of any comorbidities. To avoid the progression of the NHL, despite HCV eradication, antiviral therapy should be provided as soon as the viral infection is discovered; before that, the chronic antigenic stimulation determines the irreversible proliferation of neoplastic B cells.

Hepatitis C virus (HCV) infection is a systemic disease with hepatic and extrahepatic manifestations, including neuropsychiatric conditions. Depression is a frequent disorder, which has been reported in one-third of patients with HCV infection and has an estimated prevalence of 1.5 to

4.0 times higher than that observed in patients with chronic hepatitis B virus infection or the general population. HCV seems to play a direct and indirect role in the development of depression. Impaired quality of life and increasing health care costs have been reported for patients with HCV infection with depression. Treatment-induced HCV clearance has been associated with improvement of depression and quality of life.

The extrahepatic manifestations of hepatitis C include effects on the central nervous system, which have been associated with the ability of hepatitis C virus (HCV) to replicate in microglial and endothelial cells and the chronic inflammation induced by HCV. HCV can induce impaired neurocognition, which is clinically manifested by impaired quality of life, fatigue, and brain fog. These cognitive defects can be present even in patients with mild histologic HCV and have been confirmed by neurocognitive testing and brain imaging by magnetic resonance spectroscopy. Neurocognitive defects include loss of functioning memory and subtle changes in attention and processing speed.

Epidemiologic studies show an increased risk of mortality among hepatitis C virus (HCV)-infected individuals compared with uninfected individuals from hepatic and nonhepatic causes. This article reviews the biologic plausibility of and epidemiologic evidence for the association between HCV and five extrahepatic malignancies: cholangiocarcinoma (CCA), pancreatic adenocarcinoma, papillary thyroid cancer, oral squamous cell cancer, and renal/kidney cancer. There is sufficient evidence to suggest that HCV is associated with intrahepatic CCA. The evidence for the link between HCV and pancreatic adenocarcinoma, oral squamous cell cancer, and renal/kidney cancer is compelling but requires further study. Based on available studies, there is no significant association between HCV, extrahepatic CCA, and papillary thyroid cancer.

Chronic hepatitis C virus (HCV) infection is associated with various extrahepatic manifestations, including dermatologic involvement mostly caused by immune complexes. Mixed cryoglobulinemia has a strong relationship with HCV with 95% of these patients being infected with HCV. Lichen planus is a disease of the squamous epithelium and may affect any part of the skin, with 4% to 24% of patients with lichen planus reported to have chronic HCV infection. Porphyria cutanea tarda is the most common form of porphyria, and it is thought that HCV interferes with iron stores, which can promote porphyria cutanea tarda. Finally, necrolytic acral erythema is a rare, psoriasis-like disease closely associated with HCV.

Fatigue is a common symptom. Diagnosis is difficult. Fatigue is often a complex symptom. In the recent years, fatigue has gained considerable amount of attention. It has 2 major types, central and peripheral, which may occur together or alone. Although fatigue has many strong relations with depression and sleep disorders, it is a separate entity. For the diagnosis of fatigue, self-reports and patient-reported outcomes are highly valuable tools because these methods can reflect patients' perceptions. Treating the underlying disease with newly developed direct-acting antivirals often improves the perceived fatigue. Healthy lifestyle changes are the cornerstone of the treatment.

The economic burden of chronic hepatitis C might exceed $10 billion annually in the United States alone. This disease has a worldwide prevalence of up to 3%, making the global burden of the disease comparably tremendous. The cost of the disease includes direct medical expenses for its hepatic and extrahepatic manifestations, and also indirect costs incurred from impaired quality of life and the loss of work productivity. Recent emergence of treatment options that are not only highly effective and safe but also costly has emphasized the need to study the disease from the economic point of view.

Chronic hepatitis C virus (HCV) infection remains a leading cause of chronic liver disease in the United States. Although the hepatic impact of chronic HCV leading to cirrhosis and the need for liver transplantation is paramount, the extrahepatic manifestations of chronic HCV infection are equally important. In particular, a better understanding of the prevalence and impact of extrahepatic manifestations of chronic HCV infection in the post-liver transplant setting relies on understanding the interplay between the effects of chronic HCV infection in a posttransplant environment characterized by strong immunosuppression and the associated risks of this milieu.

Extrahepatic manifestations of hepatitis C virus (HCV) infection are a rare but serious condition. This article summarizes the current literature on the association between HCV and endocrine and pulmonary manifestations, as well as idiopathic thrombocytopenic purpura (ITP). HCV may directly infect extrahepatic tissues and interact with the immune system predisposing for obstructive and interstitial lung disease, ITP, autoimmune thyroiditis, infertility, growth hormone and adrenal deficiencies, osteoporosis, and potentially lung and thyroid cancers. However, in many cases, the current evidence is divergent and cannot sufficiently confirm a true association, which emphasizes the need for future targeted projects in this field.

Elisabetta Degasperi, Alessio Aghemo, and Massimo Colombo

Chronic infection with hepatitis C virus (HCV) is a multifaceted disease characterized by many extrahepatic manifestations (EHMs) that affect outcome and quality of life. HCV eradication by antiviral treatment has been proved beneficial in preventing the development of EHMs and is also able to improve many HCV-related severe disorders and neurocognitive outcomes and quality of life. Until recently, antiviral therapy of EHMs was limited to the presence of interferon-based treatment, and was contraindicated in many patients because of hematologic toxicity or risk of exacerbating immune-mediated disorders. The availability of interferon-free regimens solves this issue allowing for enhanced safety and efficacy to provide universal treatment of HCV-related EHMs.

CLINICS IN LIVER DISEASE

THE CLINICS ARE AVAILABLE ONLINE!
Access your subscription at:
www.theclinics.com

Preface

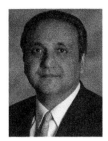

Zobair M. Younossi, MD, MPH, FACG, AGAF, FAASLD
Editor

The discovery of hepatitis C virus (HCV) in 1989 was the culmination of years of scientific efforts to identify one of the most challenging causes of chronic liver disease, the so-called non-A, non-B hepatitis. Following this discovery, efforts in the next decades focused on accurately diagnosing HCV infection, quantifying the amount of virus in the blood, determining HCV genotypes, clarifying its natural history, identifying its economic burden, and developing curative treatment regimens. In this context, the liver disease related to HCV infection has always been at the centerpiece of these efforts. Nevertheless, there is increasing evidence that HCV infection is a systemic infection with important clinical, economic, and patient-reported outcomes. Furthermore, it is now fully recognized that the clinical consequences of HCV infection include both hepatic and extrahepatic manifestations. In this issue of *Clinics in Liver Disease*, the nonhepatic, the patient-centered, and the economic consequences of HCV infection are reviewed in detail by an international group of experts. The main purpose of this issue of *Clinics in Liver Disease* is to raise awareness about the multifaceted aspects of HCV infection leading to hepatic, extrahepatic, economic, and patient-reported outcomes (PROs).

Zobair M. Younossi, MD, MPH, FACG, AGAF, FAASLD
Department of Medicine
Inova Fairfax Hospital
Inova Health System
Inova Campus
Beatty Center for Integrated Research
3300 Gallows Road
Falls Church, VA, 22042, USA

E-mail address:
zobair.younossi@inova.org

Clin Liver Dis 21 (2017) xiii
http://dx.doi.org/10.1016/j.cld.2017.05.001
1089-3261/17/© 2017 Published by Elsevier Inc.

liver.theclinics.com

Hepatitis C Infection

A Systematic Disease

 CrossMark

Zobair M. Younossi, MD, MPH[a,b,*]

KEYWORDS

- Hepatitis C virus • Hepatic complications • Extrahepatic complications

KEY POINTS

- It is critical to recognize that hepatitis C virus (HCV) infection is a multifaceted systemic disease with both hepatic and extrahepatic complications.
- The comprehensive burden of HCV should not only include its clinical burden, but also its burden on the economic and patient-reported outcomes.
- It is only through this comprehensive approach to HCV infection that we can fully appreciate its true burden, and understand the full benefit of curing HCV for the patient and the society.

Currently, it is estimated that approximately 170 million individuals carry hepatitis C virus (HCV) antibody worldwide, with more than 40% of the infected individuals living in the Asian countries.[1–8] The global distribution of HCV genotype also can vary by geography. Genotype 1 (GT1) is the predominant genotype in the United States, Europe, Australia, and Japan, whereas genotype 3 (GT3) is more common in Pakistan and genotype 4 (GT4) is the predominant HCV genotype in Egypt and North Africa.[4,8,9]

Although approximately 25% of acute HCV infection is self-limiting, 75% of these infections become chronic. This rate of chronicity can be affected by a number of factors, including the age at time of infection, gender, ethnicity, and the development of jaundice at the onset of acute infection.[2,3,5–7]

Of patients who are chronically infected with HCV, liver disease is the most common and important complication. In this context, the rate of progression to cirrhosis can also vary by geographic location. In the United States and Europe, the rate of progression to cirrhosis is approximately 15% (range 8%–24%) over 20 to 30 years with approximately 1% to 4% annual incidence of hepatocellular carcinoma

Disclosure: Dr. Z.M. Younossi has received research funding or consultation fees from BMS, Gilead, Intercept, GSK and Allergan.
[a] Betty and Guy Beatty Center for Integrated Research, Inova Health System, 3300 Gallows Road, Falls Church, VA 22042, USA; [b] Department of Medicine, Center for Liver Disease, Inova Fairfax Hospital, 3300 Gallows Road, Falls Church, VA 22042, USA
* Corresponding author. Betty and Guy Beatty Center for Integrated Research, Inova Health System, 3300 Gallows Road, Falls Church, VA 22042.
E-mail address: zobair.younossi@inova.org

(HCC).[10–17] In contrast, the rate of HCV progression to cirrhosis in Japan is higher, ranging from 30% to 46% with approximately 5% to 7% annual incidence of HCC.[18] It has been recognized that a number of host factors can influence the rate of liver disease progression in HCV, including older age, male gender, coinfection with human immunodeficiency virus or hepatitis B virus, and comorbid conditions, such as immunosuppression and insulin resistance as well as superimposed nonalcoholic steatohepatitis, hemochromatosis, and schistosomiasis.[19–24] In addition to the host factors, a number of external factors can also negatively impact the progression of HCV-related liver disease. In this context, chronic alcohol use is an important factor for the progression of chronic hepatitis C to cirrhosis and hepatocellular carcinoma.[25]

As liver disease progresses, patients with HCV can develop hepatic decompensation, leading to increased liver-related mortality.[18] The cumulative probability of an episode of hepatic decompensation is 5% at year 1, increasing to 30% at 10 years from the time of diagnosis of cirrhosis. The development of gastroesophageal varices and other signs of advanced liver disease are associated with an additive increase in the risk for mortality.[5,6,26,27] After development of decompensated cirrhosis, the 5-year survival of patients with HCV can be as low as 50%.[27] On the other hand, 3-year, 5-year, and 10-year survival rates of patients with HCV with compensated cirrhosis is estimated to be 96%, 91%, and 79%, respectively.[28–30]

Although hepatic complications of HCV infection are the primary drivers of its clinical and economic burden, a number of extrahepatic manifestations (EHMs) of HCV also can influence its clinical and economic outcomes.[31–34] The EHMs of HCV infection can be divided into those that are strongly associated with HCV and those that are possibly associated.[31–34] Unlike the large amount of data that have been published about HCV-related liver disease, our understanding of the underlying mechanisms for the EHMs of HCV and factors that contribute to their progression or regression are more limited.

In addition to the hepatic manifestations and EHMs, chronic HCV infection impairs a number of important patient-reported outcomes (PROs). These PROs can be accurately captured through the use of validated instruments for health-related quality of life and fatigue.[35–43]

Finally, the clinical (both hepatic and extrahepatic) and PRO manifestations of HCV can lead to substantial economic burden. Some of this burden is directly related to the clinical cost associated with caring for the liver and nonliver complications of patients with HCV infections.[44,45] Additionally, there are a number of important indirect economic burdens of HCV, especially those related to work productivity losses and other societal costs.[46–56]

In summary, it is critical to recognize that HCV infection is, in fact, a multifaceted systemic disease with both hepatic and extrahepatic complications. It is also important to recognize that the comprehensive burden of HCV should not only include its clinical burden but also its burden on the economic outcomes and PROs. It is only through this comprehensive approach to HCV infection that we can fully appreciate its true burden and understand the full benefit of curing HCV for the patient and the society.

REFERENCES

1. Williams IT, Bell BP, Kuhnert W, et al. Incidence and transmission patterns of acute hepatitis C in the United States, 1982-2006. Arch Intern Med 2011; 171(3):242–8.

2. Alter MJ, Margolis HS, Krawczynski K, et al. The natural history of community-acquired hepatitis C in the United States. The sentinel counties chronic non-A, non-B hepatitis study team. N Engl J Med 1992;327(27):1899–905.

3. Purcell RH, Walsh JH, Holland PV, et al. Seroepidemiological studies of transfusion-associated hepatitis. J Infect Dis 1971;123:406–13.

4. Gower E, Estes C, Blach S, et al. Global epidemiology and genotype distribution of the hepatitis C virus infection. J Hepatol 2014;61(1 Suppl):S45–57.

5. Hajarizadeh B, Grebely J, Dore GJ. Epidemiology and natural history of HCV infection. Nat Rev Gastroenterol Hepatol 2013;10(9):553–62.

6. Leone N, Rizzetto M. Natural history of hepatitis C virus infection: from chronic hepatitis to cirrhosis, to hepatocellular carcinoma. Minerva Gastroenterol Dietol 2005;51(1):31–46.

7. Westbrook RH, Dusheiko G. Natural history of hepatitis C. J Hepatol 2014;61(1 Suppl):S58–68.

8. Messina JP, Humphreys I, Flaxman A, et al. Global distribution and prevalence of hepatitis C virus genotypes. Hepatology 2015;61(1):77–87.

9. Liakina V, Hamid S, Tanaka J, et al. Historical epidemiology of hepatitis C virus (HCV) in select countries. J Viral Hepat 2015;22(Suppl 4):4–20.

10. Zalesak M, Francis K, Gedeon A, et al. Current and future disease progression of the chronic HCV population in the United States. PLoS One 2013;8(5):e63959.

11. Castells L, Vargas V, Gonzalez A, et al. Long interval between HCV infection and development of hepatocellular carcinoma. Liver 1995;15(3):159–63.

12. Donato F, Boffetta P, Puoti M. A meta-analysis of epidemiological studies on the combined effect of hepatitis B and C virus infections in causing hepatocellular carcinoma. Int J Cancer 1998;75(3):347–54.

13. Gordon SC, Bayati N, Silverman AL. Clinical outcome of hepatitis C as a function of mode of transmission. Hepatology 1998;28(2):562–7.

14. Younossi Z, Park H, Henry L, et al. Extrahepatic manifestations of hepatitis C: a meta-analysis of prevalence, quality of life, and economic burden. Gastroenterology 2016;150(7):1599–608.

15. Younossi ZM, Tanaka A, Eguchi Y, et al. The impact of hepatitis C virus outside the liver: evidence from Asia. Liver Int 2017;37(2):159–72.

16. Younossi ZM, Birerdinc A, Henry L. Hepatitis C infection: a multi-faceted systemic disease with clinical, patient reported and economic consequences. J Hepatol 2016;65(1 Suppl):S109–19.

17. Fattovich G, Stroffolini T, Zagni I, et al. Hepatocellular carcinoma in cirrhosis: incidence and risk factors. Gastroenterology 2004;127:S35–50.

18. Lee MH, Yang HI, Lu SN, et al, R.E.V.E.A.L.-HCV Study Group. Chronic hepatitis C virus infection increases mortality from hepatic and extrahepatic diseases: a community-based long-term prospective study. J Infect Dis 2012;206(4):469–77.

19. Cammà C, Bruno S, Di Marco V, et al. Insulin resistance is associated with steatosis in nondiabetic patients with genotype 1 chronic hepatitis C. Hepatology 2006;43(1):64–71.

20. Ortiz V, Berenguer M, Rayon JM, et al. Contribution of obesity to hepatitis C-related fibrosis progression. Am J Gastroenterol 2002;97(9):2408–14.

21. D'Souza R, Sabin CA, Foster GR. Insulin resistance plays a significant role in liver fibrosis in chronic hepatitis C and in the response to antiviral therapy. Am J Gastroentrol 2005;100(7):1509–15.

22. Calvaruso V, Craxì A. Immunological alterations in hepatitis C virus infection. World J Gastroenterol 2013;19(47):8916–23.

23. Hung CH, Lee CM, Lu SN. Hepatitis C virus-associated insulin resistance: pathogenic mechanisms and clinical implications. Expert Rev Anti Infect Ther 2011; 9(5):525–33.
24. Davis GL, Alter MJ, El-Serag H, et al. Aging of hepatitis C virus (HCV)-infected persons in the United States: a multiple cohort model of HCV prevalence and disease progression. Gastroenterology 2010;138(2):513–21, 521.e1-6.
25. Taylor AL, Denniston MM, Klevens RM, et al. Association of hepatitis C virus with alcohol use among U.S. adults: NHANES 2003-2010. Am J Prev Med 2016;51(2): 206–15.
26. Ly KN, Hughes EM, Jiles RB, et al. Rising mortality associated with hepatitis C virus in the United States, 2003-2013. Clin Infect Dis 2016;62(10):1287–8.
27. D'Amico G, Pasta L, Morabito A, et al. Competing risks and prognostic stages of cirrhosis: a 25-year inception cohort study of 494 patients. Aliment Pharmacol Ther 2014;39(10):1180–93.
28. Fattovich G, Giustina G, Degos F, et al. Morbidity and mortality in compensated cirrhosis type C: a retrospective follow-up study of 384 patients. Gastroenterology 1997;112(2):463–72.
29. Serfaty L, Aumaître H, Chazouillères O, et al. Determinants of outcome of compensated hepatitis C virus-related cirrhosis. Hepatology 1998;27(5): 1435–40.
30. Hu KQ, Tong MJ. The long-term outcomes of patients with compensated hepatitis C virus-related cirrhosis and history of parenteral exposure in the United States. Hepatology 1999;29(4):1311–6.
31. Younossi ZM, Singer ME, Mir HM, et al. Impact of interferon free regimens on clinical and cost outcomes for chronic hepatitis C genotype 1 patients. J Hepatol 2014;60(3):530–7.
32. Cacoub P, Comarmond C, Domont F, et al. Extrahepatic manifestations of chronic hepatitis C virus infection. Ther Adv Infect Dis 2016;3(1):3–14.
33. Petta S, Maida M, Macaluso FS, et al. Hepatitis C virus infection is associated with increased cardiovascular mortality: a meta-analysis of observational studies. Gastroenterology 2016;150:145–55.e4.
34. Domont F, Cacoub P. Chronic hepatitis C virus infection, a new cardiovascular risk factor? Liver Int 2016;36:621–7.
35. Younossi Z, Kallman J, Kincaid J. The effects of HCV infection and management on health-related quality of life. Hepatology 2007;45(3):806–16.
36. Younossi ZM. Chronic liver disease and health-related quality of life. Gastroenterology 2001;120(1):305–7.
37. Afendy A, Kallman JB, Stepanova M, et al. Predictors of health-related quality of life in patients with chronic liver disease. Aliment Pharmacol Ther 2009;30(5): 469–76.
38. Dan AA, Crone C, Wise TN, et al. Anger experiences among hepatitis C patients: relationship to depressive symptoms and health-related quality of life. Psychosomatics 2007;48(3):223–9.
39. Kallman J, O'Neil MM, Larive B, et al. Fatigue and health-related quality of life (HRQL) in chronic hepatitis C virus infection. Dig Dis Sci 2007;52(10):2531–9.
40. Bonkovsky HL, Snow KK, Malet PF, et al, HALT-C Trial Group. Health-related quality of life in patients with chronic hepatitis C and advanced fibrosis. J Hepatol 2007;46(3):420–31.
41. Younossi ZM, Boparai N, Price LL, et al. Health-related quality of life in chronic liver disease: the impact of type and severity of disease. Am J Gastroenterol 2001;96:2199–205.

42. Spiegel BM, Younossi ZM, Hays RD, et al. Impact of hepatitis C on health related quality of life: a systematic review and quantitative assessment. Hepatology 2005;41:790–800.
43. Loria A, Doyle K, Weinstein AA, et al. Multiple factors predict physical performance in people with chronic liver disease. Am J Phys Med Rehabil 2014; 93(6):470–6.
44. Younossi ZM, Jiang Y, Smith NJ, et al. Ledipasvir/sofosbuvir regimens for chronic hepatitis C infection: insights from a work productivity economic model from the United States. Hepatology 2015;61(5):1471–8.
45. Younossi Z, Brown A, Buti M, et al. Impact of eradicating hepatitis C virus on the work productivity of chronic hepatitis C (CH-C) patients: an economic model from five European countries. J Viral Hepat 2016;23(3):217–26.
46. DiBonaventura MD, Wagner JS, Yuan Y, et al. The impact of hepatitis C on labor force participation, absenteeism, presenteeism and non-work activities. J Med Econ 2011;14(2):253–61.
47. Su J, Brook RA, Kleinman NL, et al. The impact of hepatitis C virus infection on work absence, productivity, and healthcare benefit costs. Hepatology 2010; 52(2):436–42.
48. Younossi ZM, Stepanova M, Feld J, et al. Sofosbuvir and velpatasvir combination improves outcomes reported by patients with HCV infection, without or with compensated or decompensated cirrhosis. Clin Gastroenterol Hepatol 2016. http://dx.doi.org/10.1016/j.cgh.2016.10.037.
49. Younossi ZM, Stepanova M, Sulkowski M, et al. Sofosbuvir and ledipasvir improve patient-reported outcomes in patients co-infected with hepatitis C and human immunodeficiency virus. J Viral Hepat 2016;23(11):857–65.
50. Younossi ZM, Stepanova M, Sulkowski M, et al. Ribavirin-free regimen with sofosbuvir and velpatasvir is associated with high efficacy and improvement of patient-reported outcomes in patients with genotypes 2 and 3 chronic hepatitis C: results from astral-2 and -3 clinical trials. Clin Infect Dis 2016;63(8):1042–8.
51. Younossi ZM, Stepanova M, Henry L, et al. An in-depth analysis of patient-reported outcomes in patients with chronic hepatitis C treated with different anti-viral regimens. Am J Gastroenterol 2016;111(6):808–16.
52. Younossi ZM, Stepanova M, Henry L, et al. Association of work productivity with clinical and patient-reported factors in patients infected with hepatitis C virus. J Viral Hepat 2016;23(8):623–30.
53. Younossi ZM, Stepanova M, Feld J, et al. Sofosbuvir/velpatasvir improves patient-reported outcomes in HCV patients: results from ASTRAL-1 placebo-controlled trial. J Hepatol 2016;65(1):33–9.
54. Younossi ZM, Stepanova M, Chan HL, et al. Patient-reported outcomes in Asian patients with chronic hepatitis C treated with ledipasvir and sofosbuvir. Medicine (Baltimore) 2016;95(9):e2702.
55. Younossi ZM, Stepanova M, Nader F, et al. Patient-reported outcomes of elderly adults with chronic hepatitis C treated with interferon- and ribavirin-free regimens. J Am Geriatr Soc 2016;64(2):386–93.
56. Younossi ZM, Stepanova M, Pol S, et al. The impact of ledipasvir/sofosbuvir on patient-reported outcomes in cirrhotic patients with chronic hepatitis C: the SIRIUS study. Liver Int 2016;36(1):42–8.

Rheumatologic Manifestations of Hepatitis C Virus Infection

Patrice Cacoub, MD[a,b,c,d,*], Cloé Comarmond, MD, PhD[a,b,c,d], Anne Claire Desbois, MD[a,b,c,d], David Saadoun, MD, PhD[a,b,c,d]

KEYWORDS

- Hepatitis C (HCV) • Rheumatic disorders • Arthritis • Vasculitis • Arthralgia
- Sicca syndrome

KEY POINTS

- Main rheumatologic manifestations reported with hepatitis C virus (HCV) chronic infection include arthralgia, myalgia, cryoglobulinemia vasculitis, and sicca syndrome.
- Immunologic factors predisposing to develop such manifestations include stimulation of B cells, expansion of B-cell–producing immunoglobulin M with rheumatoid factor activity and of clonal marginal zone, like B cells, and a decrease of regulatory T cells.
- The treatment of HCV infection with interferon alpha has been contraindicated for a long time in many rheumatologic autoimmune/inflammatory disorders.
- New oral interferon-free combinations now offer an opportunity for patients with HCV extrahepatic manifestations, including rheumatologic autoimmune/inflammatory disorders, to be cured with a high efficacy rate and a low risk of side effects.

Approximately 130 to 170 million people are infected with hepatitis C virus (HCV) worldwide. HCV induces tremendous morbidity and mortality mainly due to liver complications (cirrhosis, hepatocellular carcinoma). This chronic viral infection has been also recognized to induce many extrahepatic manifestations and increased

Conflict of Interest: P. Cacoub has received consultancies, honoraria, advisory board, or speakers' fees from Abbvie, AstraZeneca, Bayer, Boehringer Ingelheim, Gilead, GlaxoSmithKline, Janssen, Merck Sharp and Dohme, Pfizer, Roche, Servier, and Vifor. A.C. Desbois has received speakers' fees from Gilead. D. Saadoun has received speakers' fees from Gilead. C. Commarmond has nothing to disclose.
a Inflammation-Immunopathology-Biotherapy Department (DHU i2B), UMR 7211, UPMC Université Paris 06, Sorbonne Universités, Paris F-75005, France; b INSERM, UMR_S 959, Paris F-75013, France; c CNRS, FRE3632, Paris F-75005, France; d Department of Internal Medicine and Clinical Immunology, AP-HP, Groupe Hospitalier Pitié-Salpêtrière, 83 boulevard de l'hôpital, Paris F-75013, France
* Corresponding author. Department of Internal Medicine and Clinical Immunology, AP-HP, Hôpital Pitié-Salpêtrière, 83 boulevard de l'hôpital, Paris F-75013, France.
E-mail address: patrice.cacoub@aphp.fr

Clin Liver Dis 21 (2017) 455–464
http://dx.doi.org/10.1016/j.cld.2017.03.002
1089-3261/17/© 2017 Elsevier Inc. All rights reserved.

HCV-related morbidity and mortality due to cryoglobulinemia vasculitis, B-cell non-Hodgkin lymphoma, arthralgia, myalgia, and sicca syndrome.[1,2] Interferon (IFN) alpha has long been the cornerstone of antiviral combinations in HCV-infected patients with a low rate efficacy and a poor tolerance. In patients infected by HCV and suffering of autoimmune/inflammatory rheumatic diseases, IFN was either contraindicated or reported to induce a flare of the disease. Recently, new direct-acting antiviral (DAA) IFN-free treatments led to HCV cure in most (>90%) patients with a very good safety profile and a short duration (12 weeks). Our review focuses on main rheumatologic diseases associated with chronic HCV infection.

HEPATITIS C VIRUS AND ARTHRALGIA/MYALGIA

Arthralgia is reported in 6% to 20% of HCV-infected patients.[3–5] Arthralgia involves more frequently fingers, knee, and back, and is bilateral and symmetric.[6] Synovitis is usually absent. Arthralgia is more frequent in patients with cryoglobulinemia vasculitis compared with those without vasculitis.[3] The presentation may mimic rheumatoid arthritis. The frequent rheumatoid factor positivity in HCV-infected patients may lead to a misdiagnosis; however, HCV-infected patients do not develop anticyclic citrullinated peptide antibodies (anti-CCP Abs), a feature useful to differentiate both diseases. Smoking and a previous diagnosis of arthritis are independent risk factors for self-reported joint pain (Odds ratio [OR] 5.0 and 4.25, respectively). Myalgia is less common, affecting approximately 2% to 5% of HCV-infected patients.[3,5] Arthritis, unrelated to mixed cryoglobulinemia, is less common (<5% of patient), involving small joints associated with carpal tunnel syndrome and palmar tenosynovitis.

HEPATITIS C VIRUS–RELATED MIXED CRYOGLOBULINEMIA VASCULITIS

Mixed cryoglobulinemia vasculitis (CryoVas) is a small-vessel vasculitis involving mainly the skin, the joints, the peripheral nervous system, and the kidneys.[1,2] Cryoglobulinemia is defined by the presence of circulating immunoglobulins that precipitate at cold temperature and dissolve with rewarming. CryoVas is related to HCV infection in 70% to 80% of cases, mostly associated with a type II immunoglobulin (Ig)M kappa mixed cryoglobulin. Conversely, 50% to 60% of HCV-infected patients produce a mixed cryoglobulin that will lead to a CryoVas in 15% of cases. Main symptoms include asthenia, purpura, arthralgia, myalgia, peripheral neuropathy, and glomerulonephritis.[7,8] Baseline factors associated with a poor prognosis of HCV-CryoVas were the presence of severe liver fibrosis (hazard ratio [HR] 5.31), central nervous system involvement (HR 2.74), kidney involvement (HR 1.91), and heart involvement (HR 4.2).[9] Arthralgia is reported in 40% to 80% of HCV-infected patients positive for a mixed cryoglobulin.[10–12] Joint pains are bilateral, symmetric, and nondeforming and involve mainly the knees and hands, and less commonly the elbows and ankles. A rheumatoid factor (RF) activity is found in 70% to 80% of patients with CryoVas, not correlated with the occurrence of joint disease. Anti-CCP Abs are usually absent in patients with HCV. There is no evidence of joint destruction. Some clinical features might be confusing for clinicians when IFN-based treatment used for HCV led to exacerbation of arthralgia and myalgia.

HEPATITIS C VIRUS AND SICCA SYNDROME

Sicca symptoms of either the mouth or eyes have been reported in 10% to 30% of HCV-infected patients. Conversely, fewer than 5% of patients with a defined Sjögren syndrome (SS) are HCV-positive.[10] In a recent literature review, Younossi and colleagues[13] reported an SS prevalence of 11.9% in patients with HCV (risk ratio 2.29). However, the criteria for SS diagnosis were based on a clinical questionnaire in some studies and were not well detailed. Although sicca symptoms are frequent in HCV-infected patients, a characterized SS defined by the presence of anti-SSA or anti-SSB antibodies and a typical salivary gland histology is uncommon. A large cohort study of patients with a definite SS (1993 international criteria) showed that patients with HCV-associated SS compared with those with a primary form were older, more frequently male individuals, and presented more frequently vasculitis, peripheral neuropathy, and neoplasia. They also had more frequently a positive RF, a cryoglobulinemia, and less frequently anti-SSA or SSB antibodies.[14,15] Of note, only 23% of HCV-associated patients with SS had positive anti-ENA. The possibility of a direct impact of HCV itself on the development of sialadenitis is supported by the detection of HCV-RNA and HCV core antigen in epithelial cells of patients with HCV-associated SS and the development of SS-like exocrinopathy in transgenic mice carrying the HCV envelope genes.[16,17]

HEPATITIS C VIRUS AND FIBROMYALGIA/FATIGUE

In a large prospective study, 19% of 1614 HCV-infected patients fulfilled the main diagnostic criteria of fibromyalgia (fatigue, arthralgia, and myalgia).[3] Fatigue, with or without fibromyalgia, was the most frequent extrahepatic manifestation (35%–67%). Many underlying factors were independently associated with fatigue, such as older age, female gender, the presence of arthralgia/myalgia, and neuropsychological factors. Conversely, there was no link with alcohol consumption, HCV genotype or viral load, the presence of cryoglobulin, and thyroid dysfunction. Of note, after IFN-based treatment, only the group of patients with a sustained virological response showed a benefit impact on fatigue. The benefit of treatment on arthralgia/myalgia was found in approximately 50% of patients, independently of the virological response.

HEPATITIS C VIRUS AND THE PRODUCTION OF AUTOANTIBODIES

The prevalence of circulating autoantibodies is high in patients with chronic HCV infection. This may induce diagnostic difficulties in patients with miscellaneous rheumatic manifestations.[3,10] The most frequent immunologic abnormalities include mixed cryoglobulins (50%–60%), RF activity (40%), and antinuclear (20%–35%), anticardiolipin (10%–15%), antithyroid (10%), and anti–smooth muscle antibodies (7%).[3,18,19] At least one immunologic abnormality is found in up to 53% of HCV-infected patients. The presence of such antibodies (ie, RF, antinuclear, or anticardiolipin) is usually not associated with specific clinical symptoms related to autoimmune disease.[3,20] The most frequent risk factors for the presence of such biological extrahepatic manifestations are the presence of extensive liver fibrosis and older age.[3,19]

UNDERLYING MECHANISMS LEADING TO RHEUMATOLOGIC MANIFESTATIONS IN HEPATITIS C VIRUS–INFECTED PATIENTS

There are multiple immunologic factors predisposing HCV-infected patients to develop CryoVas or other systemic rheumatologic manifestations. Chronic stimulation of B cells by HCV directly modulates B-cell and T-cell function and results in polyclonal activation and expansion of B-cell–producing IgM with RF activity. There is an expansion of clonal $CD21^{-/low}IgM^{+}CD27^{+}$ marginal zone–like B cells,[21] and a decrease of regulatory T cells.[22] In a genome-wide association study, significant associations were identified on chromosome 6.[23] It has been shown a higher percentage of a particular allele of the promoter of the B-cell–activating factor.[24] In contrast, specific virological factors (viral load, genotype) have not yet been identified. Other factors are related to the peripheral blood mononuclear cell infection, including peripheral dendritic cells, monocytes, and macrophages.[25] Persistent viral stimulation enhances expression of lymphomagenesis-related genes, particularly the activation-induced cystidine deaminase, which is critical for somatic hypermutation and could lead to polyclonal and later monoclonal expansion of B cells.[26] Under this trigger effect, oligoclonal or monoclonal IgM, which shares rheumatoid activity, is produced by a permanent clone of B cells, which favors the appearance of immune-complexes, formed by circulating HCV, anti-HCV polyclonal IgG, and the monoclonal IgM itself.

IMPACT OF HEPATITIS C VIRUS INFECTION ON RHEUMATOLOGIC DISEASES

Studies analyzing the impact of HCV infection on the prognosis of patients with chronic inflammatory rheumatologic disorders are scarce. In a recent prospective cohort of US veterans, HCV-positive patients reported higher pain scores, had higher tender joint counts, and higher patient global scores contributing to higher disease activity scores (DAS)28, after adjustment for age, gender, race, smoking status, and days from enrollment.[27] After further adjustments for differences in the use of methotrexate, prednisone, and anti–tumor necrosis factor (TNF) therapies, DAS28 scores remained significantly higher in HCV-positive patients over all study visits. There was no difference in physician-reported outcomes (swollen joints or physician global scores). After adjusting for age, gender, and race, HCV-positive patients were more likely to use prednisone (OR 1.41) and anti-TNF therapies (OR 1.51), and far less likely to use methotrexate (OR 0.27).[27]

INCREASED CARDIOMETABOLIC MORBIDITY AND MORTALITY IN HEPATITIS C VIRUS–INFECTED PATIENTS

Autoimmune rheumatic diseases are now well recognized as independent risk factors for major cardiovascular events. A strong relationship between HCV infection and major adverse cardiovascular events has been reported. Such risk has been shown to be higher in HCV-infected patients compared with non-HCV controls, independently of the severity of the liver disease or the common cardiovascular risk factors. Patients with HCV chronic infection have an increased prevalence of carotid atherosclerosis and increased intima-media thickness compared with healthy controls, or patients with hepatitis B or nonalcoholic steatohepatitis. Active chronic HCV infection appears as an independent risk factor for ischemic cerebrovascular accidents and ischemic heart disease.[28,29] Successful IFN-based therapy showed a beneficial impact on cardiovascular risk, underlining the link between HCV and the occurrence of major cardiovascular events.[30–32] Consistently, HCV infection has been associated with higher rates of diabetes mellitus and insulin resistance compared with healthy volunteers and patients with hepatitis B. In addition, glucose abnormalities in patients with HCV is associated with poor liver outcomes defined by advanced liver fibrosis, lack of sustained virologic response to IFN-based treatment, and a higher risk of hepatocellular carcinoma development.[33–36] In the context of chronic inflammatory rheumatologic disorders, which already lead to an increased cardiovascular risk (related to chronic inflammation), the presence of HCV infection should be taken into account to assess the global cardiovascular risk.

TREATMENT OF HEPATITIS C VIRUS INFECTION AND ASSOCIATED RHEUMATOLOGIC MANIFESTATIONS

The cornerstone of HCV-CryoVas therapy is the capacity of treatments to achieve a sustained virologic response. Introduced in the early 1980s as a monotherapy, IFN was found to be both poorly tolerated and poorly effective with virologic cure ("sustained virologic response" [SVR]) in fewer than 10%. During the decade 2000 to 2010, pegylated (Peg)-IFN plus ribavirin combination as compared with IFN plus ribavirin showed higher rates of complete clinical and virological responses, regardless of HCV genotype and viral load.[37,38] However, the safety profile was not satisfactory and such therapies often led to many severe adverse events, such as severe cytopenia, disabling fatigue, fever, and depression. Fatigue, arthralgia, and myalgia were frequently reported, a particular concern in rheumatology patients in whom distinction of drug side effects from underlying disease was often difficult.[39] Some investigators reported cases of rheumatoid arthritis occurrence with anti-CCP Abs after IFN-based treatment, despite HCV cure.[40,41] Other autoimmune exacerbations in SS and systemic lupus erythematosus have been reported after IFN treatments.[42] In patients with CryoVas, cases of peripheral neuropathy induced or flared after IFN-based treatment have been reported.[43]

In the early 2010s, a new era was characterized by the development of DAAs. In combination with Peg-IFN/ribavirin, first-generation HCV protease inhibitors (boceprevir, telaprevir) improved the efficacy of antiviral combination, leading to approximately 70% SVR rate in genotype 1 infection. However, these agents worsened toxicity of IFN-based treatments and thus limited their use in all patients with HCV as well as in patients with rheumatic diseases.[44,45]

More recently, new all oral IFN-free, as well as and ribavirin-free, regimens have been approved. They are characterized by a dramatic efficacy leading to cure rates of 90% to 100% in all HCV genotypes, with minimal side effects and short duration (12–24 weeks).[46–49] Although such treatments remain today highly expensive, they now offer a "therapeutic revolution" for HCV-infected patients, particularly those with rheumatic diseases in whom IFN-based treatment has failed, was not well tolerated, or was contraindicated. For the treatment of HCV-CryoVas, the Vascuvaldic study enrolled 24 patients (median age 56.5 years, 54% males, 50% cirrhotic) who received sofosbuvir plus ribavirin for 24 weeks.[12] Seven patients also received immunosuppressive therapy; that is, rituximab, corticosteroids, and plasmapheresis. Eighty-seven percent of patients were complete clinical responders and SVR was obtained in 74%. The complete clinical response was very rapid, as it was noted at treatment week 12 in two-thirds of patients. Kidney involvement with membranoproliferative glomerulonephritis improved in 4 of 5 patients. Only 2 (8%) serious adverse events were observed. Sise and colleagues[50] reported a retrospective case series of 12 patients with HCV-CryoVas (median age 61 years, 58% men, 50% cirrhotic) treated with sofosbuvir plus simeprevir (n = 8) or sofosbuvir plus ribavirin (n = 4). Seven patients had evidence of renal involvement, including 5 membranoproliferative glomerulonephritis. Four patients received rituximab concurrent with DAA therapy. An SVR was achieved in 83% of patients. Cryoglobulin levels decreased in most patients (from 1.5% to 0.5%), and completely disappeared in 4 of 9 cases. Only 2 (17%) patients experienced serious adverse events. The Italian experience reported an overall 100% rate of clinical response of vasculitis in 44 patients with HCV-CryoVas who received DAAs.[51] Ten percent of patients also received immunosuppressants. A response on CryoVas symptoms was defined as complete in 18 (49%), partial in 13 (35%), and no response was noted in 6 (16%) patients. The Birmingham

Vasculitis Activity Score decreased from 5.41 to 1.27, and the mean cryocrit value fell from 7.2% to 1.8%.

Immunosuppression remains a major treatment in patients with HCV-CryoVas with a severe presentation (renal, digestive, or cardiac involvements), failure, or contraindication to antivirals. Randomized controlled trials showed that rituximab has a better efficacy than conventional immunosuppressive treatments (ie, glucocorticoids, azathioprine, cyclophosphamide, or plasmapheresis) or placebo.[52,53] Two other controlled trials showed that addition of rituximab to Peg-IFN/ribavirin led to a shorter time to clinical remission, better renal response rate, and higher rates of cryoglobulin clearance.[54,55] Of note, paradoxic worsening of vasculitis has been described after rituximab in such patients. Rituximab may form a complex with IgMk mixed cryoglobulin and lead to severe exacerbation of vasculitis involvements.[56] Considering the very rapid and potent virological efficacy of new DAA combination and the well-demonstrated correlation between SVR and clinical response, the exact place of rituximab, plasmapheresis, or other immunosuppressive drugs remains to be defined.[56] Other treatments for CryoVas have a limited place. Corticosteroids, used alone or in addition to IFN, did not favorably affect the response of HCV-CryoVas manifestations in controlled studies.[57] Plasmapheresis, which offers the advantage of removing the pathogenic cryoglobulins from the circulation, should be considered for rapidly progressive glomerulonephritis or life-threatening involvements. Immunosuppressive therapy is usually needed associated with plasma exchange to avoid the rebound increase in cryoglobulin serum level seen after discontinuation of apheresis.[58] There are no available data to date with DAA.

The impact of new DAAs on other rheumatologic manifestations (ie, arthralgia, myalgia, and sicca syndrome) are lacking. For fibromyalgia, Younossi and colleagues[59] recently reported major benefits of sofosbuvir-based DAAs on most patient-reported outcomes, including mental and physical fatigue, at week 12 and week 24 posttreatment. A benefit of DAAs was also suggested on cerebral magnetic resonance signal in basal ganglia correlated to the virological response.[60]

SUMMARY

HCV chronic infection is frequently associated with clinical and biological rheumatologic autoimmune/inflammatory manifestations. Treatment of HCV infection with IFN-alpha has for a long time excluded most patients with rheumatisms because of the poor virological efficacy, high rates of side effects, and the risk of exacerbation of autoimmune and rheumatic disorders. New oral IFN-free combinations offer the opportunity for HCV-infected patients with extrahepatic manifestations, such as rheumatic disorders, to be cured with great efficacy, low risk of side effects, and a short treatment duration.

REFERENCES

1. Cacoub P, Gragnani L, Comarmond C, et al. Extrahepatic manifestations of chronic hepatitis C virus infection. Dig Liver Dis 2014;46(Suppl 5):S165–73.

2. Ferri C, Sebastiani M, Giuggioli D, et al. Hepatitis C virus syndrome: a constellation of organ- and non-organ specific autoimmune disorders, B-cell non-Hodgkin's lymphoma, and cancer. World J Hepatol 2015;7:327–43.

3. Cacoub P, Poynard T, Ghillani P, et al. Extrahepatic manifestations of chronic hepatitis C. MULTIVIRC Group. Multidepartment Virus C. Arthritis Rheum 1999;42:2204–12.

4. Cheng Z, Zhou B, Shi X, et al. Extrahepatic manifestations of chronic hepatitis C virus infection: 297 cases from a tertiary medical center in Beijing, China. Chin Med J (Engl) 2014;127:1206–10.

5. Mohammed RH, ElMakhzangy HI, Gamal A, et al. Prevalence of rheumatologic manifestations of chronic hepatitis C virus infection among Egyptians. Clin Rheumatol 2010;29:1373–80.

6. Ogdie A, Pang WG, Forde KA, et al. Prevalence and risk factors for patient-reported joint pain among patients with HIV/hepatitis C coinfection, hepatitis C monoinfection, and HIV monoinfection. BMC Musculoskelet Disord 2015;16:93.

7. Landau DA, Scerra S, Sene D, et al. Causes and predictive factors of mortality in a cohort of patients with hepatitis C virus-related cryoglobulinemic vasculitis treated with antiviral therapy. J Rheumatol 2010;37:615–21.

8. Ferri C, Sebastiani M, Giuggioli D, et al. Mixed cryoglobulinemia: demographic, clinical, and serologic features and survival in 231 patients. Semin Arthritis Rheum 2004;33:355–74.

9. Terrier B, Semoun O, Saadoun D, et al. Prognostic factors in patients with hepatitis C virus infection and systemic vasculitis. Arthritis Rheum 2011;63:1748–57.

10. Cacoub P, Renou C, Rosenthal E, et al. Extrahepatic manifestations associated with hepatitis C virus infection. A prospective multicenter study of 321 patients. The GERMIVIC. Groupe d'Etude et de Recherche en Medecine Interne et Maladies Infectieuses sur le Virus de l'Hepatite C. Medicine (Baltimore) 2000;79: 47–56.

11. Lee YH, Ji JD, Yeon JE, et al. Cryoglobulinaemia and rheumatic manifestations in patients with hepatitis C virus infection. Ann Rheum Dis 1998;57:728–31.

12. Saadoun D, Thibault V, Si Ahmed SN, et al. Sofosbuvir plus ribavirin for hepatitis C virus-associated cryoglobulinaemia vasculitis: VASCUVALDIC study. Ann Rheum Dis 2016;75(10):1777–82.

13. Younossi Z, Park H, Henry L, et al. Extra-hepatic manifestations of hepatitis C—a meta-analysis of prevalence, quality of life, and economic burden. Gastroenterology 2016;150(7):1599–608.

14. Brito-Zerón P, Gheitasi H, Retamozo S, et al. How hepatitis C virus modifies the immunological profile of Sjögren syndrome: analysis of 783 patients. Arthritis Res Ther 2015;17:250.

15. Ramos-Casals M, Loustaud-Ratti V, De Vita S, et al. Sjögren syndrome associated with hepatitis C virus: a multicenter analysis of 137 cases. Medicine (Baltimore) 2005;84:81–9.

16. Arrieta JJ, Rodríguez-Iñigo E, Ortiz-Movilla N, et al. In situ detection of hepatitis C virus RNA in salivary glands. Am J Pathol 2001;158:259–64.

17. Koike K, Moriya K, Ishibashi K, et al. Sialadenitis histologically resembling Sjogren syndrome in mice transgenic for hepatitis C virus envelope genes. Proc Natl Acad Sci U S A 1997;94:233–6.

18. Khairy M, El-Raziky M, El-Akel W, et al. Serum autoantibodies positivity prevalence in patients with chronic HCV and impact on pegylated interferon and ribavirin treatment response. Liver Int 2013;33:1504–9.

19. Hsieh MY, Dai CY, Lee LP, et al. Antinuclear antibody is associated with a more advanced fibrosis and lower RNA levels of hepatitis C virus in patients with chronic hepatitis C. J Clin Pathol 2008;61:333–7.

20. Himoto T, Masaki T. Extrahepatic manifestations and autoantibodies in patients with hepatitis C virus infection. Clin Dev Immunol 2012;2012:871401.

21. Terrier B, Joly F, Vazquez T, et al. Expansion of functionally anergic CD21-/low marginal zone-like B cell clones in hepatitis C virus infection-related autoimmunity. J Immunol 1950;2011(187):6550–63.

22. Saadoun D, Rosenzwajg M, Joly F, et al. Regulatory T-cell responses to low-dose interleukin-2 in HCV-induced vasculitis. N Engl J Med 2011;365:2067–77.

23. Zignego AL, Wojcik GL, Cacoub P, et al. Genome-wide association study of hepatitis C virus- and cryoglobulin-related vasculitis. Genes Immun 2014;15:500–5.

24. Gragnani L, Piluso A, Giannini C, et al. Genetic determinants in hepatitis C virus-associated mixed cryoglobulinemia: role of polymorphic variants of BAFF promoter and Fcγ receptors. Arthritis Rheum 2011;63:1446–51.

25. Caussin-Schwemling C, Schmitt C, Stoll-Keller F. Study of the infection of human blood derived monocyte/macrophages with hepatitis C virus in vitro. J Med Virol 2001;65:14–22.

26. Muramatsu M, Kinoshita K, Fagarasan S, et al. Class switch recombination and hypermutation require activation-induced cytidine deaminase (AID), a potential RNA editing enzyme. Cell 2000;102:553–63.

27. Patel R, Mikuls TR, Richards JS, et al. Disease characteristics and treatment patterns in veterans with rheumatoid arthritis and concomitant hepatitis C infection. Arthritis Care Res 2015;67:467–74.

28. Domont F, Cacoub P. Chronic hepatitis C virus infection, a new cardiovascular risk factor? Liver Int 2016;36:621–7.

29. Maruyama S, Koda M, Oyake N, et al. Myocardial injury in patients with chronic hepatitis C infection. J Hepatol 2013;58:11–5.

30. Hsu YH, Hung PH, Muo CH, et al. Interferon-based treatment of hepatitis C virus infection reduces all-cause mortality in patients with end-stage renal disease: an 8-year nationwide cohort study in Taiwan. Medicine (Baltimore) 2015;94:e2113.

31. Hsu YC, Lin JT, Ho HJ, et al. Antiviral treatment for hepatitis C virus infection is associated with improved renal and cardiovascular outcomes in diabetic patients. Hepatology 2014;59:1293–302.

32. Hsu CS, Kao JH, Chao YC, et al. Interferon-based therapy reduces risk of stroke in chronic hepatitis C patients: a population-based cohort study in Taiwan. Aliment Pharmacol Ther 2013;38:415–23.

33. Elkrief L, Chouinard P, Bendersky N, et al. Diabetes mellitus is an independent prognostic factor for major liver-related outcomes in patients with cirrhosis and chronic hepatitis C. Hepatol Baltim Md 2014;60:823–31.

34. Huang YW, Yang SS, Fu SC, et al. Increased risk of cirrhosis and its decompensation in chronic hepatitis C patients with new-onset diabetes: a nationwide cohort study. Hepatology 2014;60:807–14.

35. Hung CH, Lee CM, Wang JH, et al. Impact of diabetes mellitus on incidence of hepatocellular carcinoma in chronic hepatitis C patients treated with interferon-based antiviral therapy. Int J Cancer 2011;128:2344–52.

36. Eslam M, Aparcero R, Kawaguchi T, et al. Meta-analysis: insulin resistance and sustained virological response in hepatitis C. Aliment Pharmacol Ther 2011;34:297–305.

37. Mazzaro C, Zorat F, Caizzi M, et al. Treatment with peg-interferon alfa-2b and ribavirin of hepatitis C virus-associated mixed cryoglobulinemia: a pilot study. J Hepatol 2005;42:632–8.

38. Saadoun D, Resche-Rigon M, Thibault V, et al. Antiviral therapy for hepatitis C virus–associated mixed cryoglobulinemia vasculitis: a long-term followup study. Arthritis Rheum 2006;54:3696–706.

39. Cacoub P, Comarmond C, Domont F, et al. Cryoglobulinemia vasculitis. Am J Med 2015;128:950–5.
40. Yang D, Arkfeld D, Fong TL. Development of anti-CCP-positive rheumatoid arthritis following pegylated interferon-α2a treatment for chronic hepatitis C infection. J Rheumatol 2010;37:1777.
41. Cacopardo B, Benanti F, Pinzone MR, et al. Rheumatoid arthritis following PEG-interferon-alfa-2a plus ribavirin treatment for chronic hepatitis C: a case report and review of the literature. BMC Res Notes 2013;6:437.
42. Onishi S, Nagashima T, Kimura H, et al. Systemic lupus erythematosus and Sjögren's syndrome induced in a case by interferon-alpha used for the treatment of hepatitis C. Lupus 2010;19:753–5.
43. Stübgen JP. Interferon alpha and neuromuscular disorders. J Neuroimmunol 2009;207:3–17.
44. Gragnani L, Fabbrizzi A, Triboli E, et al. Triple antiviral therapy in hepatitis C virus infection with or without mixed cryoglobulinaemia: a prospective, controlled pilot study. Dig Liver Dis 2014;46:833–7.
45. Saadoun D, Resche Rigon M, Pol S, et al. PegIFNα/ribavirin/protease inhibitor combination in severe hepatitis C virus-associated mixed cryoglobulinemia vasculitis. J Hepatol 2015;62:24–30.
46. Afdhal N, Zeuzem S, Kwo P, et al. Ledipasvir and sofosbuvir for untreated HCV genotype 1 infection. N Engl J Med 2014;370:1889–98.
47. Sulkowski MS, Gardiner DF, Rodriguez-Torres M, et al. Daclatasvir plus sofosbuvir for previously treated or untreated chronic HCV infection. N Engl J Med 2014;370:211–21.
48. Sulkowski MS, Vargas HE, Di Bisceglie AM, et al. Effectiveness of simeprevir plus sofosbuvir, with or without ribavirin, in real-world patients with HCV genotype 1 infection. Gastroenterology 2016;150:419–29.
49. Pol S, Corouge M, Vallet-Pichard A. Daclatasvir-sofosbuvir combination therapy with or without ribavirin for hepatitis C virus infection: from the clinical trials to real life. Hepat Med 2016;8:21–6.
50. Sise ME, Bloom AK, Wisocky J, et al. Treatment of hepatitis C virus–associated mixed cryoglobulinemia with direct-acting antiviral agents. Hepatology 2016;63:408–17.
51. Gragnani L, Visentini M, Fognani E, et al. Prospective study of guideline-tailored therapy with direct-acting antivirals for hepatitis C virus-associated mixed cryoglobulinemia. Hepatology 2016;64(5):1473–82.
52. De Vita S, Quartuccio L, Isola M, et al. A randomized controlled trial of rituximab for the treatment of severe cryoglobulinemic vasculitis. Arthritis Rheum 2012;64:843–53.
53. Sneller MC, Hu Z, Langford CA. A randomized controlled trial of rituximab following failure of antiviral therapy for hepatitis C virus-associated cryoglobulinemic vasculitis. Arthritis Rheum 2012;64:835–42.
54. Saadoun D, Resche Rigon M, Sene D, et al. Rituximab plus Peg-interferon-alpha/ribavirin compared with Peg-interferon-alpha/ribavirin in hepatitis C-related mixed cryoglobulinemia. Blood 2010;116:326–34 [quiz: 504–5].
55. Dammacco F, Tucci FA, Lauletta G, et al. Pegylated interferon-alpha, ribavirin, and rituximab combined therapy of hepatitis C virus-related mixed cryoglobulinemia: a long-term study. Blood 2010;116:343–53.
56. Sène D, Ghillani-Dalbin P, Amoura Z, et al. Rituximab may form a complex with IgMkappa mixed cryoglobulin and induce severe systemic reactions in patients with hepatitis C virus-induced vasculitis. Arthritis Rheum 2009;60:3848–55.

57. Dammacco F, Sansonno D, Han JH, et al. Natural interferon-alpha versus its combination with 6-methyl-prednisolone in the therapy of type II mixed cryoglobulinemia: a long-term, randomized, controlled study. Blood 1994;84:3336–43.

58. Hausfater P, Cacoub P, Assogba U, et al. Plasma exchange and interferon-alpha pharmacokinetics in patients with hepatitis C virus-associated systemic vasculitis. Nephron 2002;91:627–30.

59. Younossi ZM, Stepanova M, Marcellin P, et al. Treatment with ledipasvir and sofosbuvir improves patient-reported outcomes: results from the ION-1, -2, and -3 clinical trials. Hepatol Baltim Md 2015;61:1798–808.

60. Byrnes V, Miller A, Lowry D, et al. Effects of anti-viral therapy and HCV clearance on cerebral metabolism and cognition. J Hepatol 2012;56:549–56.

Cardiovascular Manifestations of Hepatitis C Virus

Nicolas Goossens, MD, MSc[a], Francesco Negro, MD[a,b],*

KEYWORDS

- Hepatitis C virus • Carotid atherosclerosis • Coronary artery disease
- Cardiovascular mortality • Stroke • Peripheral artery disease

KEY POINTS

- Hepatitis C virus (HCV) infection is a prevalent condition associated with numerous extra-hepatic manifestations, including cardiovascular manifestations.
- Epidemiologic studies have found that HCV is associated with cardiovascular mortality.
- HCV is also associated with carotid atherosclerosis, an increased risk of cerebrovascular events, coronary heart disease, and acute coronary events.
- Sustained virological response with interferon-based regimens is associated with reduced cardiovascular events, although this must be validated with newer direct-acting antivirals.
- The association between HCV and cardiovascular events may have significant economic and public health implications if cardiovascular risk prevention becomes a validated indication for therapy.

INTRODUCTION

Approximately 1% of the world's population, or 71 million people, are infected with the hepatitis C virus (HCV).[1] HCV is a major cause of chronic liver disease, culminating in cirrhosis, hepatocellular carcinoma, and increased hepatic-related mortality.[2] However, in addition to hepatic manifestations of HCV, multiple cohort longitudinal studies have underlined the important morbidity of extrahepatic manifestations of HCV.[3] The

Disclosure: Dr F. Negro is advising Bristol Myers Squibb, Gilead, Merck, and AbbVie, and has received unrestricted educational grants from Gilead and AbbVie. Dr N. Goossens has nothing to disclose.
Financial Support: The authors' work reported in the present article is supported by grant 314730-166609 from the Swiss National Science Foundation, the Nuovo-Soldati foundation (N. Goossens), the FLAGS Foundation, and by an unrestricted educational grant from Roche Pharma (Schweiz) AG.
[a] Division of Gastroenterology and Hepatology, Geneva University Hospitals, 4 Rue Gabrielle-Perret-Gentil, Geneva 4 1211, Switzerland; [b] Division of Clinical Pathology, Geneva University Hospitals, 4 Rue Gabrielle-Perret-Gentil, Geneva 4 1211, Switzerland
* Corresponding author. Divisions of Clinical Pathology and Gastroenterology and Hepatology, Geneva University Hospitals, 4 Rue Gabrielle-Perret-Gentil, Geneva 4 1211, Switzerland.
E-mail address: Francesco.Negro@hcuge.ch

Clin Liver Dis 21 (2017) 465–473
http://dx.doi.org/10.1016/j.cld.2017.03.003
1089-3261/17/© 2017 Elsevier Inc. All rights reserved.
liver.theclinics.com

spectrum of extrahepatic manifestations of HCV is wide, ranging from cryoglobuline-mia to neurologic manifestations but among the more intriguing associations that has been unraveled in the past decades is the association with metabolic alterations and with increased cardiovascular diseases.[3]

HCV, in particular genotype 3, induces steatosis, morphologically similar to that found in other causes of steatosis but with differing pathogenic mechanisms and prognostic implications.[4,5] In addition, the relationship between insulin resistance and HCV is equally complex with an increased risk of insulin resistance in HCV patients.[5] However, despite seemingly a more metabolic profile in HCV subjects, HCV infection is associated with reduced cholesterol serum levels or a more protective lipid profile,[6] further confusing the association between HCV and cardiovascular risk factors.

In recent years, the association between HCV infection and cardiovascular disease has been further examined in several epidemiologic studies. Due to the high prevalence of both cardiovascular disease and HCV, evidence connecting the 2 has occasionally been challenging to tease out. This article discusses the epidemiologic evidence and potential mechanisms linking the 2 and the impact of antiviral therapy on cardiovascular disease (**Fig. 1**).

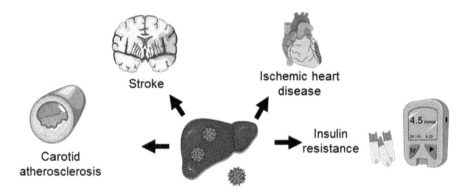

HCV: Increased cardiovascular mortality

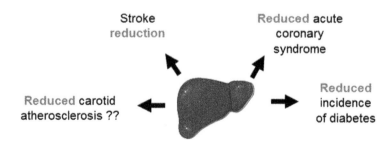

Post SVR: Improved cardiovascular outcomes

Fig. 1. Spectrum of the current understanding of cardiovascular manifestations of HCV infection before (*top panel*) and after (*bottom panel*) sustained virological response (SVR). (*Courtesy of* Servier Medical Art, Suresnes, France [www.servier.fr].)

HEPATITIS C VIRUS AND CARDIOVASCULAR MORTALITY

When dealing with the interaction between HCV and cardiovascular disease, the most pressing question remains whether HCV infection is associated with increased cardiovascular mortality. Surprisingly, a limited number of studies have attempted to answer this question and the results are somewhat contradictory. A retrospective cohort of more than 10,000 HCV-positive blood donors noted an increase in cardiovascular mortality in the HCV-positive group (hazard ratio [HR] 2.2, 95% CI 1.41–3.46).[7] An Asian cohort of more than 1000 HCV-positive individuals, the Risk Elevation of Viral Load Elevation and Associated Liver Disease/Cancer in HCV (REVEAL-HCV) study based in Taiwan, similarly found an increased risk of mortality for extrahepatic disease, when compared with HCV-negative individuals and, in particular, a higher risk of death from circulatory disease (HR 2.77, 95% CI 1.49–5.15).[2] In contrast, an Australian cohort of nearly 30,000 opioid substitution therapy recipients did not find increased cardiovascular mortality in HCV-positive individuals, although it may be argued that the population examined was different in this case to the other studies.[8] A systematic review and meta-analysis of these 3 studies nonetheless found a significant association between cardiovascular mortality and HCV infection (odds ratio [OR], 1.65; 95% CI 1.07 to 2.56, $P = .02$), although the investigators noted significant heterogeneity in the studies, suggesting that additional confounders or factors are yet to be identified in the link between HCV infection and cardiovascular mortality.[9] Similarly, in dialysis subjects a systematic review of 14 observational studies also identified an increased risk of cardiovascular mortality in HCV-positive individuals compared with HCV-negative controls (risk ratio 1.26, 95% CI 1.10–1.45).[10]

HEPATITIS C VIRUS AND SPECIFIC CARDIOVASCULAR DISEASE MANIFESTATIONS
Hepatitis C Virus Infection and Carotid Atherosclerosis

Japanese investigators were the first to identify a link between HCV infection and carotid atherosclerosis.[11–14] For instance, a cross-sectional study of 4784 individuals, including 2.2% positive for HCV, found that HCV seropositivity was associated with an increased risk of carotid-artery plaque (odds ratio [OR] 1.92, 95% CI 1.56–2.38, $P = .002$) and carotid intima-media thickening (IMT; OR 2.85, 95% CI 2.28–3.57, $P<.0001$).[12] These findings were confirmed in another Japanese study finding that HCV, but not hepatitis B virus infection, was associated with increased pulse wave velocity, a measure of arterial stiffness, in 7514 subjects.[13] More recently, the association between carotid atherosclerosis and HCV infection has also been reported in non-Asian populations. A prospective study in Italy by Petta and colleagues[15] in 174 consecutive genotype 1 HCV subjects found that HCV subjects had significantly more carotid atherosclerotic plaques and increased IMT when compared with controls. In addition, degree of liver fibrosis and more advanced age were independently associated with carotid plaques in multivariable regression.[15] Similarly, a cross-sectional Egyptian study in 329 HCV-positive subjects, found increased IMT in HCV-infected subjects when compared with individuals never infected with HCV using multivariable regression.[16] Finally, a large study based in Taiwan, including 7641 HCV-positive subjects and more than 30,000 controls based on health insurance claims data, found that that the excess risk of peripheral arterial disease development in HCV-infected subjects is 1.43-fold higher (95% CI 1.23–1.67) compared with non-HCV subjects.[17]

Although the association between coronary atherosclerosis and HCV has been validated in a wide variety of clinical settings, some conflicting studies have not identified this association. For instance, in the United States, a cross-sectional study based in HCV–human immunodeficiency virus (HIV) coinfected and HCV-monoinfected subjects from the Women's Interagency HIV Study found that HCV infection was associated with increased IMT and presence of carotid plaques in univariable analysis but not in multivariable analysis when adjusted for other factors.[18] Despite a few negative studies displaying the lack of association, a systematic review has recently clarified that HCV infection was associated with carotid atherosclerotic plaques (pooled OR 2.27, 95% CI 1.76–2.94, $P<.001$) without significant heterogeneity between studies.[9] In addition, when pooling 7 case-control studies, this systematic review identified increased IMT in HCV subjects albeit in the presence of significant heterogeneity.[9]

Hepatitis C Virus Infection and Cerebrovascular Events

In light of the significant association between HCV infection and carotid atherosclerotic plaques, it would be expected that this would lead to an increased number of cerebrovascular events in HCV-positive subjects. For instance, in a community-based prospective cohort study, Lee and colleagues[19] found that during 382,011 person-years of follow-up the cumulative risk of cerebrovascular deaths was 1.0% and 2.7% for HCV-negative and HCV-positive, respectively ($P<.001$). This result was confirmed in multivariable cox regression and, interestingly, an association with HCV RNA levels was noted, although no significant association between HCV genotype and cerebrovascular death was identified.[19] Conversely, Younossi and colleagues[20] assessed the relationship between HCV and cardiovascular risk factors and outcomes using the US National Health and Nutrition Examination Surveys (NHANES), and they found that, although HCV infection was independently associated with certain cardiovascular outcomes, it was not associated with stroke. The systematic review cited previously nevertheless confirmed that HCV infection was associated with cerebrovascular events (pooled OR 1.35, 95% CI 1.00–1.82, $P = .05$), although the significance threshold was barely met.[9] Of note, although the bulk of the data linking HCV and cerebrovascular events relate to ischemic events, some data suggest that HCV may also be linked to increased risk of intracerebral hemorrhage.[21]

Hepatitis C Virus Infection and Coronary Artery Disease

In an Italian cohort of subjects with coronary artery disease (CAD) and controls, HCV seropositivity was found to be associated with the presence of CAD (OR 3.2, 95% CI 1.1–9.2, $P<.05$) even after adjustment for confounding risk factors.[22] Although this study was a case-control study and, therefore, potentially biased, the investigators noted increased proportions of HCV-positive subjects with increasing number of coronary vessels affected ranging from 4.5% for 1-vessel disease to 8.4% for 3-vessel disease ($P<.05$).[22] These results were later confirmed in a national, observational United States cohort of more than 82,000 HCV-infected veterans and nearly 90,000 uninfected controls in which HCV infection was associated, in multivariable analysis, with a higher risk of CAD (HR 1.25, 95% CI 1.20–1.30).[23] Yet another retrospective cohort study, at the University of Arkansas in the United States, compared 8251 HCV-positive individuals with 14,799 HCV-negative subjects and found an increased incidence of CAD events compared with controls (4.9% vs 3.2%, $P<.001$).[24] In the HCV cohort, subjects with detectable HCV RNA had a significantly higher incidence of CAD events compared with subjects who had no detectable RNA (5.9% vs 4.7%, $P = .04$), further reinforcing the association between CAD and HCV infection. Recent data from the HIV-HCV coinfection literature also underline this association. For instance, a study found that when comparing men with or without HIV and HCV infection, HCV infection was significantly associated with a higher prevalence of coronary artery calcium (prevalence ratio 1.29, 95% CI 1.02–1.63) and, although HCV infection and HIV infection were independently associated with the finding of any plaque, there was no evidence of a synergistic effect due to HIV-HCV coinfection.[25] In addition, a retrospective study in HIV-HCV coinfected subjects found that coinfected subjects had a greater incidence of cardiovascular disease events and/or death than HIV-monoinfected individuals (4% vs 1.2%, P = .004), further underlining the importance of a holistic, non–liver-centric approach to HCV monoinfected and HIV-HCV coinfected subjects.[26]

Some studies did not find a relationship between HCV and CAD. For instance, a retrospective cohort study among general practices in the United Kingdom, including 4809 HCV subjects and 71,668 matched controls with a median follow-up of 3.2 years, did not find a significant difference in the rates of myocardial infarction between HCV-positive and HCV-negative subjects (1.02 vs 0.92 events per 1000 person-years, P = .7).[27] Nevertheless, a systematic review of the available literature confirmed that the risk of an HCV-positive person to develop coronary atherosclerosis is about triple the risk in uninfected persons (OR 3.06, 95% CI 1.99–4.72),[28] whereas another systematic review found that HCV infection was associated with increased cardiovascular events (OR 1.20, 95% CI 1.03–1.40, P = .02).[9]

HEPATITIS C VIRUS INFECTION AND INSULIN RESISTANCE

Insulin resistance and/or type 2 diabetes is a known cardiovascular risk factor linked to cardiovascular morbidity and mortality. Although the evidence is complex and has been reviewed elsewhere,[5,29] multiple lines of evidence converge to suggest that there is a link between HCV and insulin resistance that may, in susceptible patients, lead to type 2 diabetes.

The epidemiologic evidence linking HCV to type 2 diabetes is multifaceted and complex to interpret because it is derived from retrospective and prospective clinical data often not collected primarily to assess for the effect of insulin resistance. A systematic review pooling 34 studies and a total of more than 300,000 subjects analyzed the risk of type 2 diabetes in subjects with HCV and found an OR of approximately 1.7 for type 2 diabetes in HCV patients (adjusted OR 1.68, 95% CI 1.15–2.20 for retrospective studies for instance).[30] This was later confirmed in another systematic review pooling 35 observational studies with a pooled OR of 1.7 for type 2 diabetes in HCV subjects compared with uninfected controls and a pooled OR of 1.9 when comparing to hepatitis-B infected controls.[31] In a longitudinal study of more than 1000 adults, HCV-positive patients at high risk of developing diabetes based on metabolic risk factors were 11 times more likely to develop diabetes than HCV-negative individuals, although this effect was not found in subjects at low risk of developing diabetes,[32] suggesting that HCV increases the risk of diabetes especially in predisposed individuals. Despite the clear epidemiologic link between HCV and insulin resistance, it remains unclear whether the magnitude of the increased cardiovascular risk in HCV patients is linked to the presence of insulin resistance, although type 2 diabetes is clearly associated with cerebrovascular events in HCV subjects, especially when the prevalence of type 2 diabetes is greater than 10%.[9]

IMPACT OF HEPATITIS C VIRUS SUSTAINED VIROLOGICAL RESPONSE ON CARDIOVASCULAR DISEASE

In the past years, direct-acting antivirals (DAAs) have revolutionized the management of HCV infection by achieving high rates of sustained virological response (SVR) with low rates of side effects and ever-shortening therapy duration. However, due to high costs, the effect of these therapies on hepatic but also extrahepatic and, in particular, cardiovascular, outcomes has been scrutinised.[33] For instance, in a retrospective cohort study of 3113 HCV-positive individuals, interferon-based therapy use was associated with a significant reduction of stroke in HCV subjects (HR 0.39, 95% CI 0.16–0.95, $P = .039$) after adjusting for known prognostic factors, suggesting a potential benefit for interferon-based therapy to reduce cardiovascular events in HCV.[34] Another Taiwanese study, including 1411 HCV diabetic subjects treated with pegylated interferon and ribavirin matched by propensity-score to the same number of controls, found that HCV therapy was associated with less ischemic strokes (HR 0.53, 95% CI 0.30–0.93) and reduced rates of acute coronary syndrome (HR 0.64, 95% CI 0.39–1.06) in the specific population of HCV-infected diabetics.[35] In a Scottish cohort of HCV subjects, SVR was also associated with reduced cardiovascular disease (adjusted HR, 0.70, $P = .001$).[36] Finally, a recent French study in 1323 HCV subjects with compensated cirrhosis followed up for a median of 58 months found that subjects who had achieved SVR had a lower risk of cardiovascular events (HR 0.42, 95% CI 0.25–0.69, $P = .001$) and major adverse cardiac events, although there was no association with viral genotype.[37] Therefore, although there is a clear lack of data for the effect of DAA-based therapy on cardiovascular events, the evidence for interferon-based therapy points toward reduced cardiovascular risk after achieving SVR. This might be an important public health consideration to address the current prevalent DAA reimbursement strategies that limit payment only for patients with advanced liver disease and disregarding metabolic and cardiovascular risk factors.

PATHOGENESIS OF HEPATITIS C VIRUS–INDUCED CARDIOVASCULAR INJURY

The potential association between HCV infection and cardiovascular risk raises the question of the mechanism underlying this association. Metabolic factors may play a role. The insulin resistance associated with HCV leads to hyperglycemia, endothelial dysfunction, and inflammation, all of which produce vessel damage and unstable plaques. A recent study showed an increased cardiac left ventricular mass in normotensive HCV-positive individuals, similar to hypertensive subjects.[38] In addition, the investigators noted a significant correlation between insulin resistance and left ventricular mass among HCV-infected subjects, and a strong relationship between HCV viral load and both left ventricular mass and insulin resistance.[38] The presence of HCV may also induce a chronic, systemic inflammatory state with effects in distant organs and tissues. The immune response to HCV induces the upregulation of proinflammatory cytokines and chemokines, such as tumor necrosis factor-α (TNF-α), interleukin (IL)-6 and IL8, and chemokine ligand 2 (CCL2), which are released in the bloodstream and may amplify and worsen the inflammatory lesions outside of the liver.[39–41] Maruyama and colleagues[42] performed a myocardial scintigraphy study of HCV-infected subjects and found that 87% had myocardial perfusion defects. Interestingly, these myocardial defects seemed to fluctuate and improve after successful HCV eradication with interferon-based therapy.[42] The proinflammatory, profibrogenic milieu that characterizes long-standing, severe liver damage may be more prone to systemic effects. Consistent with this suggestion, in genotype 1 HCV subjects, severe hepatic fibrosis (F3/F4 vs F1/F2) was independently associated with the development of carotid plaque, according to a study by Petta and colleagues,[15] even among subjects younger than 55 years old. Finally, a direct colonization of atherosclerotic lesions cannot be excluded, in keeping with the observation that cardiovascular damage may correlate with viral load.[41,42] A single report identified HCV RNA sequences within plaque tissue[43] but this has not been independently confirmed.

SUMMARY

Increasing epidemiologic evidence suggests that there is a link between cardiovascular disease and HCV infection (see **Fig. 1**). Earlier studies showed an association between surrogate markers of cardiovascular disease, such as IMT and HCV infection[44]; however, this was not confirmed in other studies.[16] Subsequently, HCV infection has been associated with cerebrovascular disease[19] and CAD.[45] Although imperfect, numerous studies suggest a link between HCV infection and increased cardiovascular mortality independently of other known risk factors.[2,7] Although, there seems to be converging evidence underlying a possible association between chronic HCV infection and cardiovascular events, such as carotid atherosclerosis, cerebrovascular events, CAD, and other cardiovascular manifestations, the evidence is complex and other studies have not found such an association.[46] Far from being a purely academic discussion, further well-conducted prospective trials are required to answer this question. If validated, the improvement of cardiovascular outcomes by curing HCV, especially in individuals at high-risk for cardiovascular events, could represent an important future indication for HCV therapy regardless of liver disease staging. This would, of course, have important economic and public health implications, and could become the predominant indication for HCV therapy in the near future.

REFERENCES

1. Collaborators TPOH. Global prevalence and genotype distribution of hepatitis C virus infection in 2015: a modelling study. Lancet Gastroenterol Hepatol 2017; 2(3):161–76.
2. Lee MH, Yang HI, Lu SN, et al. Chronic hepatitis C virus infection increases mortality from hepatic and extrahepatic diseases: a community-based long-term prospective study. J Infect Dis 2012;206:469–77.
3. Negro F, Forton D, Craxì A, et al. Extrahepatic morbidity and mortality of chronic hepatitis C. Gastroenterology 2015;149(6):1345–60.
4. Goossens N, Negro F. Is genotype 3 of the hepatitis C virus the new villain? Hepatology 2014;59(6):2403–12.
5. Goossens N, Negro F. Insulin resistance, non-alcoholic fatty liver disease and hepatitis C virus infection. Rev Recent Clin Trials 2014;9(3):204–9.
6. Hofer H, Bankl HC, Wrba F, et al. Hepatocellular fat accumulation and low serum cholesterol in patients infected with HCV-3a. Am J Gastroenterol 2002;97(11):2880–5.
7. Guiltinan AM, Kaidarova Z, Custer B, et al. Increased all-cause, liver, and cardiac mortality among hepatitis C virus-seropositive blood donors. Am J Epidemiol 2008;167(6):743–50.
8. Vajdic CM, Pour SM, Olivier J, et al. The impact of blood-borne viruses on cause-specific mortality among opioid dependent people: an Australian population-based cohort study. Drug Alcohol Depend 2015;152:264–71.
9. Petta S, Maida M, Macaluso FS, et al. Hepatitis C virus infection is associated with increased cardiovascular mortality: a meta-analysis of observational studies. Gastroenterology 2016;150(1):145–55.e4.
10. Fabrizi F, Dixit V, Messa P. Impact of hepatitis C on survival in dialysis patients: a link with cardiovascular mortality? J Viral Hepat 2012;19(9):601–7.
11. Ishizaka Y, Ishizaka N, Takahashi E, et al. Association between hepatitis C virus core protein and carotid atherosclerosis. Circ J 2003;67(1):26–30.
12. Ishizaka N, Ishizaka Y, Takahashi E, et al. Association between hepatitis C virus seropositivity, carotid-artery plaque, and intima-media thickening. Lancet 2002; 359(9301):133–5.

13. Tomiyama H, Arai T, Hirose K, et al. Hepatitis C virus seropositivity, but not hepatitis B virus carrier or seropositivity, associated with increased pulse wave velocity. Atherosclerosis 2003;166(2):401–3.
14. Fukui M, Kitagawa Y, Nakamura N, et al. Hepatitis C virus and atherosclerosis in patients with type 2 diabetes. JAMA 2003;289(10):1245–6.
15. Petta S, Torres D, Fazio G, et al. Carotid atherosclerosis and chronic hepatitis C: a prospective study of risk associations. Hepatology 2012;55(5):1317–23.
16. Mostafa A, Mohamed MK, Saeed M, et al. Hepatitis C infection and clearance: impact on atherosclerosis and cardiometabolic risk factors. Gut 2010;59(8): 1135–40.
17. Hsu YH, Muo CH, Liu CY, et al. Hepatitis C virus infection increases the risk of developing peripheral arterial disease: a 9-year population-based cohort study. J Hepatol 2015;62(3):519–25.
18. Tien PC, Schneider MF, Cole SR, et al. Association of hepatitis C virus and HIV infection with subclinical atherosclerosis in the women's interagency HIV study. AIDS 2009;23(13):1781.
19. Lee MH, Yang HI, Wang CH, et al. Hepatitis C virus infection and increased risk of cerebrovascular disease. Stroke 2010;41(12):2894–900.
20. Younossi ZM, Stepanova M, Nader F, et al. Associations of chronic hepatitis C with metabolic and cardiac outcomes. Aliment Pharmacol Ther 2013;37(6): 647–52.
21. Tseng CH, Muo CH, Hsu CY, et al. Increased risk of intracerebral hemorrhage among patients with hepatitis C virus infection. Medicine 2015;94(46):e2132.
22. Vassalle C, Masini S, Bianchi F, et al. Evidence for association between hepatitis C virus seropositivity and coronary artery disease. Heart 2004;90(5):565–6.
23. Butt AA, Xiaoqiang W, Budoff M, et al. Hepatitis C virus infection and the risk of coronary disease. Clin Infect Dis 2009;49(2):225–32.
24. Pothineni NV, Delongchamp R, Vallurupalli S, et al. Impact of hepatitis C seropositivity on the risk of coronary heart disease events. Am J Cardiol 2014;114(12): 1841–5.
25. McKibben RA, Haberlen SA, Post WS, et al. A cross-sectional study of the association between chronic hepatitis C virus infection and subclinical coronary atherosclerosis among participants in the multicenter AIDS cohort study. J Infect Dis 2016;213(2):257–65.
26. Fernández-Montero J, Barreiro P, Mendoza C, et al. Hepatitis C virus coinfection independently increases the risk of cardiovascular disease in HIV-positive patients. J Viral Hepat 2016;23(1):47–52.
27. Forde KA, Haynes K, Troxel AB, et al. Risk of myocardial infarction associated with chronic hepatitis C virus infection: a population-based cohort study. J Viral Hepat 2012;19(4):271–7.
28. Olubamwo O, Aregbesola A, Miettola J, et al. Hepatitis C and risk of coronary atherosclerosis–A systematic review. Public Health 2016;138:12–25.
29. Gastaldi G, Goossens N, Clément S, et al. Current level of evidence on causal association between Hepatitis C virus and type 2 diabetes: a review. J Adv Res 2017;8(2):149–59.
30. White DL, Ratziu V, El-Serag HB. Hepatitis C infection and risk of diabetes: a systematic review and meta-analysis. J Hepatol 2008;49(5):831–44.
31. Naing C, Mak JW, Ahmed SI, et al. Relationship between hepatitis C virus infection and type 2 diabetes mellitus: meta-analysis. World J Gastroenterol 2012; 18(14):1642–51.

32. Mehta SH, Brancati FL, Strathdee SA, et al. Hepatitis C virus infection and incident type 2 diabetes. Hepatology 2003;38(1):50–6.
33. Vernaz N, Girardin F, Goossens N, et al. Drug pricing evolution in hepatitis C. PLoS One 2016;11(6):e0157098.
34. Hsu CS, Kao JH, Chao YC, et al. Interferon-based therapy reduces risk of stroke in chronic hepatitis C patients: a population-based cohort study in Taiwan. Aliment Pharmacol Ther 2013;38(4):415–23.
35. Hsu YC, Lin JT, Ho HJ, et al. Antiviral treatment for hepatitis C virus infection is associated with improved renal and cardiovascular outcomes in diabetic patients. Hepatology 2014;59(4):1293–302.
36. Innes HA, McDonald SA, Dillon JF, et al. Toward a more complete understanding of the association between a hepatitis C sustained viral response and cause-specific outcomes. Hepatology 2015;62(2):355–64.
37. Nahon P, Bourcier V, Layese R, et al. Eradication of hepatitis C virus infection in patients with cirrhosis reduces risk of liver and non-liver complications. Gastroenterology 2017;152(1):142–56.e2.
38. Perticone M, Miceli S, Maio R, et al. Chronic HCV infection increases cardiac left ventricular mass index in normotensive patients. J Hepatol 2014;61(4):755–60.
39. Tsui JI, Whooley MA, Monto A, et al. Association of hepatitis C virus seropositivity with inflammatory markers and heart failure in persons with coronary heart disease: data from the Heart and Soul study. J Card Fail 2009;15(5):451–6.
40. Balasubramanian A, Munshi N, Koziel MJ, et al. Structural proteins of Hepatitis C virus induce interleukin 8 production and apoptosis in human endothelial cells. J Gen Virol 2005;86(Pt 12):3291–301.
41. Adinolfi LE, Restivo L, Zampino R, et al. Chronic HCV infection is a risk of atherosclerosis. Role of HCV and HCV-related steatosis. Atherosclerosis 2012; 221(22385985):496–502.
42. Maruyama S, Koda M, Oyake N, et al. Myocardial injury in patients with chronic hepatitis C infection. J Hepatol 2013;58(1):11–5.
43. Boddi M, Abbate R, Chellini B, et al. Hepatitis C virus RNA localization in human carotid plaques. J Clin Virol 2010;47(1):72–5.
44. Targher G, Bertolini L, Padovani R, et al. Differences and similarities in early atherosclerosis between patients with non-alcoholic steatohepatitis and chronic hepatitis B and C. J Hepatol 2007;46(17335930):1126–32.
45. Alyan O, Kacmaz F, Ozdemir O, et al. Hepatitis C infection is associated with increased coronary artery atherosclerosis defined by modified Reardon severity score system. Circ J 2008;72(12):1960–5.
46. Negro F. Facts and fictions of HCV and comorbidities: steatosis, diabetes mellitus, and cardiovascular diseases. J Hepatol 2014;61(1S):S69–78.

Metabolic Manifestations of Hepatitis C Virus
Diabetes Mellitus, Dyslipidemia

Lawrence Serfaty, MD

KEYWORDS

- Hepatitis C • Steatosis • Hypobetalipoproteinemia
- Microsomal triglyceride transfer protein • Insulin resistance • Tumor necrosis factor

KEY POINTS

- Out of excessive alcohol consumption, steatosis should be classified into 2 types according to hepatitis C virus (HCV) genotypes: metabolic steatosis, which is associated with features of metabolic syndrome and insulin resistance in patients infected with nongenotype 3, and viral steatosis, which is correlated with viral load and hyperlipemia in patients infected with genotype 3.
- HCV interacts with host lipid metabolism by several mechanisms, such as promotion of lipogenesis, reduction of fatty acid oxidation, and decreases of lipids export, leading to hepatic steatosis and hypolipidemia.
- A strong link between HCV infection and diabetes mellitus has been found in subject-based studies and, to a lesser degree, in population-based studies.
- HCV-mediated insulin resistance may be promoted through multiple pathogenic mechanisms, such as direct inhibition of insulin signaling pathway by HCV core protein in the liver, overproduction of tumor necrosis factor-alpha, oxidative stress, modulation of incretins, or pancreatic ß-cells dysfunction.

Metabolic disorders are common in patients with chronic hepatitis C (CHC) virus (HCV) infection. In a nationwide population-based register study conducted in Sweden, type 2 diabetes was the second cause of extrahepatic disease among patients with CHC and its prevalence was twice higher than that reported in the general population (10.6 vs 5.5%, $P<.05$).[1] According to a meta-analysis on extrahepatic manifestations of hepatitis C, conservative estimates suggest that as many 402,000 patients in the

Disclosure: Dr L. Serfaty serves on consulting committees, advisory committees, or review panels for AbbVie, Janssen, Merck Sharp & Dohme (MSD), Roche, Bristol-Meyers Squibb (BMS), Gilead, and performs speaking and teaching for Roche, AbbVie, MSD, Gilead, BMS, and Janssen.
Hepatology Department, INSERM UMR_S 938, APHP, Saint-Antoine Hospital, UPMC Univ Paris 06, Paris, France
E-mail address: lawrence.serfaty@aphp.fr

Clin Liver Dis 21 (2017) 475–486
http://dx.doi.org/10.1016/j.cld.2017.03.004
1089-3261/17/© 2017 Elsevier Inc. All rights reserved.

United States have HCV-associated diabetes mellitus.[2] Several experimental and clinical studies have provided evidence that HCV itself is able to promote insulin resistance (IR) through multiple pathogenic mechanisms, including impairment of the insulin signaling pathway.[3] There is also considerable evidence for an overprevalence of lipid disorders and steatosis in patients with CHC, suggesting close relationship with HCV infection.[3] In this setting, chronic HCV infection can be considered a metabolic disease in view of its interaction with lipid metabolism leading to steatosis, as well as its impairment of glucose metabolism leading to IR and diabetes. This article examines the relationship between HCV, lipid abnormalities, steatosis, IR, and diabetes, as well as the pathogenic mechanisms accounting for these events in persons infected with HCV. The impact of these metabolic disorders on the natural course of CHC will not be discussed.

HEPATITIS C VIRUS, LIPID METABOLISM, AND HEPATIC STEATOSIS
Hepatitis C Virus–Related Steatosis: Prevalence and Risk Factors

In CHC patients, the prevalence of steatosis ranges from 40% to 86% (mean 55%), which is higher than in the general population (20%–30%) or in patients with other chronic liver disease (19%–50%), including chronic hepatitis B.[4,5] Most patients have mild steatosis affecting less than 30% of hepatocytes with a pattern of distribution in the periportal region of the liver, whereas the centrilobular region is mainly affected in nonalcoholic steatohepatitis patients.[6] Out of excessive alcohol consumption, steatosis should be classified into 2 types according to HCV genotypes: metabolic steatosis, which is associated with features of metabolic syndrome and IR in patients infected with nongenotype 3, and viral steatosis, which is correlated with viral load and hypolipidemia in patients infected with genotype 3.[7] Compared with other genotypes, infection with genotype 3 is associated with higher prevalence and more severe steatosis in 73% versus 50%, and moderate to severe steatosis in 40% versus 10% to 15%, respectively.[4] Furthermore, the severity of steatosis in patients infected with genotype 3 is inversely related with cholesterol and apolipoprotein B lipoprotein serum levels, defining in some cases hypobetalipoproteinemia.[5] Antiviral treatment is able to reverse this hypobetalipoproteinemia concomitantly with significant reduction of steatosis.[4,5,8] In patients infected with nongenotype 3, genetic background, such as interleukin and patatin-like phospholipase-3 (PNPLA3) polymorphisms, is associated with HCV-related steatosis.[9,10] In the era of new direct antiviral agents (DAAs) regimen, the role of viral-related steatosis has been suggested for the lower efficacy of antiviral treatment in patients infected with genotype 3.[11] In this setting, intrahepatic fat sequestration by the replicating virus may reduce access to DAAs and reduce their efficacy. Specific studies are needed to evaluate the impact of HCV-related steatosis on the efficacy of DAAs.

Pathogenic Mechanisms of Hepatitis C Virus–Related Steatosis

The HCV life cycle is closely associated with lipid droplets and lipoprotein metabolism in hepatocytes.[12,13] HCV interacts with host lipid metabolism by several mechanisms, such as promotion of lipogenesis, reduction of fatty acid oxidation, and decreases of lipids export, leading to hepatic steatosis and hypolipidemia. In transgenic mouse model, it has been shown that HCV core protein that promotes steatosis is able to inhibit both the microsomal triglyceride transfer protein (MTTP) activity and very low density lipoprotein secretion,[14] to impair the expression of peroxisome proliferator-activated receptor (PPAR)$_\gamma$,[15] and to induce hepatic gene expression and transcriptional activity of sterol response element binding protein (SREBP)-1.[16] Elevated lipogenesis and reduced cholesterol synthesis have been confirmed in patients with CHC compared with healthy controls.[17] In HCV-infected human hepatoma (Huh)-7.5 cells, mitochondrial lipid β-oxidation is significantly attenuated, which results in low lipid combustion.[18] Lipids accumulation seems depend on HCV genotype, as demonstrated in experimental models. Triglycerides accumulation only occurs in genotypes 1 or 3 transfected cells,[19] although it is the greatest with genotype 3 core protein in transgenic mouse.[20] SREBP-1–dependent fatty acid synthase promoter activity and PPAR$_\gamma$ impairment are also greater with HCV genotype 3.[20,21] In subjects receiving antiviral therapy, it has been shown that genotype 3 but not genotype 2 selectively interferes with the late cholesterol synthesis pathway and this distal interference was resolved with systemic vascular resistance.[22] Finally, MTTP may play a central role in HCV-related steatosis, mainly through hyperinsulinemia in nongenotype 3 infected patients, and by direct virus-related effects in patients infected with genotype 3.[23]

HEPATITIS C VIRUS, TYPE 2 DIABETES, AND INSULIN RESISTANCE
Prevalence and Risk Factors

IR has been clinically defined as a condition in which cells become resistant to the action of insulin, such that the typical response to a defined amount of insulin is markedly diminished. The net result is that higher levels of insulin are needed to evoke the same cellular response. In humans, IR is thus evaluated by the ability of insulin to control glycemia. Methods used to estimate IR include (1) fasting insulin concentration; (2) quantitative insulin sensitivity check index, which is calculated as 1/(log [fasting insulin]1log [fasting glucose]); and (3) the homoeostasis model assessment (HOMA)-IR, calculated as insulin (mU/m) $\times$ (fasting glucose [mmol/L]/22.5); a 12-hour overnight fast is essential for the assessment of IR.[24] HOMA-IR is easily calculated using fasting insulin and fasting glucose but is poorly related to IR data obtained by the gold standard euglycemic hyperinsulinemic clamp.[25] The presence of IR has been defined as a HOMA value of greater than 4.65 or a value of greater than 3.60 in persons with a body mass index (BMI) of 4 27.5 kg/m^2.[26]

The link between HCV infection and type 2 diabetes has been evaluated in several studies with conflicting results according to the study population; that is, subject-based versus population-based study. In subjects with chronic liver disease, the prevalence of diabetes ranges between 13.6% and 67.4% in case of HCV infection, which is higher than that reported for subjects with other chronic liver diseases, such as chronic hepatitis B, independent of the stage of liver fibrosis (**Table 1**).[27–33] In 2 meta-analyses, a significant relationship between HCV and diabetes was reported when compared with hepatitis B virus (HBV)-infected controls, with an adjusted odds ratio (OR) of 1.8 (95% CI 1.2–2.4) and 1.9 (95% CI 1.4–2.6), respectively.[34,35] Among 462 nondiabetic CHC subjects, IR assessed by HOMA-IR greater than 3 was present in 32.4%, which was greater when compared with patients with chronic HBV matched for age, sex, BMI, and fibrosis score (35 vs 5%, $P<.0001$).[36] Multivariate analysis revealed that infection with genotypes 1 and 4 was a significant factor associated with IR in nondiabetic chronic HCV subjects (OR 2.984, $P<.001$). Other significant factors included age greater than 40 years, the presence of metabolic syndrome, extensive fibrosis, and severe steatosis. Moreover, IR was associated with a high serum viral load and HOMA-IR correlated significantly with serum HCV RNA level and necroinflammation, in this subgroup of subjects. The genotype specific association with IR has been found in another study.[37] The dose-dependent relationship between HCV viral load and IR, independent of visceral fat in one study, has been

Table 1
Prevalence of type 2 diabetes in hepatitis C virus–positive versus hepatitis C virus–negative subjects

Author (Reference)	Study Population (N)	HCV+ (%)	HCV− (%)
Alison et al,[28] 1994	Cirrhosis (100)	50	9
Grimbert et al,[29] 1996	Chronic viral disease (304)	24	9
Mason et al,[27] 1999	Viral hepatitis (1117)	21	12
Caronia et al,[30] 1999	Virus-related cirrhosis (1232)	24	9
Arao et al,[31] 2003	Viral hepatitis (866)	21	12
	Cirrhosis	31	12
Imazeki et al,[32] 2008	Viral hepatitis (952)	13.6	6.3
	HCV-cleared	—	9
Rouabhia et al,[33] 2010	Viral hepatitis (416)	39.1	5
	Cirrhosis	67.4	20
Metha et al,[52] 2000	General population (9841) (Prevalence of HCV+: 2.1%) (Prevalence of diabetes: 8.4%)	NA Age >40 y: adjusted OR 3.77	NA
Montenegro et al,[53] 2013	General population (2472) (Prevalence of HCV+: 26.2%)	10.1	7.5
Stepanova et al,[54] 2012	General population (39,506) 1988–94 (15,866, HCV+ 1.95%) 1999–2004 (13,970, HCV+ 1.97%) 2005–2008 (9670, HCV+ 1.68%)	7.7 7.9 10.1	5.5 7.9 9.1
Younossi et al,[55] 2013	General population (19,741) (Prevalence of rHCV+: 0.88%)	12.66	7.36
Ruhl et al,[56] 2014	General population (15,128) (Prevalence of HCV+: 1.7%)	10.5	10.2
Schnier et al,[57] 2016	General population (HCV+: 21,929) (Matched HCV−: 65,074)	2.9	2.9

confirmed in 2 additional studies.[38,39] Conversely, the prevalence of HCV infection in diabetic subjects is higher than in the general population, ranging from 5% to 12% (**Table 2**).[27,40–42] This statistical relationship could be the result of nosocomial risk in diabetic subjects. However, long-term follow-up population-based studies assessing the incidence of diabetes in large cohorts of subjects have shown the risk of developing diabetes was significantly higher in HCV subjects with risk factors such as age or obesity.[43,44] In a longitudinal study of liver transplant recipients who were followed for 1 year, HCV-positive subjects were 4 times more likely to become diabetic after transplant than were HCV-negative subjects. In addition, HCV RNA levels correlated with a more rapid development of IR.[45] Steatosis, which is highly prevalent in CHC, may be another explanation for the link between HCV and IR. The absence of IR in subjects with viral steatosis indirectly suggests that steatosis is the consequence rather than the cause of IR in chronic HCV.[6,7] Moderate iron overload is frequent in chronic HCV but there is no association between intrahepatic iron concentration and HOMA index.[7] Association of IR with oxidative stress has been found in 1 study.[46] The association of IL-28 B polymorphism with IR has been suggested in HCV patients but with conflicting results.[47,48] Finally, the improvement of IR in patients with HCV clearance following antiviral therapy suggests that HCV infection itself may promote IR.[49,50] In this setting, a long-term follow-up study in nondiabetic HCV subjects receiving antiviral therapy has shown that SVR was associated with lower incidence of type 2 diabetes onset compared with non-SVR.[51]

However, despite the evidence in subject-based studies that HCV may promote IR and diabetes, the link between HCV and diabetes was not fully confirmed in population-based studies, mainly cross-sectional. The prevalence of type 2 diabetes in HCV-positive persons ranges between 2.9% and 12.6%, which was globally similar to that reported for HCV-negative persons and far lower than that reported for HCV subjects with chronic liver disease (see **Table 1**).[52–57] In a study using National Health and Nutrition Examination Survey (NHANES) data, the relationship between HCV infection and diabetes was found significant among persons greater than 40 years of age.[52] In another study using NHANES cycles, no association was found in NHANES 1999 to 2004 (OR 0.9, 95% CI 0.6–1.6) or NHANES 2005 to 2008 (OR 1.3, 95% CI 0.7–2.3), despite increased prevalence of diabetes in the later cycle.[54] In a second study using NHANES 1999 to 2010, the risk of having diabetes was twice higher compared with noninfected persons.[55] However, in an NHANES-based study using recent data for the diagnosis of diabetes, diabetes or IR were no longer associated with HCV infection but with alanine transferase (ALT) elevation.[56] In a large matched population-based study from Scotland, the prevalence of diabetes was low and not different between HCV-positive or HCV-negative persons.[57] The lack of

Table 2
Prevalence of hepatitis C virus infection among diabetics and controls

Author (Reference)	Study Population (n)	Diabetics (%)	Controls (%)
Mason et al,[27] 1999	Diabetics (594) Thyroid (377)	4.2	1.6
Okan et al,[40] 2002	Diabetics (692) Blood donors (1014)	7.5	0.1
Sangiorno et al,[41] 2000	Diabetics (1514)	7.6	—
Simo et al,[42] 1996	Diabetics (176) Blood donors (6172)	11.5	2.5

association between HCV and diabetes or IR in these population-based studies may be explained by their cross-sectional design and the rather low prevalences of HCV infection, liver disease, or diabetes. In this setting, longitudinal population-based studies have found a significant association between the risk of incident diabetes and HCV infection in most cases.[43,44,53]

Taken together, these results suggest a direct link between HCV infection and IR, independent of BMI and visceral adiposity. They also stress the important role of HCV genotypes and high viral load in this setting.

Mechanisms of Hepatitis C Virus–Induced Insulin Resistance

Experimental and clinical studies have suggested that HCV may interact with glucose metabolism and promote IR through multiple pathogenic mechanisms: direct inhibition of insulin signaling pathway, overproduction of proinflammatory cytokines, oxidative stress, modulation of incretins, or pancreatic ß-cells dysfunction.

Hepatitis C virus effects on insulin signaling pathway in the liver

A defect in postreceptor insulin signaling is involved in the HCV-induced IR. The comparison of liver biopsy of nondiabetic or nonobese chronic HCV subjects with matched noninfected controls showed a marked decrease in the ability of ionotropic receptor (IRS)-1 to associate with the insulin receptor, and a corresponding disruption of downstream signaling pathways, including reductions in insulin-stimulated tyrosine phosphorylation and phosphatidylinositol 3-kinase (PI3-K) enzymatic activity.[58] In transgenic mice, genotype 1 HCV core protein is able to suppress IRS-1 tyrosine phosphorylation leading to IR and overt diabetes.[59] Subsequent study has shown downregulation of hepatic expression of both IRS-1 and IRS-2 by the HCV core protein-mediated induction of suppressor of cytokine signaling protein (SOCS)-3 via a mechanism that involves proteosomal degradation through ubiquitination, the net result of which is compensatory increases in fasting insulin levels and hepatic IR.[60] In addition, the core protein of genotype 1 has been shown to promote IRS-1 degradation through mammalian target of rapamycin (mTOR) activation and to suppress phosphorylation of tyrosine on IRS-1, as well as the production of IRS-2, through modulation of a proteasome activator 28_γ-dependent pathway.[61,62] The core protein of HCV genotype 3 can also promote IRS-1 degradation, and this effect is mediated by its effects on $PPAR_\gamma$ that lead to upregulation of SOCS-7.[63] HCV may also promote dephosphorylation of Akt by endoplasmic reticulum stress signal, leading to reduction of insulin signaling.[64] Interestingly, clearance of HCV infection has been shown to improve IR and restore the hepatic expression of IRS-1 and IRS-2.[49] These latter findings indicate a direct role for HCV infection in promoting IR through a reduction in insulin signaling mechanisms and a beneficial effect of anti-viral therapy on restoring insulin sensitivity in persons with HCV.

Proinflammatory cytokines and hepatitis C virus–mediated insulin resistance

Among the proinflammatory cytokines that have been associated with HCV infection in the liver, tumor necrosis factor (TNF)-alpha and its soluble receptor molecules, sTNFR1 and sTNFR2, may be most important. The levels of TNF-α in patients with CHC is strongly associated with both hepatic and systemic IR[48,65] and the development of diabetes.[66] Levels of sTNFR1 and sTNFR2, which are considered reliable and stable indicators of TNF activation, also are significantly associated with IR, in diabetic as well in nondiabetic HCV patients.[48,65,66] In transgenic mice, the hepatic IR caused by HCV core gene expression was principally mediated by increased TNF-α expression, whereas administration of an antibody to TNF could restore insulin levels to normal and return insulin sensitivity to normal.[59] TNF-α can also have indirect effects on IR and adipokines in persons with HCV. In a study conducted in chronic HCV subjects, serum TNF-α levels were positively correlated with steatosis grades and HOMA-IR values, whereas serum levels of adiponectin were inversely correlated with steatosis grades, serum TNF-α levels, and HOMA-IR values.[67] These findings support the close association of TNF-α, adiponectin, steatosis, and IR in chronic HCV patients. In a study comparing proinflammatory cytokine expression in liver tissues, intrahepatic expression of the cytokine IL-18, a potent inducer of gamma-IFN, was significantly upregulated in subjects with CHC versus controls, with a concordant increase in gamma-IFN expression.[68] HCV-infected patients develop IR in peripheral tissues (mainly skeletal muscle), as well as the liver, although the molecular mechanism remains unclear.[69] In another study, CHC was even associated with peripheral, rather than hepatic, IR.[70] Although mechanisms remain unknown, humoral factors such as TNF-α might be necessary for the development of IR in peripheral tissues that are distant from the HCV-infected liver, as demonstrated in a non-HCV experimental model.[71] Taken together, these data provide evidence that increased expression of TNF-α in the liver results in a suppression of insulin action in the liver and, likely, peripheral tissue, leading to IR and eventual progression to overt diabetes.

Reactive oxygen species and hepatitis C virus–mediated insulin resistance
Given the importance of reactive oxygen species (ROS) in the development of IR, it is noteworthy that HCV has been shown to be a potent inducer of ROS. In vitro and in vivo studies have demonstrated that HCV core protein was able to increase the production of ROS, without hepatic inflammation in some cases.[72,73] In subjects with CHC, serum and hepatic levels of thioredoxin, which are markers of oxidative stress, were significantly correlated with HOMA-IR and hepatic mRNA levels independently predicted HOMA-IR.[46] Both thioredoxin level and HOMA-IR were significantly reduced after phlebotomy. These findings argue for a role of oxidative stress, which may be directly induced by HCV core protein, in the development of IR.

Incretin and hepatitis C virus–mediated insulin resistance
Few reports to date have addressed the relationship between incretin and HCV infection. One study in HCV subjects found that the level of serum incretin hormones glucagon-like peptide (GLP)-1, which promote insulin biosynthesis, insulin secretion, and ß-cell survival, was significantly decreased compared with HBV or inflammatory bowel disease (IBD) subjects, or healthy controls. This decrease of GLP-1 level was associated with upregulation of liver and ileum dipeptidyl peptidase (DPP)-IV expression, which inactivate GLP-1, and with a significant decrease of hepatic glycogen content. The investigators concluded the altered expressions of GLP-1 and DPP-IV may be involved in the development of HCV-associated glucose intolerance.[74]

Effect of hepatitis C virus on pancreatic ß-cells
In vitro studies have demonstrated that HCV infection of human ß-cells leads to a reduction in the cells' glucose-stimulated insulin release and induces apoptosis-like death through an endothelial reticulum (ER) stress-involved, caspase 3-dependent, specific pathway.[75,76] However, in transgenic mice, the HCV core protein had no substantial effects on pancreas-related insulin, due to a compensatory increase of islet mass.[59] Further studies are needed to elucidate how HCV affects pancreatic ß-cells and their production or release of insulin.

In conclusion, there is considerable evidence that HCV through its interactions with lipid metabolism promotes steatosis and hypolipidemia. The epidemiologic link between HCV and diabetes mellitus in patients with chronic liver disease rather than in the general population suggests that inflammation play a major role in HCV-induced IR. In this setting, proinflammatory cytokines such as TNF-α have a central role, likely in liver but also in peripheral IR. Although host-related metabolic steatosis is likely involved in the promotion of IR, the role of viral-related steatosis is not evident. Therapies to reduce inflammation, HCV viral load, steatosis, and TNF-α activity can be expected to improve metabolic parameters and reduce DM risk in patients with chronic HCV.

REFERENCES

1. Büsch K, Waldenström J, Lagging M, et al. Prevalence and comorbidities of chronic hepatitis C: a nationwide population-based register study in Sweden. Scand J Gastroenterol 2017;52:61–8.
2. Younossi Z, Park H, Henry L, et al. Extrahepatic manifestations of hepatitis C: a meta-analysis of prevalence, quality of life, and economic burden. Gastroenterology 2016;150:1599–608.
3. Serfaty L, Capeau J. Hepatitis C, insulin resistance and diabetes: clinical and pathogenic data. Liver Int 2009;29:13–25.
4. Lonardo A, Loria P, Adinolfi LE, et al. Hepatitis C and steatosis: a reappraisal. J Viral Hepat 2006;13:73–80.
5. Serfaty L, Andreani T, Giral P, et al. Hepatitis C virus induced hypobetalipoproteinemia: a possible mechanism for steatosis in chronic hepatitis C. J Hepatol 2001; 34:428–34.
6. Bedossa P, Moucari R, Chelbi E, et al. Evidence for a role of nonalcoholic steatohepatitis in hepatitis C: a prospective study. Hepatology 2007;46:380–7.
7. Fartoux L, Poujol-Robert A, Guéchot J, et al. Insulin resistance is a cause of steatosis and fibrosis progression in chronic hepatitis C. Gut 2005;54:1003–8.
8. Poynard T, Ratziu V, McHutchison J, et al. Effect of treatment with peginterferon or interferon alfa-2b and ribavirin on steatosis in patients infected with hepatitis C. Hepatology 2003;38:75–85.
9. Cai T, Dufour JF, Muellhaupt B, et al, Swiss Hepatitis C Cohort Study Group. Viral genotype-specific role of PNPLA3, PPARG, MTTP, and IL28B in hepatitis C virus-associated steatosis. J Hepatol 2011;55:529–35.
10. Clark PJ, Thompson AJ, Zhu Q, et al. The association of genetic variants with hepatic steatosis in patients with genotype 1 chronic hepatitis C infection. Dig Dis Sci 2012;57:2213–21.
11. Hsu CS. Sofosbuvir for previously untreated chronic hepatitis C infection (Letter). N Engl J Med 2013;369:678–9.
12. Miyanari Y, Atsuzawa K, Usuda N, et al. The lipid droplet is an important organelle for hepatitis C virus production. Nat Cell Biol 2007;9:1089–97.
13. Alvisi G, Madan V, Bartenschlager R. Hepatitis C virus and host cell lipids: an intimate connection. RNA Biol 2011;8:258–69.
14. Perlemuter G, Sabile A, Letteron P, et al. Hepatitis C virus core protein inhibits microsomal triglyceride transfer protein activity and very low density lipoprotein secretion: a model of viral-related steatosis. FASEB J 2002;16:185–94.
15. Dharancy S, Malapel M, Perlemuter G, et al. Impaired expression of the peroxisome proliferator-activated receptor alpha during hepatitis C virus infection. Gastroenterology 2005;128:334–42.
16. Kim KH, Hong SP, Kim K, et al. HCV core protein induces hepatic lipid accumulation by activating SREBP1 and PPARgamma. Biochem Biophys Res Commun 2007;355:883–8.

17. Lambert JE, Bain VG, Ryan EA, et al. Elevated lipogenesis and diminished cholesterol synthesis in patients with hepatitis C viral infection compared to healthy humans. Hepatology 2013;57:1697–704.
18. Amako Y, Munakata T, Kohara M, et al. Hepatitis C virus attenuates mitochondrial lipid β-oxidation by downregulating mitochondrial trifunctional-protein expression. J Virol 2015;89:4092–101.
19. Abid K, Pazienza V, de Gottardi A, et al. An in vitro model of hepatitis C virus genotype 3a-associated triglycerides accumulation. J Hepatol 2005;42:744–51.
20. Jackel-Cram C, Babiuk LA, Liu Q. Up-regulation of fatty acid synthase promoter by hepatitis C virus core protein: genotype-3a core has a stronger effect than genotype-1b core. J Hepatol 2007;46:999–1008.
21. de Gottardi A, Pazienza V, Pugnale P, et al. Peroxisome proliferator-activated receptor-alpha and -gamma mRNA levels are reduced in chronic hepatitis C with steatosis and genotype 3 infection. Aliment Pharmacol Ther 2006;23:107–14.
22. Clark PJ, Thompson AJ, Vock DM, et al. Hepatitis C virus selectively perturbs the distal cholesterol synthesis pathway in a genotype-specific manner. Hepatology 2012;56:49–56.
23. Mirandola S, Realdon S, Iqbal J, et al. Liver microsomal triglyceride transfer protein is involved in hepatitis C liver steatosis. Gastroenterology 2006;130:1661–9.
24. Katsuki A, Sumida Y, Gabazza EC, et al. Homeostasis model assessment is a reliable indicator of insulin resistance during follow-up of patients with type 2 diabetes. Diabetes Care 2001;24:362–5.
25. Matthews DR, Hosker JP, Rudenski AS, et al. Homeostasis model assessment: insulin resistance and beta-cell function from fasting plasma glucose and insulin concentrations in man. Diabetologia 1985;28:412–9.
26. Stern SE, Williams K, Ferrannini E, et al. Identification of individuals with insulin resistance using routine clinical measurements. Diabetes 2005;54:333–9.
27. Mason AL, Lau JY, Hoang N, et al. Association of diabetes mellitus and chronic hepatitis C virus infection. Hepatology 1999;29:328–33.
28. Allison ME, Wreghitt T, Palmer CR, et al. Evidence for a link between hepatitis C virus infection and diabetes mellitus in a cirrhotic population. J Hepatol 1994;21:1135–9.
29. Grimbert S, Valensi P, Levy-Marchal C, et al. High prevalence of diabetes mellitus in patients with chronic hepatitis C. A case–control study. Gastroenterol Clin Biol 1996;20:544–8.
30. Caronia S, Taylor K, Pagliaro L, et al. Further evidence for an association between non-insulin-dependent diabetes mellitus and chronic hepatitis C virus infection. Hepatology 1999;30:1059–63.
31. Arao M, Murase K, Kusakabe A, et al. Prevalence of diabetes mellitus in Japanese patients infected chronically with hepatitis C virus. J Gastroenterol 2003;38:355–60.
32. Imazeki F, Yokosuka O, Fukai K, et al. Prevalence of diabetes mellitus and insulin resistance in patients with chronic hepatitis C: comparison with hepatitis B virus-infected and hepatitis C virus-cleared patients. Liver Int 2008;28:355–62.
33. Rouabhia S, Malek R, Bounecer H, et al. Prevalence of type 2 diabetes in Algerian patients with hepatitis C virus infection. World J Gastroenterol 2010;16:3427–31.
34. White DL, Ratziu V, El-Serag HB. Hepatitis C infection and risk of diabetes: a systematic review and meta-analysis. J Hepatol 2008;49:831–44.
35. Naing C, Mak JW, Ahmed SI, et al. Relationship between hepatitis C virus infection and type 2 diabetes mellitus: meta-analysis. World J Gastroenterol 2012;18:1642–51.

36. Moucari R, Asselah T, Cazals-Hatem D, et al. Insulin resistance in chronic hepatitis C: association with genotypes 1 and 4, serum HCV RNA level, and liver fibrosis. Gastroenterology 2008;134:416–23.

37. Mihm S. Hepatitis C virus, diabetes and steatosis: clinical evidence in favor of a linkage and role of genotypes. Dig Dis 2010;28:280–4.

38. Hsu CS, Liu CJ, Liu CH, et al. High hepatitis C viral load is associated with insulin resistance in patients with chronic hepatitis C. Liver Int 2008;28:271–7.

39. Yoneda M, Saito S, Ikeda T, et al. Hepatitis C virus directly associates with insulin resistance independent of the visceral fat area in nonobese and nondiabetic patients. J Viral Hepat 2007;14:600–7.

40. Okan V, Araz M, Aktaran S, et al. Increased frequency of HCV but not HBV infection in type 2 diabetic patients in Turkey. Int J Clin Pract 2002;56:175–7.

41. Sangiorgio L, Attardo T, Gangemi R, et al. Increased frequency of HCV and HBV infection in type 2 diabetic patients. Diabetes Res Clin Pract 2000;48:147–51.

42. Simo R, Hernandez C, Genesca J, et al. High prevalence of hepatitis C virus infection in diabetic patients. Diabetes Care 1996;19:998–1000.

43. Mehta SH, Brancati FL, Strathdee SA, et al. Hepatitis C virus infection and incident type 2 diabetes. Hepatology 2003;38:50–6.

44. Wang CS, Wang ST, Yao WJ, et al. Hepatitis C virus infection and the development of type 2 diabetes in a community-based longitudinal study. Am J Epidemiol 2007;166:196–203.

45. Delgado-Borrego A, Liu Y-S, Jordan SH, et al. Prospective study of liver transplant recipients with HCV infection: evidence for a causal relationship between HCV and insulin resistance. Liver Transpl 2008;14:193–201.

46. Mitsuyoshi H, Itoh Y, Sumida Y, et al. Evidence of oxidative stress as a cofactor in the development of insulin resistance in patients with chronic hepatitis C. Hepatol Res 2008;38:348–53.

47. Stättermayer AF, Rutter K, Beinhardt S, et al. Association of the IL28B genotype with insulin resistance in patients with chronic hepatitis C. J Hepatol 2012;57:492–8.

48. Lemoine M, Chevaliez S, Bastard JP, et al. Association between IL28B polymorphism, TNFα and biomarkers of insulin resistance in chronic hepatitis C-related insulin resistance. J Viral Hepat 2015;22:890–6.

49. Kawaguchi T, Ide T, Taniguchi E, et al. Clearance of HCV improves insulin resistance, beta-cell function, and hepatic expression of insulin receptor substrate 1 and 2. Am J Gastroenterol 2007;102:570–6.

50. Sanchez-Tapias JM, Diago M, Escartín P, et al, Diago MTeraViC-4 Study Group. Peginterferon-alfa2a plus ribavirin for 48 versus 72 weeks in patients with detectable hepatitis C virus RNA at week 4 of treatment. Gastroenterology 2006;131:451–60.

51. Arase Y, Suzuki F, Suzuki Y, et al. Sustained virological response reduces incidence of onset of type 2 diabetes in chronic hepatitis C. Hepatology 2009;49:739–44.

52. Mehta SH, Brancati FL, Sulkowski MS, et al. Prevalence of type 2 diabetes mellitus among persons with hepatitis C virus infection in the United States. Ann Intern Med 2000;133:592–9.

53. Montenegro L, De Michina A, Misciagna G, et al. Virus C hepatitis and type 2 diabetes: a cohort study in southern Italy. Am J Gastroenterol 2013;108:1108–11.

54. Stepanova M, Lam B, Younossi Y, et al. Association of hepatitis C with insulin resistance and type 2 diabetes in US general population: the impact of the epidemic of obesity. J Viral Hepat 2012;19:341–5.

55. Younossi ZM, Stepanova M, Nader F, et al. Associations of chronic hepatitis C with metabolic and cardiac outcomes. Ali Ment Pharmacol Ther 2013;37:647–52.
56. Ruhl CE, Menke A, Cowie CC, et al. Relationship of hepatitis C virus infection with diabetes in the U.S. population. Hepatology 2014;60:1139–49.
57. Schnier C, Wild S, Kurdi Z, et al. Matched population-based study examining the risk of type 2 diabetes in people with and without diagnosed hepatitis C virus infection. J Viral Hepat 2016;23:596–605.
58. Aytug S, Reich D, Sapiro LE, et al. Impaired IRS-1/PI3-kinase signaling in patients with HCV: a mechanism for increased prevalence of type 2 diabetes. Hepatology 2003;38:1384–92.
59. Shintani Y, Fujie H, Miyoshi H, et al. Hepatitis C virus infection and diabetes: direct involvement of the virus in the development of insulin resistance. Gastroenterology 2004;126:840–8.
60. Kawaguchi T, Yoshida T, Harada M, et al. Hepatitis C virus down-regulates insulin receptor substrates 1 and 2 through up-regulation of suppressor of cytokine signaling 3. Am J Pathol 2004;165:1499–508.
61. Pazienza V, Clément S, Pugnale P, et al. The hepatitis C virus core protein of genotypes 3a and 1b downregulates insulin receptor substrate 1 through genotype-specific mechanisms. Hepatology 2007;45:1164–71.
62. Miyamoto H, Moriishi K, Moriya K, et al. Involvement of the PA28gamma-dependent pathway in insulin resistance induced by hepatitis C virus core protein. J Virol 2007;81:1727–35.
63. Pazienza V, Vinciguerra M, Andriulli A, et al. Hepatitis C virus core protein genotype 3a increases SOCS-7 expression through PPAR-{gamma} in Huh-7 cells. J Gen Virol 2010;91:1678–86.
64. Christen V, Treves S, Duong FH, et al. Activation of endoplasmic reticulum stress response by hepatitis viruses up-regulates protein phosphatase 2A. Hepatology 2007;46:558–65.
65. Lecube A, Hernández C, Genescà J, et al. Proinflammatory cytokines, insulin resistance, and insulin secretion in chronic hepatitis C patients: a case-control study. Diabetes Care 2006;29:1096–101.
66. Knobler H, Zhornicky T, Sandler A, et al. Tumor necrosis factor-alpha-induced insulin resistance may mediate the hepatitis C virus-diabetes association. Am J Gastroenterol 2003;98:2751–6.
67. Durante-Mangoni E, Zampino R, Marrone A, et al. Hepatic steatosis and insulin resistance are associated with serum imbalance of adiponectin/tumour necrosis factor-alpha in chronic hepatitis C patients. Aliment Pharmacol Ther 2006;24:1349–57.
68. McGuinness PH, Painter D, Davies S, et al. Increases in intrahepatic CD68 positive cells, MAC387 positive cells, and proinflammatory cytokines (particularly interleukin 18) in chronic hepatitis C infection. Gut 2000;46:260–9.
69. Vanni E, Abate ML, Gentilcore E, et al. Sites and mechanisms of insulin resistance in nonobese, nondiabetic patients with chronic hepatitis C. Hepatology 2009;50:697–706.
70. Milner KL, van der Poorten D, Trenell M, et al. Chronic hepatitis C is associated with peripheral rather than hepatic insulin resistance. Gastroenterology 2010;138:932–41.
71. Hotamisligil GS, Budavari A, Murray D, et al. Reduced tyrosine kinase activity of the insulin receptor in obesity-diabetes. Central role of tumor necrosis factor-alpha. J Clin Invest 1994;94:1543–9.

72. Okuda M, Li K, Beard MR, et al. Mitochondrial injury, oxidative stress, and antioxidant gene expression are induced by hepatitis C virus core protein. Gastroenterology 2002;122:366–75.

73. Lerat H, Honda M, Beard MR, et al. Steatosis and liver cancer in transgenic mice expressing the structural and nonstructural proteins of hepatitis C virus. Gastroenterology 2002;122:352–65.

74. Itou M, Kawaguchi T, Taniguchi E, et al. Altered expression of glucagon-like peptide-1 and dipeptidyl peptidase IV in patients with HCV-related glucose intolerance. J Gastroenterol Hepatol 2008;23:244–51.

75. Masini M, Campani D, Boggi U, et al. Hepatitis C virus infection and human pancreatic beta-cell dysfunction. Diabetes Care 2005;28:940–1.

76. Wang Q, Chen J, Wang Y, et al. Hepatitis C virus induced a novel apoptosis-like death of pancreatic beta cells through a caspase 3-dependent pathway. PLoS One 2012;7:e38522.

Renal Manifestations of Hepatitis C Virus

Clodoveo Ferri, MD*, Dilia Giuggioli, MD, Michele Colaci, MD

KEYWORDS

- Hepatitis C virus • Kidney • Renal involvement • Glomerulonephritis • Autoimmunity
- Cryoglobulinemia • Cryoglobulinemic vasculitis • Lymphoma

KEY POINTS

- Hepatitis C virus (HCV) is both a hepatotropic and lymphotropic virus responsible for a spectrum of hepatic and extrahepatic immune-mediated and neoplastic disorders, including renal involvement.
- HCV-infected patients should undergo careful clinicoserologic assessment at the first referral followed by constant monitoring to detect possible organ involvement early, including renal involvement.
- HCV-related nephropathy may show different histopathologic patterns, more often a membranoproliferative glomerulonephritis, which may appear at any time during the natural history of HCV infection.
- Renal involvement may develop as isolated manifestation or in association with other HCV-related disorders, mainly mixed cryoglobulinemia syndrome (MCS).
- New direct-acting viral agents (DAAs) represent the first-line treatment of HCV-related nephropathy; other pathogenetic therapies (steroids/immunosuppressors/plasmapheresis) may be usefully used for rapidly progressive glomerulonephritis.

INTRODUCTION

HCV is a hepatotropic and lymphotropic virus responsible for a wide spectrum of both hepatic and extrahepatic diseases.[1–3] The HCV-related extrahepatic manifestations (HCV-EHMs) include nonorgan and organ-specific autoimmune/lymphoproliferative and neoplastic disorders (**Fig. 1**).[2,3] MCS, also termed cryoglobulinemic vasculitis, represents the prototype of extrahepatic systemic immune-mediated disorder characterized by multiple organ involvement.[1–3] The authors previously introduced the term, *HCV syndrome* (see **Fig. 1**), to refer to the multiform complex of HCV-related diseases.[1,3] In this scenario, HCV- related renal involvement is one of the most severe

The authors have nothing to disclose.
Rheumatology Unit, University of Modena and Reggio Emilia, Azienda Ospedaliero-Universitaria Policlinico di Modena, Via del Pozzo, 71, Modena 41100, Italy
* Corresponding author.
E-mail address: clferri@unimore.it

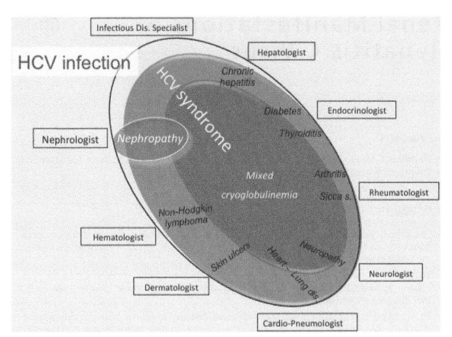

Fig. 1. Renal involvement and HCV infection. The figure schematically reproduces the spectrum of HCV infection and diseases. HCV is a hepatotropic and lymphotropic virus responsible for a wide spectrum of both hepatic and extrahepatic diseases. The term HCV syndrome refers to the multiform complex of all HCV-related diseases. Besides HCV-infected patients without clinical manifestations or isolated liver involvement, HCV-EHMs may include a variety of nonorgan and organ-specific autoimmune/lymphoproliferative and neoplastic disorders; therefore, HCV-positive patients are commonly referred to different specialists according the prevalent clinical manifestation(s). MCS, also termed cryoglobulinemic vasculitis, represents the prototype of extrahepatic systemic immune-mediated disorder characterized by multiple organ involvement. In this scenario, HCV-related renal involvement is one of the most severe HCV-EHMs; it may present as apparently isolated condition or in association with other HCV-EHMs, mainly MCS. dis, diseases; sicca s, sick syndrome/Sjogren's syndrome.

HCV-EHMs; it includes a broad spectrum of kidney histopathologic lesions, mostly the membrane-proliferative glomerulonephritis (MPGN).

Clinically, patients with HCV nephropathy may be totally asymptomatic, showing only mild urinary abnormalities; on the other hand, renal insufficiency, up to end-stage renal failure requiring kidney transplant, may represent a possible harmful evolution.[4–6] Overall, HCV infection per se has been clearly recognized as an independent risk factor for kidney damage, even if some possible comorbidities, such as diabetes mellitus or other metabolic disorders, may be also involved.[7]

The actual prevalence of renal involvement in HCV-infected patients is difficult to estimate, because of the large heterogeneity of reported case series, in terms of both geographic provenience and subspecialty referral (see **Fig. 1**); in the setting of HCV-related MCS, previous cohort studies showed a fairly constant percentage of approximately a third of patients with complicating nephropathy.[8,9]

HEPATIATIS C VIRUS–ASSOCIATED RENAL DISEASE
Histopathologic Features

HCV-related renal damage may include several histopathologic patterns, with possible glomerular and/or interstitial lesions.[4,10,11] As shown in **Table 1**, MPGN type 1 is the most typical and frequent pathologic entity. This renal manifestation may be in the context of the clinical picture of MCS; on the other hand, MPGN may appear as unique or clinically relevant organ involvement as part of the HCV syndrome, regardless of the presence/absence of detectable serum mixed cryoglobulins.

Etiopathogenesis

Kidney injury may be the result of 2 main processes, not mutually exclusive: immune-mediated tissue damage and HCV direct effects (**Fig. 2**). Moreover, other unknown environmental and/or host factors, such as genetic background, and/or other concomitant severe manifestations (decompensated cirrhosis, widespread cryoglobulinemic vasculitis, and/or comorbidities, such as diabetes) may contribute to renal damage.[4–11]

The renal deposition of cryoprecipitable and noncryoprecipitable immune complexes containing HCV antigens is the main pathogenetic mechanism of the glomerular inflammation, even if the virus may directly contribute to tissue damage by infecting the endothelium, tubular epithelial cells, and infiltrating leukocytes.[6,10,11]

Table 1
Histopathological features of hepatitis C virus–related renal involvement

Renal Disease Pattern	Histologic Features	Frequency
Diffuse or focal MPGN	Mesangial cells proliferation plus deposits of immune complexes, including HCV particles, complement fragments, immunoglobulins with/without cryoprecipitation capability; frequently, double contour appearance of the capillary wall	Typically found
Mesangial proliferative GN	Diffuse mild mesangial matrix expansion and mesangial cells proliferation	Occasionally found
Tubulointerstitial nephritis[a]	Interstitial fibrosis and infiltrating leukocytes, usually focal, with negative immunofluorescence	Rare
Membranous GN	Subepithelial deposits of immune complexes and C3	Rare
IgA nephropathy	Mesangial IgA deposits	Rare
Thrombotic microangiopathy[b]	Arterioles showed intimal thickening, swollen endothelium, narrowed glomerular capillary lumen, and thrombi that may extend into afferent arterioles	Rare
Focal segmental glomerulosclerosis	Sclerosed glomeruli and tubular atrophy, negative immunofluorescence, deletion of podocytes of epithelial cells (electronic microscopy)	Anecdotal
Immunotactoid glomerulopathy fibrillary GN	Extracellular deposits of microfibrils within the mesangium and glomerular capillary walls; Ig (mainly IgG4) and C3 immunofluorescence	Anecdotal

Abbreviation: GN, glomerulonephritis.
 [a] Interstitial fibrosis and infiltrating leukocytes are associated with greater than 60% MPGN, whereas an isolated interstitial nephritis is rare.
 [b] Endoluminal thrombi are frequently associated with other pathologic patterns (>50% of MPGN); besides, a peculiar form in the context of a hemolytic uremic syndrome was rarely described in renal transplanted patients.

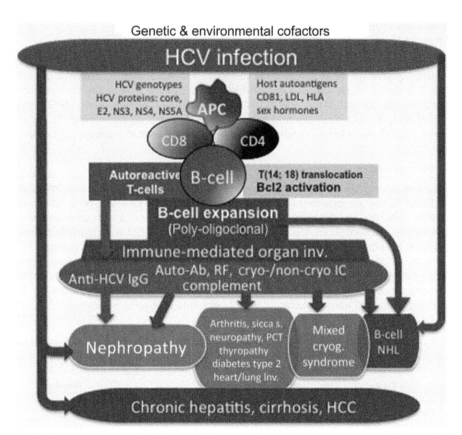

Fig. 2. Etiopathogenesis of HCV-related diseases. Kidney involvement may be the result of 2 main processes, not mutually exclusive: immune-mediated tissue damage and HCV direct injury. In addition, other unknown environmental and/or host predisposing factors (genetic background, and/or concomitant severe manifestations, such as decompensated cirrhosis or diabetes) may contribute to renal damage. The HCV lymphotropism represents the main pathogenetic mechanism of HCV-related clinical manifestation, including the nephropathy, in the setting of HCV syndrome (see **Fig. 1**). HCV antigens are responsible for both T-lymphocyte and B-lymphocyte activation with production of different autoantibodies and cryoprecipitable and noncryoprecipitable immune complexes, potentially involved in the pathogenesis of HCV-related nephropathy. Moreover, the HCV infection of B-lymphocytes is responsible for lymphoproliferative manifestations, including frank B-cell NHL. HCV-related nephropathy is the result of glomerular deposition of immune complexes, anti-HCV IgG, and/or antiendothelial antibodies and complement responsible for the inflammatory process. On the other hand, HCV may directly contribute to tissue damage by infecting the endothelium, tubular epithelial cells, and infiltrating leukocytes. Ab, antibodies; APC, antigen-presenting cells; cryo, cryoprecipitable; cryog, cryoglobulinemia; HCC, hepatocellular carcinoma; HLA, human leukocyte antigen; IC, immune complexes; inv, involvement; LDL, low-density lipoprotein; NHL, non-Hodgkin lymphoma; PCT, porphyria cutanea tarda; RF, rheumatoid factor; s, syndrome.

Mixed cryoglobulins that circulate in the arteriolar vessels may deposit in the mesangium after the active crossing through the endothelial barrier, during the macromolecular trafficking in the glomeruli. Immunofluorescence reveals subendothelial IgM deposits; sometimes, immune complexes also occlude capillary lumen as dense eosinophilic deposits.[6,10,11] The strong affinity of the IgM with rheumatoid activity for cellular fibronectin in the mesangium is considered a cause of nephrotoxicity.[11] Moreover, the immune complexes produce vasculitis, via complement activation, with fibrinoid necrosis of the glomerular vessels. On the other hand, endothelial cells overexpress adhesion molecules that recruit inflammatory cells; platelet activation and aggregation complete this pathologic process. Finally, if capillary damage results, cryoglobulins may pass into the urinary space, contributing to the development of crescents and tubular casts.

In cases of noncryoglobulinemic immune complexes, anti-HCV IgG deposits and complement fragments may be found in the mesangium, leading to MPGN.[6,10,11] Furthermore, immunoglobulins with antiendothelial activity may also stimulate cell activation and injury.

Endothelial damage may be determined by the direct effect of HCV, as observed in the hepatic sinusoids where cell apoptosis is induced by the virus. Also, epithelial cells from the Bowman capsule may be infected by HCV that eventually causes the loss of podocytes as well as the cells of renal tubules.[6,10,11] Finally, a direct effect of the virus on mesangial cells cannot be excluded.

Clinical Aspects

Patients with HCV-related nephropathy may present a variety of clinical features, including both typical renal symptoms and 1 or more possible extrarenal manifestations[4-11]; in particular, they may be totally asymptomatic with occult urinary abnormalities or with the multiform manifestations of cryoglobulinemic vasculitis (see **Figs. 1** and **2**). For descriptive purposes, the following main clinical patterns can be identified.

Isolated hepatitis C virus–related renal disease

Patients with isolated MPGN or other less frequent renal conditions[4] generally present with microscopic hematuria and mild proteinuria, associated with variable impairment of renal function; the latter is reported in approximately 10% of HCV-infected individuals in a large US cohort.[12] In more severe cases, higher amounts of proteinuria led to nephrotic syndrome or, less commonly, to acute nephritic syndrome, acute renal failure, and/or oligo-anuria in a few instances. These conditions may be responsible for a variable degree of edema, pericardial or pleural effusion, and/or hypertension with possible end-organ damage.

Renal involvement plus other hepatitis C virus extrahepatic manifestations

The clinical pattern, renal involvement plus other HCV extra-hepatic manifestations, encompasses a heterogeneous group of extrarenal disorders, namely different organ-specific and non–organ-specific autoimmune diseases or neoplastic complications that characterize the HCV syndrome (see **Fig. 1**; discussed previously).[3] HCV may persistently infect several cell types, including lymphocytes and epithelial and glandular cells, triggering autoimmune processes that may lead to thyroiditis, arthritis, sialadenitis, diabetes, myocarditis, and so forth. On the other hand, HCV may facilitate lymphomagenesis as a consequence of its persistent antigenic stimulation and/or direct oncogenic potential.[1-3,13] The more frequent types of hematological malignancy are diffuse large B-cell, lymphoplasmacytic, and marginal zone non-Hodgkin lymphomas.

In this scenario, it is often difficult to completely define the exact clinical pattern of a single patient because of the complex overlap between different HCV-related disorders; in these instances, a multidisciplinary approach is opportune for a comprehensive patient assessment and tailored treatment (**Fig. 3**). Therefore, a systematic

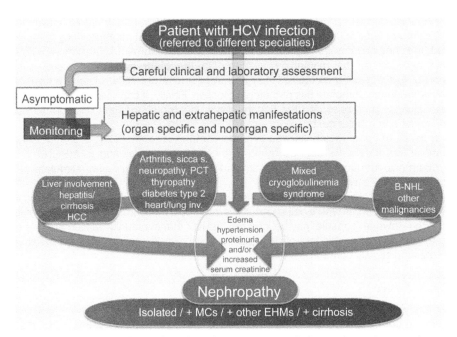

Fig. 3. HCV-related nephropathy: clinical assessment and diagnosis. Patients with HCV infection should be systematically investigated with regards to both hepatic and extrahepatic autoimmune/lymphoproliferartive and neoplastic disorders, regardless of the specialty of the referral centers. In addition, asymptomatic HCV-infected subjects should be monitored to detect possible hepatic and HCV-EHMs early, including urinalysis and sediment evaluation. Nephropathy may be easily suspected in the presence of urinary abnormalities, edema, hypertension, proteinuria and/or increased serum creatinine, ultrasound kidney evaluation, and if opportune renal needle-biopsy. Clinically, renal manifestations, mainly the MPGN, can be observed as isolated manifestation or more frequently in association with MCS or other HCV-EHMs; alternatively, it may complicate severe hepatic (decompensated cirrhosis), metabolic (diabetes), and/or cardiopulmonary manifestations. inv, involvement; HCC, hepatocellular carcinoma; MCs, mixed cryoglobulinemia syndrome; NHL, non-Hodgkin lymphoma; PCT, porphyria cutanea tarda; s, syndrome.

clinicoserologic evaluation of HCV patients is mandatory, according to proposed guidelines (discussed later).[14]

Renal involvement and cryoglobulinemic vasculitis

In the setting of HCV-EHMs, the MCS (cryoglobulinemic vasculitis) represents one of the most complex and harmful manifestations that may be complicated by renal involvement.[1–3,8]

MCS is the prototype of systemic autoimmune disease related to chronic HCV infection.[1–3,8] It is classically characterized by cutaneous leukocytoclastic vasculitis; the classic clinical triad of palpable orthostatic purpura, asthenia, and arthralgias; and possible multiorgan involvement.[1–3,8] The MC-associated nephropathy, mainly MPGN due to glomerul deposition of cryoprecipitable immune complexes (see **Table 1**), may represent the main clinical feature in approximately one-third of cases. In these patients, other autoimmune disorders can be clinically relevant, including the increased risk of non-Hodgkin lymphoma; they may contribute to renal damage and may severely affect the overall prognosis.[6,8]

Renal dysfunction in hepatitis C virus–related liver cirrhosis

Patients with advanced lived damage, mainly decompensated cirrhosis, may develop acute renal failure, the classic hepatorenal syndrome, a life-threatening condition that may require dialysis and liver transplant.[15] The hepatorenal syndrome is considered a consequence of splanchnic vasodilation due to portal hypertension with renal hypoperfusion. The activation of the renin-angiotensin-aldosterone system ultimately produces prerenal azotemia, which may progress to acute or chronic tubular necrosis.[6,15] The renal involvement secondary to decompensated cirrhosis may also precipitate a contemporary/preexisting immune-mediated glomerulonephritis in HCV-infected patients.

Other comorbidities, such as diabetes or ongoing treatments (immunosuppressors/corticosteroids), may contribute to renal injury.

DIAGNOSIS

All HCV-infected patients should routinely undergo urinalysis, including sediment evaluation, to identify the clinical onset of possible renal disease early (see **Fig. 3**).[4,14] Renal involvement in HCV patients may be easily suspected in the presence of urinary abnormalities, edema, hypertension, proteinuria, and/or increased serum creatinine (see **Fig. 3**).[4,14] Patients with these presenting symptoms are firstly referred to a nephrologist (see **Figs. 1** and **3**). Ultrasound kidney evaluation often reveals cortical hyperechogenicity and loss of cortical-medullar differentiation, whereas urinary sediment may contain dysmorphic erythrocytes due to their crossing through damaged glomeruli. Renal needle biopsy is mandatory to histologically assess glomerular/interstitial patterns, including the immunofluorescence studies (see **Table 1**). Glomerulonephritis may complicate the clinical pattern in MC patients or subjects affected by other autoimmune or neoplastic HCV-related disorders, requiring a multidisciplinary patient assessment (see **Fig. 3**).

PROGNOSIS

It is difficult to evaluate the prognosis of HCV-related nephropathy because of the complexity of the clinical spectrum of HCV syndrome and possible comorbidities.[1–3] Besides the careful evaluation of the severity/activity of histopathologic alterations, the prognostic value of renal involvement should be contextualized in the entire clinical pattern presented by a single patient.

Moreover, the impact of chronic kidney disease in HCV patients with increased risk of cardiovascular complications (severe arrhythmia, congestive heart failure, and death) has been evaluated in a large US population diagnosed between 2004 and 2014.[16] Negative prognostic factors were the higher rates of hypertension and diabetes observed in HCV patients with renal involvement compared with those without.[12] In this context, a direct pathogenetic role of the virus in the development of endothelial dysfunction has been hypothesized; HCV may induce a chronic inflammation that in turn may induce the development of diffuse atherosclerosis.[17]

The impact of persistent HCV infection per se on chronic kidney disease is relevant; lower survival rates in dialyzed populations[5,7] were reported, with hepatocellular carcinoma and liver cirrhosis frequent causes of death. A review, including 18 observational studies, showed that HCV-infected renal transplant recipients have worse outcomes (mortality and graft loss) than HCV-negative recipients with HCV infection as an independent risk factor for graft loss and increased mortality.[18] Overall, the survival of patients with kidney transplant was significantly lower in the HCV-positive patients than in the HCV-negative patients.[19]

For patients with HCV-related renal disease, the risk of progression to end-stage renal failure is correlated with patient age, serum creatinine level, and proteinuria at the time of histologic diagnosis.[4]

Finally, renal involvement is one of the most harmful complications in MCS and may severely affect a patient's clinical outcome; a survival study demonstrated that renal failure caused by chronic glomerulonephritis was responsible for death in one-third of deceased MC patients.[8]

TREATMENT

Considering the complex, multistep etiopathogenesis of HCV-related disorders, the therapeutic strategy of HCV-related nephropathy, as well as of other HCV-EHMs, is essentially based on 3 main levels of intervention (see **Fig. 1**): the etiologic treatment by means of antivirals directed at HCV eradication, the pathogenetic therapies with immunomodulating-immunosuppressive agents, and the pathogenetic/symptomatic therapies, such as corticosteroids, plasmapheresis, and antinflammatory/analgesic drugs.[20]

The antiviral therapy for HCV, formerly based on the association of pegylated interferon alpha and ribavirin, has been recently revolutionized by the availability of new DAAs.[21–23] These agents, variably combined, with or without ribavirin, permit avoiding the harmful side effects of interferon, mainly in patients affected by autoimmune disorders (ie, neuropathy and thyroiditis). The stronger antiviral activity of DAAs and better adherence to therapeutic protocols have permitted high successful eradication rates. Therefore, the eradication of HCV is considered a mainstay of the treatment of patients affected by virus-related hepatic or extrahepatic disorders.[1,20] It can be assumed that the elimination of the principal etiologic factor may interrupt the complex autoimmune process underlying different manifestations of HCV syndrome (**Fig. 4**).

The actual role of DAAs in HCV-related kidney disease needs to be further studied. Among the currently approved DAAs, sofosbuvir is the only one that has significant renal elimination. The other DAAs (simeprevir, ledipasvir, daclatasvir, paritaprevir/ritonavir, ombitasvir, dasabuvir, grazoprevir, and elbasvir) are not eliminated by the kidneys and thus do not need dose adjustment, even in patients with severe renal impairment.

Besides the etiologic therapy, various pathogenetic/symptomatic treatments mat be used to control different HCV-EHMs, alone or in concomitance (see **Fig. 4**).[2,20]

The immunologic/pathogenetic therapies include the use of rituximab, a monoclonal anti-CD20 antibody, to reduce B-lymphocyte overexpression.[24] This biologic agent was revealed as particularly effective in HCV-related extrahepatic autoimmune manifestations, including glomerulonephritis, showing a generally safe profile, particularly at a dose of 375 mg/m^2 a week for 4 consecutive weeks (see **Fig. 4**).[23,24]

Other immunosuppressive agents potentially effective for HCV-related renal disease are corticosteroids, cyclophosphamide, and plasma exchange, alone or as combination therapy (see **Fig. 4**). This approach may represent a prompt, useful treatment of recent-onset, rapidly progressive glomerulonephritis; sensory-motor peripheral neuropathy; and/or severe life-threatening vasculitis.[20] Corticosteroids may be used in a wide range of dosages; low-dose corticosteroids may be sufficient for mild to moderate HCV-EHMs, such as purpura, arthralgias/arthritis, and so forth.[20] Finally, plasma exchange (or double-filtration plasmapheresis for patients with cryoglobulinemic vasculitis) still represents an effective and safe therapeutic approach, usually in association with other immunosuppressors, to avoid the possible rebound of circulating cryoprecipitable and noncryoprecipitable immune complex levels.

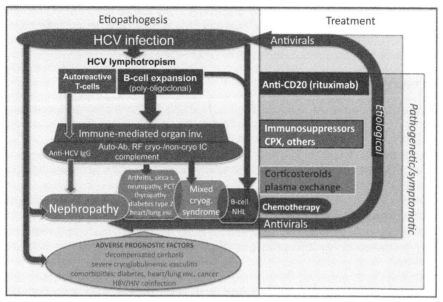

Fig. 4. Therapeutic strategies of HCV-related diseases. Therapeutic strategies of HCV-related diseases, including the nephropathy, are essentially based on 3 main levels of intervention: (1) etiologic treatment by means of antivirals directed at HCV eradication, (2) pathogenetic therapies with immunomodulating-immunosuppressive agents, and (3) pathogenetic/symptomatic therapies, such as corticosteroids, plasmapheresis, antinflammatory/analgesic drugs (see text). The antiviral therapy might represent the gold standard in all HCV-infected patients regardless the presence of HCV-EHMs. Besides the etiologic therapy, various pathogenetic/symptomatic treatments mat be used to control different HCV-EHMs, alone or in concomitance. HCV-related renal disease, mainly recent-onset, rapidly progressive acute nephritic syndrome; sensory-motor peripheral neuropathy; and/or severe life-threatening vasculitic may be usefully treated with high-dose corticosteroids, cyclophosphamide, and plasma exchange, alone or as combination therapy (see **Fig. 4**). The presence of some adverse prognostic factors should be carefully evaluated in all cases before the therapeutic decisions. Ab, antibodies; CPX, cyclophosphamide; cryo, cryoprecipitable; cryiog, cryoglobulinemia; HBV, hepatitis B virus; IC, immune complexes; inv, involvement; NHL, non-Hodgkin lymphoma; PCT, porphyria cutanea tarda; RF, rheumatoid factor.

In all cases, the presence of some adverse prognostic factors should be carefully evaluated before the therapeutic decisions; in particular, the severity of liver involvement with decompensated cirrhosis, diffuse cryoglobulinemic vasculitis with multiple-organ damage, and some important comorbidities, such as diabetes, heart/lung involvement, cancer, and possible HBV/HIV coinfection.

In conclusion, the etiologic treatment with DAAs, alone or in combination with immunosuppressors, may represent the gold standard therapy that may lead to HCV eradication and possible improvement or complete resolution of HCV-EHMs. Preliminary trials regarding small patients series with short clinical follow-up after HCV eradication showed somewhat discordant results.[21–23] Unfortunately, there are not available predictive factors for therapeutic effects of antivirals in the single patient; the unpredictable results might be related to different steps of the HCV-related immune-system condition underlying the HCV-EHMs in a given subject at the time of antiviral therapy; it is possible to hypothesize that in some individuals lymphoproliferative alterations might have passed the point of no return and are not yet reversible despite virus eradication. Therefore, the actual role of antivirals in the natural history of HCV-EHMs can be clarified in the near future by means of clinical trials on wider patients' series with homogeneous clinicoimmunologic patterns, including HCV-related glomerulonephritis alone or in association with MCS or other HCV-EHMs.

REFERENCES

1. Ferri C, Sebastiani M, Giuggioli D, et al. Hepatitis C virus syndrome: a constellation of organ- and non-organ specific autoimmune disorders, B-cell non-Hodgkin's lymphoma, and cancer. World J Hepatol 2015;7:327–43.

2. Zignego AL, Gragnani L, Piluso A, et al. Virus-driven autoimmunity and lymphoproliferation: the example of HCV infection. Expert Rev Clin Immunol 2015;11: 15–31.

3. Ferri C, Antonelli A, Mascia MT, et al. HCV-related autoimmune and neoplastic disorders: the HCV syndrome. Dig Liver Dis 2007;39(Suppl 1):S13–21.

4. Roccatello D, Fornasieri A, Giachino O, et al. Multicenter study on hepatitis C virus-related cryoglobulinemic glomerulonephritis. Am J Kidney Dis 2007;49: 69–82.

5. Cacoub P, Desbois AC, Isnard-Bagnis C, et al. Hepatitis C virus infection and chronic kidney disease: time for reappraisal. J Hepatol 2016;65(1 Suppl):S82–94.

6. Barsoum RS, William EA, Khalil SS. Hepatitis C and kidney disease: a narrative review. J Adv Res 2017;8:113–30.

7. Fabrizi F, Martin P, Dixit V, et al. Hepatitis C virus infection and kidney disease: a meta-analysis. Clin J Am Soc Nephrol 2012;7:549–57.

8. Ferri C, Sebastiani M, Giuggioli D, et al. Mixed cryoglobulinemia: demographic, clinical, and serologic features and survival in 231 patients. Semin Arthritis Rheum 2004;33:355–74.

9. Terrier B, Cacoub P. Renal involvement in HCV-related vasculitis. Clin Res Hepatol Gastroenterol 2013;37:334–9.

10. Ozkok A, Yildiz A. Hepatitis C virus associated glomerulopathies. World J Gastroenterol 2014;20:7544–54.

11. Fabrizi F, Plaisier E, Saadoun D, et al. Hepatitis C virus infection, mixed cryoglobulinemia, and kidney disease. Am J Kidney Dis 2013;61:623–37.

12. Moorman AC, Tong X, Spradling PR, et al. Prevalence of renal impairment and associated conditions among HCV-infected persons in the chronic hepatitis cohort study (CHeCS). Dig Dis Sci 2016;61:2087–93.

13. Vannata B, Arcaini L, Zucca E. Hepatitis C virus-associated B-cell non-Hodgkin's lymphomas: what do we know? Ther Adv Hematol 2016;7:94–107.

14. Ferri C, Ramos-Casals M, Zignego AL, et al, ISG-EHCV coauthors. International diagnostic guidelines for patients with HCV-related extrahepatic manifestations. A multidisciplinary expert statement. Autoimmun Rev 2016;15:1145–60.

15. Pipili C, Cholongitas E. Renal dysfunction in patients with cirrhosis: where do we stand? World J Gastrointest Pharmacol Ther 2014;5:156–68.

16. Tartof S, Arduino JM, Wei R, et al. The additional impact of chronic kidney disease on cardiovascular outcomes and death among HCV patients. Poster presented at the EASL Meeting. Barcelona, Spain, April 15, 2016.

17. Oyake N, Shimada T, Murakami Y, et al. Hepatitis C virus infection as a risk factor for increased aortic stiffness and cardiovascular events in dialysis patients. J Nephrol 2008;21:345–53.

18. Rostami Z, Nourbala MH, Alavian SM, et al. The impact of Hepatitis C virus infection on kidney transplantation outcomes: a systematic review of 18 observational studies: the impact of HCV on renal transplantation. Hepat Mon 2011;11:247–54.

19. Amir AA, Amir RA, Sheikh SS. Hepatitis C infection in kidney transplantion. In: Rath T, editor. Current issues and future direction in kidney transplantation. In-Tech; 2013. Available at: https://www.intechopen.com/books/current-issues-and-future-direction-in-kidney-transplantation/hepatitis-c-infection-in-kidney-transplantion. Accessed April 11, 2017.

20. Pietrogrande M, De Vita S, Zignego AL, et al. Recommendations for the management of mixed cryoglobulinemia syndrome in hepatitis C virus-infected patients. Autoimmun Rev 2011;10:444–54.

21. Sise ME, Bloom AK, Wisocky J, et al. Treatment of hepatitis C virus-associated mixed cryoglobulinemia with direct-acting antiviral agents. Hepatology 2016; 63:408–17.

22. Gragnani L, Visentini M, Fognani E, et al. Prospective study of guideline-tailored therapy with direct-acting antivirals for hepatitis C virus-associated mixed cryoglobulinemia. Hepatology 2016;64:1473–82.

23. Fabrizi F, Martin P, Cacoub P, et al. Treatment of hepatitis C-related kidney disease. Expert Opin Pharmacother 2015;16:1815–27.

24. Ferri C, Cacoub P, Mazzaro C, et al. Treatment with rituximab in patients with mixed cryoglobulinemia syndrome: results of multicenter cohort study and review of the literature. Autoimmun Rev 2011;11:48–55.

Hepatitis C Virus–Associated Non-Hodgkin Lymphomas

Biology, Epidemiology, and Treatment

Gabriele Pozzato, MD[a],*, Cesare Mazzaro, MD[b],
Valter Gattei, MD[b]

KEYWORDS

- Hepatitis C virus • Marginal zone lymphoma • Non-Hodgkin lymphoma
- Direct antiviral agents

KEY POINTS

- Eradication of hepatitis C virus (HCV) in indolent non-Hodgkin lymphomas (NHLs), especially in marginal zone lymphomas (MZLs), determines the regression of the hematological disorder in a significant fraction of cases.
- Because direct antiviral agents (DAAs) show an excellent profile in terms of efficacy, safety, and rapid onset of action, these drugs can be used in any clinical situation and the presence of any comorbidities.
- To avoid the progression of the NHL, despite HCV eradication, antiviral therapy should be provided as soon as the viral infection is discovered; before that, the chronic antigenic stimulation determines the irreversible proliferation of neoplastic B cells.

INTRODUCTION

A few years after its discovery, it became evident that HCV was able to cause not only acute liver diseases and chronic liver diseases (CLDs) but also several extrahepatic disorders. The chronic HCV infection is often associated with several rheumatological and autoimmune diseases,[1–6] among them the most common is mixed cryoglobulinemia (MC).[7,8] This disease is characterized, clinically, by the presence of fatigue, palpable purpura (usually on the legs), and arthralgia and, biologically, by detectable serum levels of immunoglobulins able to precipitate at a low temperature. For years,

The authors have nothing to disclose.
[a] Department of Clinical and Surgical Sciences, University of Trieste, Ematologia Clinica, Ospedale Maggiore, Piazza Ospedale 1, Trieste 34121, Italy; [b] Clinical and Experimental Onco-Hematology Unit, Centro di Riferimento Oncologico, I.R.C.C.S., Aviano 33081, Italy
* Corresponding author.
E-mail address: g.pozzato@fmc.units.it

MC had been considered a rheumatic disease because the histologic lesions are secondary to vasculitis, which is determined by the deposition of immunocomplexes in small and medium vessels.[9–11] After the availability of anti-HCV antibodies tests, more than 90% of patients affected by MC resulted were carriers of HCV infection,[12–14] whereas only an insignificant fraction of the anti-HCV antibodies tests was positive for HBV infection[15] or without any virologic markers and, therefore, considered as "essential". During 1990, accurate studies on the clinical aspects and the biological characteristics of MC revealed that this disease could be regarded as a small lymphoproliferative disease because a monoclonal B-cell population was detectable in each case, including peripheral mononuclear cells.[16] The B-cell monoclonality was present not only in cryoglobulinemic patients but also in a small fraction of cases of HCV hepatitis without any clinical feature of the syndrome and dosable level of cryoglobulins. This indicates that these cases show an intermediate or prodromic phase of the disease and, therefore, that the virus seems the true culprit of the MC. How an RNA virus, unable to integrate into DNA of the host, is capable of determining a lymphoproliferative disease was an intriguing question for researchers worldwide.

BIOLOGY OF HEPATITIS C VIRUS–POSITIVE LYMPHOPROLIFERATIVE DISORDERS

The HCV genome consists of a positive single-stranded RNA molecule enveloped by a lipid bilayer within which 2 different glycoproteins are anchored.[17] The viral genome has 3 regions: (1) a short 5' noncoding region with 2 domains: a loop structure involved in HCV replication and the internal ribosome entry site, the region responsible for attachment of the ribosome and polyprotein translation[18]; (2) a large, single open reading frame of approximately 9000 nucleotides, which encodes a single polyprotein precursor that is subsequently processed by host and viral proteases into at least 3 structural and 7 nonstructural proteins with various enzymatic activities; and (3) the 3' nontranslated region endowed with high variability in the length and structure. The virus shows a high genetic diversity because, like other RNA viruses, the RNA-dependent RNA polymerase lacks a 3'-5' exonuclease with proofreading activity for removal of the misincorporated bases. Therefore, the viral replication is error-prone, and this determines a large number of variants in the same host (quasispecies virus population) with unsolvable problems for the host immune system.[19] The taxonomy of HCV is complicated because the virus, by the nucleotide sequence, is classified into 6 genotypes, which show different geographic distribution, and, in addition, each genotype contains a variable number of subtypes. At the nucleotide level, the genotypes differ from each other by 31% to 33%, whereas subtypes differ from each other by 20% to 25%.[20] The peculiar characteristic of HCV is the ability to infect not only the liver cells but also the lymphocytes[21] and, likely, other cells and tissues. This characteristic is due to liver cells and lymphocytes sharing the same HCV receptor, the CD81.[22,23] This transmembrane molecule is a tetraspanin expressed on the surface of various cell types, including B cells, T cells, and natural killer (NK) cells. On human B cells, CD81 forms a costimulatory complex with CD19 and CD21, and the coligation of the B-cell antigen receptor (BCR) with any of the components of this costimulatory complex lowers the threshold for BCR-mediated B-cell activation/proliferation.[24] CD81-mediated activation differs from any other B-cell stimuli because it induces preferential proliferation of naïve B cells. Also, the chemokine receptor CXCR3 is up-regulated on B lymphocytes activated by CD81, whereas it is expressed at low levels after different stimulating substances.[25,26] This interaction between HCV and the immune system could be the basis to explain the immunologic and lymphoproliferative disorders frequently found in chronic HCV infections. The potential mechanisms of a virus for determining the lymphomas are 3: (1) active replication of the virus in the lymphocytes with abnormal regulation of several cellular genes, (2) a hit-and-run mechanism, and (3) chronic antigenic stimulation.

Whether HCV can replicate inside B cells is still a matter of debate. Some investigators found HCV-RNA–negative strands (ie, the viral replicative intermediates) in peripheral mononuclear cells,[27] in neutrophils,[28] and in CD34$^+$ stem cells,[29] but not all researchers obtained the same results.[30] The HCV replication in vitro has been demonstrated in cell lines of NHL infected by the virus.[31] Because there is in vitro evidence that some viral proteins can induce NHL in transgenic mice,[32] the active viral replication in B cells could be the main mechanism of lymphomagenesis of HCV. There are, however, some perplexities on this mechanism: all studies agree on the absence of viral replication in the tissue of HCV-positive NHL.[29] Moreover, the transgenic mice developed follicular or large cell lymphomas, 2 histologic subtypes not usually found in HCV-related NHL.

There is some evidence that viral replication inside the cells is not necessary for determining their neoplastic transformation.[33] Vial genomes either inserted into the cellular DNA or co-replicating with it in episomal form can be lost from neoplastic cells.[34] The hit-and-run mechanism indicates that the transient acquisition of a complete or incomplete viral genome may be sufficient to induce malignant conversion of host cells.[34] Viral oncoproteins can also cause epigenetic dysregulation, thereby reprogramming cellular gene expression in a heritable manner and, after determining these changes in the gene expression pattern, the genomes of viruses may be completely lost. Two herpesviruses (Epstein-Barr virus and the Kaposi sarcoma herpesvirus) are involved in human neoplastic diseases. Epstein-Barr virus is associated with nasopharyngeal carcinoma, with post-transplant lymphoproliferative diseases, and with a subset of Hodgkin lymphoma.[35] Kaposi sarcoma herpesvirus is associated not only with the Kaposi sarcoma but also with primary effusion lymphoma[36] and with a fraction of Castleman disease.[37] These 2 viruses persist as episomes in the tumor cells and the episomes, although bound to cellular chromatin, are not continuous with cellular DNA. These episomes can be lost during cellular replication, but their loss has not been associated with the loss of the malignant phenotype.[34] It is likely that chromosomal translocations and point mutations, induced by the virus, are the driving force for the neoplastic proliferation independently from the presence of the virus. This hit-and-run mechanism has been suggested for HCV; some investigators found that HCV in vitro is able to induce mutations in several genes involved in cellular replication, such as p53, bcl-6, and β-catenin.[38,39] The possibility that HCV could be able to induce a mutator phenotype was not confirmed by other researchers either in vitro or in lymphocytes obtained from patients chronically infected by HCV.[40]

The possibility that chronic antigen stimulation could be able to determine NHL is indicated by the well-established pathogenetic link between the chronic *Helicobacter pylori* (HP) infection and the development of mucosa-associated lymphoid tissue (MALT) gastric lymphoma[41]; in addition, the regression of the MALT lymphoma after HP eradication makes this possibility appealing.[42] Similarly, several reports showed the regression of B-cell monoclonality after HCV eradication with antiviral therapy.[43,44] Not only clinical but also molecular data are in accord with the theory of the chronic antigen stimulation as the driving force for the development of the HCV-associated NHL. Because NHL arises after a long-lasting time of infection, it is likely that persistence of the virus determines chronic stimulation of B cells through the CD81, leading to polyclonal expansion of these cells that can evolve into an oligoclonal and finally monoclonal expansion. The binding of HCV E2 protein with

CD81 is able to activate the JNK pathway and, as a consequence, B-cell proliferation.

The findings of somatic hypermutations in immunoglobulin genes in some HCV-positive immunocytomas is in line with this theory. The report of preferential expression of VH51p1 associated with the VLkv325 gene combination indicates that a subtype of B lymphocytes seems implicated in chronic HCV infection, thus explaining the association between HCV and some specific low-grade or intermediate-grade NHLs.[45] Throughout the years, several studies supported the hypothesis that some viral proteins could act as antigens, leading to B-cell proliferation and the development of NHL. Some investigators, sequencing clonal variable regions of the immunoglobulin genes, demonstrated nonrandom use of the VH segments.[46] Other investigators found restricted expression of VH and VL genes in both MC and NHL.[47] Moreover, Quinn and coworkers[48] were able to demonstrate that the BCR obtained from 2 cases of HCV-positive diffuse large B-cell lymphomas was able to bind the E2 protein of HCV. Even a single rare case of HCV-positive plasma cell leukemia showed a monoclonal IgG against an HCV protein.[49] Altogether these findings support the hypothesis that HCV-NHLs are antigen-driven, as occurs in HP-triggered gastric MALT lymphomas.[50]

Why a fraction of HCV-positive patients develop MC that evolves to NHL is not clear. There might be additional factors able to transform the benign lymphoproliferation of MC toward an overt NHL. In this field, it can only be assumed that several pathways can mediate the oncogenetic transformation. Some investigators[51] indicated interleukin 6 as a potential element able to contribute to the development of NHL. This interleukin has a strong stimulatory effect on B cells, and it is released in several infections or inflammatory conditions.[52] Therefore, other stochastic factors (bacterial or viral infections, traumas, and additional diseases) could determine the progression of the HCV-related lymphoproliferation toward an NHL. Other investigators found that B-lymphocyte stimulatory factor (B-Lys) is overexpressed in HCV-MC and in NHL.[53,54] B-Lys is a good candidate as oncogenetic factor because this substance has many actions on B cells and not only increases the immunoglobulins production but also is able to activate several pathways involved in B-cell survival and proliferation, such as nuclear factor κB (NF-κB)[55] and extracellular signal–regulated kinases (ERK).[56] At present, however, it is not clear whether B-Lys overexpression is a mere consequence of HCV replication or is an independent cause of the progression of HCV lymphoproliferative disorders. The overexpression of bcl-2 protein could be considered the second hit, able to transform the lymphoproliferation in overt lymphoma because high levels of this antiapoptotic protein have been found in liver or marrow lymphocytes of patients affected by HCV-positive MC.[57,58] The overexpression of bcl-2 is a common finding in follicular lymphomas, where it is generally (80%) due to a reciprocal 14:18 rearrangement. In these cases, the bcl-2 gene on chromosome 18q21 is coupled with the immunoglobulin heavy chain gene on chromosome 14q32.[59] Thus, bcl-2 is activated, and the cells bearing this translocation express high levels of bcl-2 protein. As expected, the 14:18 translocation was found in the peripheral mononuclear cells of a significant fraction of patients with MC (75%), especially in patients with type II MC (85%). This cytogenetic alteration, as well as bcl-2 overexpression, was not more detectable in the patients responding to interferon antiviral therapy. In the relapsers, however, the 14:18 translocation was again found after a variable time after the interruption of treatment, showing a behavior overlapping with HCV-RNA.[60]

Recently, the mutation in the MYD88 gene, resulting in a substitution of leucine with proline at amino acid 265, has been identified in a fraction of patients affected by HCV-positive MC (Pozzato G and colleagues, 2017, unpublished data). The L265P MYD88 mutation is detected in almost all cases of Waldenström macroglobulinemia[61] and in lymphoplasmacytic lymphomas with an IgM monoclonal gammopathy.[62] In MC, the serum immunocomplexes are formed by polyclonal IgG and by monoclonal IgM (endowed with rheumatoid factor activity). Therefore, it is not surprising to find the MYD88 mutation, especially in the cases of a high level of monoclonal IgM. Many years ago, however, the possible relationship between HCV and Waldenström macroglobulinemia had been hypothesized.[63–65] The L265P MYD88 mutant enhances NF-κB signaling through increased binding to phosphorylated Bruton tyrosine kinase (BTK).[66] Finding this mutation could be important regarding therapeutic approaches because recently an inhibitor targeting factors downstream of L265P MYD88 signaling has become available the BTK inhibitor ibrutinib.[67] This new drug, developed for chronic lymphocytic leukemia (CLL), was shown to have an excellent efficacy in Waldenström macroglobulinemia[68] and it is likely that it could be useful even in refractory MC bearing the MYD88 mutation.

THE EPIDEMIOLOGY OF HEPATITIS C VIRUS–NON-HODGKIN LYMPHOMA

The first studies describing the possible association of HCV with NHL were published in 1994. These studies recorded the prevalence of anti-HCV antibodies in small unselected series of patients affected by NHL[69] or described the hematological characteristics and the long-term follow-up of cases affected by MC.[70] These findings were not a novelty because the first historical cases of MC reported by Melzer and colleagues[9] and by Brouet and colleagues[11] were considered malignant lymphoproliferative disorders, given the presence of lymphadenopathy at presentation, whereas others developed lymphomas several years after the onset of purpura.[71] The possibility, however, that a virus could be the cause of hematological, neoplastic disorders was an outstanding finding. Following this line of thinking, in the next years, many investigators addressed the possible association between HCV and NHLs in studies, including a large number of cases with proper control groups in the general population.[72,73] These first epidemiologic data supporting the association of HCV and NHLS originated mainly from Italy, where the prevalence of HCV infection is high, especially in the South.[74,75] Because these findings were not confirmed by researchers of other European countries,[76–78] the relationship between HCV and NHL was thought secondary to the high prevalence of HCV in the general population and, therefore, confined to the less industrialized areas of the world. In addition to the HCV prevalence in the general population, the different results should be secondary to different enrollment modalities. The presentation of HCV-NHL is different from standard NHL, because these NHLs are usually extranodal lymphomas, involving the peripheral blood, bone marrow, spleen, and liver, thus complicating the diagnostic procedures and pathologic interpretation of histology or the imaging methods findings. In the past 20 years, many articles have been published from Europe, America, and Asia on this topic. At present, more than 10,000 cases of NHL have been evaluated for HCV infection worldwide, and several meta-analyses have been published.[79–81]

As some investigators suggested after the first epidemiologic articles, HCV and NHL seem closely associated in some countries, independently from the crude HCV prevalence in the general population. In Italy, 18 full-length articles have been published of 2668 NHL cases, showing a prevalence of HCV infection ranging from 8.9% to 37.1%, with a mean of 19.8%.[82–91] At least 3 of them were multicenter (21 cities involved) or case-control studies were showing an odds ratio (OR) ranging from 2.6 to 4.3. On the contrary, in Northern Europe (United Kingdom and Scandinavia) the epidemiologic studies[77,92,93] did not find any HCV-positive patients (0%). Because in those countries the HCV prevalence is low (0.34%–1.0%) but not zero, a small amount of NHLs positive for HCV should have been found. These findings could indicate that the ability of HCV to cause NHL shows a different geographic distribution with higher prevalence in the countries of the Mediterranean basin compared with Northern Europe.

The reports from North America confirm these finding because the 2 articles from Canada show a low incidence of HCV infection (2.3% and 0%),[94,95] mirroring the findings from the United Kingdom, whereas 2 studies performed in Los Angeles, where more than 50% of the cases are in Hispanic people, the prevalence of HCV infection is high (11.5% and 21.7% in 312 NHLs and 120 NHLs, respectively).[96,97]

The results of the epidemiologic studies coming from Japan are particularly difficult to compare with those performed in Western countries because in that clustered population the distribution of NHL subtypes is different (low prevalence of follicular lymphomas) whereas other B-cell neoplastic diseases, like CLL, are nearly absent. Despite this, at least 7 articles from 1996 to 2002[98–104] documented a prevalence of HCV infection, ranging from 5.7% to 22.2% in 771 NHLs (mean 11.3%). Because 3 studies were case control, the OR was calculated, indicating a value from 2.0 to 3.1. These findings are in contrast to the absence of the B-cell monoclonality usually found in European cases affected by HCV[105]; no cases of MC type II have been found in Japanese HCV-infected patients. The absence of the prodromic phase characterized by a small monoclonal population of B lymphocytes in peripheral blood argues against the possibility of the relationship between HCV infection and NHL, in contrast with the epidemiologic studies.

In China, the HCV prevalence in the general population ranges from 1.6% to 0.4%,[106–108] whereas in NHL it seems to be 1.8%. In aggressive NHL, the prevalence is similar to that found in the general population (1.35%) whereas it is higher in indolent NHL (1.9%). In China, MC is a rare entity and only sporadic cases of type II MC have been described.[109]

The authors recently published an updated meta-analysis on HCV and NHL,[110] including not only published studies but also those with at least 1 of the following fulfilled conditions: (1) gender-adjusted and age-adjusted relative risk (RR), (2) cases and controls matched by age and gender, and (3) measures of age (mean or median or distribution) and gender ratio in cases and controls with evidence of good comparability of the 2 groups. According to these criteria, 19 case-control studies on HCV and NHL were selected, including 9038 cases and 12,224 controls. The pooled RR was 2.4 (95% CI, 2.0–3.0), and significantly elevated RRs were found in 11 studies. Overall RR estimation was 2.3 (95% CI, 1.8–2.9) with no significant heterogeneity between study designs. The authors concluded that HCV infection might be associated with an approximately 2.5-fold increase in risk of B-cell NHL.

THE TREATMENT OF HEPATITIS C VIRUS–ASSOCIATED NON-HODGKIN LYMPHOMA

The HCV-positive NHLs are heterogeneous in terms of histologic features: the most common HCV-related NHLs are the MZLs (indolent), but several diffuse large cell lymphomas (aggressive) and some mantle cell lymphomas (very aggressive) are reported. When an HCV-NHL is referred to a hematologist, several questions should be addressed. First, is NHL secondary to HCV infections or is the virus only a comorbidity? The second question is, which is the best therapeutic approach: antiviral therapy or chemotherapy?

To answer the first question, hematologists should consider that HCV-related NHLs show some histologic, clinical, laboratory, and molecular characteristics. Histologically, the most common types of HCV-NHL are lymphoplasmacytic, primary nodal marginal zone, splenic marginal zone, and MALT marginal zone, whereas other histo-types are less closely associated with HCV.[111] Clinically, the course of the HCV-NHLs are indolent and often linked to the longstanding presence of MC.[70] From a biological point of view, the HCV-NHLs often show a monoclonal IgMk (IgM with k light chain) component and the presence of several autoantibodies. From a molecular point of view, some investigators describe the presence of the bcl-2/IgH translocation (although not confirmed by others)[57,58] and others the MYD88 mutation.

To choose the best therapeutic strategy, several factors should be taken into consideration. The first factor is the tumor burden: in the presence of large nodal or extranodal masses, chemotherapy becomes the first choice; on the contrary, when the tumor burden is low (usually mild bone marrow lymphoid infiltration associated with an enlarged spleen), antiviral therapy could be more appropriate. A second factor is the course of the disease: when the course is indolent and the lymphoma is discovered incidentally, antiviral therapy could be more attractive, whereas if a patient shows progressive and rapid node or spleen enlargement, chemotherapy is again the best choice. A third important factor is the presence and the quality of clinical symptoms: in the case of the symptoms that are traditionally NHL related (nocturnal sweating, weight loss, and fever), chemotherapy is indicated, while in the case of the symptoms that are MC related (purpura, vasculitis, arthralgia, and so forth), antiviral treatment could be more indicated.

Before starting any therapy, HCV-related NHL should always be investigated for the possible presence of an underlying CLD. This means that these patients should undergo a complete hepatological evaluation, including ultrasonography and, if indicated, endoscopy and liver biopsy. In patients showing advanced CLD or with severe portal hypertension or showing impending liver failure, chemotherapy as well as interferon-based antiviral therapy is contraindicated. In these cases, the immunotherapy with anti-CD20 antibodies could be the only therapeutic option. The presence of HCV replication, that is, detectable levels of HCV-RNA, without CLD, cannot be considered a contraindication for chemotherapy. In fact, when HCV-MC patients undergo intensive immunosuppressive therapies, including anti-CD20 therapy, liver function never worsens despite increased HCV-RNA levels.[112,113] Some articles confirm this point of view, in that acute hepatitis due to the reactivation of HCV has been noticed in a very small group of Italian HCV-RNA–positive NHL after chemotherapy,[114] and these data have been confirmed in larger cohorts of patients.[115,116]

The traditional antiviral therapy for HCV infection had been based for decades on the use of interferon-alfa (IFN) and ribavirin (RBV). From 1996 to 2013, approximately 110 cases of HCV-NHL had been treated with the combination therapy, but different outcomes are reported by various investigators. These differences can be explained by the very small number of enrolled patients: 8 articles reported a single case and only 4 articles had more than 10 cases (**Table 1**). In addition, different histotypes were enrolled with obvious different response rates. Moreover, several investigators included cases of liver disease whereas others excluded these cases, and, finally, the presence of MC is not recorded by all the investigators. To increase the complexity of the results, a fraction was treated with IFN as monotherapy, another fraction with IFN and RBV, and another group with pegylated IFN (PEG-IFN) and RBV. The different antiviral efficacy of these 3 regimens increases the difficulty to interpret these results. At least 3 studies reported rather homogeneous results because all the patients were treated with the same antiviral regimen (PEG-IFN and RBV), allowing better interpretation of the data. In all 3 articles, the hematological response significantly ($P<.005$) correlated with the disappearance of HCV-RNA, and the cases of virologic relapse

Table 1
Main studies concerning interferon-based antiviral treatments in patients with hepatitis C virus–associated lymphomas (studies with fewer than 10 cases are not reported)

Investigators	Cases (no.)	Type of Therapy	Histology of Non-Hodgkin Lymphomas	Mixed Cryoglobulinemia	Virologic Response	Non-Hodgkin Lympomas Response
Tursi et al,[117] 2004	16	IFN + RBV	MZL	Not reported	11 SVR (69%)	13 CR (81%) 2 PR (11%)
Saadoun et al,[118] 2005	18	IFN + RBV (8) PEG-IFN + RBV (10)	SPVL (18)	18	14 SVR (78%)	14 CR (78%) 4 PR (22%)
Mazzaro et al,[119] 2009	18	IFN + RBV (8)	SPVL (1), LPL (16) FL(1)	13	3 SVR (38%)	3 CR (38%) 2 PR (25%)
		PEG-IFN + RBV (10)			6 SVR (60%)	6 CR (60%) 2 PR (20%)
Vallisa et al,[120] 2005	13	PEG-IFN + RBV	FL (1) LPL (4) MZL (8)	5	7 SVR (54%)	7 CR (54%) 2 PR (15%)

Abbreviations: CR, complete response; FL, follicular lymphoma; LPL, lymphoplasmacytic lymphoma; PR, partial response; SPVL, splenic MZL with villous lympho-cytes; SVR, sustained virologic response.

also had NHL recurrence a few months later. Given better antiviral efficacy of these treatment regimens, the relapse rates were lower in these 3 studies (30%) than those of the previously reported relapse rates.[117–120]

The development of HCV therapy has progressed significantly, however, in the past few years. The traditional association of PEG-IFN and RBV has now been abandoned after the introduction of the new DAAs. These drugs include inhibitors of the HCV NS4/4A protein (simeprevir, paritaprevir, and grazoprevir) of the NS5A protein (ledipasvir, daclatasvir, ombitasvir, and elbasvir) or the viral polymerases (sofosbuvir and dasabuvir).[121] Although with different mechanisms of action, all these drugs share the same profile of high efficacy associated with low side effects. The published studies of these new DAAs indicate a remarkable eradication rate, ranging from 90% to 100% in any stage of the liver disease, with the exception of rare cases of decompensated cirrhosis. The efficacy of these new DAAs regarding the extrahepatic manifestations of HCV infection is largely unknown because few publications were available on this topic. Until now, a small series of articles has reported single cases of MC or NHL regression after HCV eradication with the new DAAs,[122–124] whereas only 3 articles have shown a large number of cases.[125–127] In these articles, despite the eradication of HCV in near the totality of cases, not all HCV-RNA–negative patients obtained the complete recovery from the clinical symptoms together with the persistence, although attenuated, of the biological characteristics of the MC. Zignego and coworkers[128] noticed that in 2 cases of a small monoclonal B-cell population in peripheral blood, the HCV eradication did not determine the disappearing of the B-cell monoclonality. Similar findings are described in another case report.[129] Recently, Arcaini and colleagues[130] described the efficacy and safety of the therapy with the new DAAs in a significant number of indolent NHLs collected in several centers of Italy and France. This report confirms the high efficacy of DAAs on HCV, because the totality of cases (except 1 single patient with decompensated cirrhosis) obtained the sustained virologic response, including in patients who had undergone previous chemotherapy and/ or previous interferon-based antiviral treatments. The hematological response seems less satisfactory because only a fraction of patients obtained the complete remission of the NHL and most patients who obtained a partial remission relapsed or had a progression of the disease requiring chemotherapy or immunotherapy. Although the methods for determining the responses are lacking, the results are interesting, confirming the good response rate of the MZLs both nodal and extranodal. On the contrary, no response was observed in the 4 cases of small lymphocytic lymphoma (SLL)/CLL. These findings support the hypothesis of different pathophysiologic events between SLL/CLL and MZL. As a consequence, the presence of HCV in SLL/CLL should be considered fortuitous without any pathogenetic correlation. The DAA therapy was well tolerated and its toxicity was negligible. The absence of side effects is crucial in this setting, especially in cases already treated or prone to undergo chemotherapy or immunochemotherapy. The efficacy of DAAs in eradicating NHL as well as HCV-RNA, at least in MZL, confirms the pathogenetic role of HCV and supports the hypothesis of a lymphomagenesis induced by the chronic antigenic stimulation. Unfortunately, in a large fraction of patients, the neoplastic hematological disease progresses despite the disappearance of HCV-RNA. It is likely that in these cases, the B-cell proliferation became independent from virus replication. As suggested by Zignego and colleagues,[128] the persistence of MC after HCV eradication is conceivable because the DAAs lack any immunomodulatory or antiproliferative effect. Alternatively, the persistence of the symptoms can be due to the short follow-up of these patients.

In conclusion, eradication of HCV in indolent NHL, especially in MZL, determines the regression of the hematological disorder in a significant fraction of cases. Because DAAs show an excellent profile in terms of efficacy, safety, and rapid onset of action, these drugs can be used in any clinical situation and presence of any comorbidities. To avoid the progression of the NHL, despite HCV eradication, antiviral therapy should be provided as soon as the viral infection is discovered; before that, the chronic antigenic stimulation determines the irreversible proliferation of neoplastic B cells.

REFERENCES

1. Mazzaro C, Panarello G, Tesio G, et al. Hepatitis C virus risk: a hepatitis C virus related syndrome. J Intern Med 2000;247(5):535–45.
2. Cossarat J, Cacoub P, Bletry O. Immunological disorders in C virus chronic hepatitis. Nephrol Dial Transplant 1996;11(Suppl 4):31–5.
3. Andreone P, Gramenzi A, Cursaro C, et al. Monoclonal gammopathy in patients with chronic hepatitis C virus infection. Blood 1996;88:11–22.
4. Ganne-Carrie N, Medini A, Coderc E, et al. Latent autoimmune thyroiditis in untreated patients with HCV chronic hepatitis: a casecontrol study. J Autoimmun 2000;14:189–93.
5. Ramos-Casals M, García-Carrasco M, Cervera R, et al. Hepatitis C virus infection mimicking primary Sjögren syndrome. A clinical and immunologic description of 35 cases. Medicine (Baltimore) 2001;80:1–8.
6. Pilli M, Penna A, Zerbini A, et al. Oral lichen planus pathogenesis: a role for the HCV-specific cellular immune response. Hepatology 2002;36:1446–52.
7. Agnello G, Chung RT, Kaplan LM. A role for hepatitis C virus infection in type II cryoglobulinemia ? N Engl J Med 1992;327:1490–6.
8. Ferri C, Greco F, Longobardo G, et al. Association between hepatitis C virus and mixed cryoglobulinemia. Clin Exp Rheumatol 1991;9:95–6.
9. Meltzer M, Franklin E, McClusckey RT, et al. Cryoglobulinemia: a clinical and laboratory study II. Cryoglobulins with rheumatoid factor activity. Am J Med 1966;40:837–56.
10. Grey HM, Kohler PF. Cryoglobulins. Semin Hematol 1977;10:87–92.
11. Brouet JC, Clauvel J, Damon F, et al. Biological and clinical significance of cryoglobulins. Am J Med 1974;57:775–8.
12. Misiani R, Bellavita P, Fenili D, et al. Hepatitis C virus infection in patients with essential mixed cryoglobulinemia. Ann Intern Med 1992;117(7):573–7.
13. Ferri C, La Civita L, Longombardo G, et al. Hepatitis C virus and mixed cryoglobulinaemia. Eur J Clin Invest 1993;23(7):399–405.
14. Mazzaro C, Santini GF, Tulissi P, et al. Clinical and virological findings in mixed cryoglobulinemia. J Intern Med 1995;238:153–60.
15. Mazzaro C, Dal Maso L, Urraro T, et al. Hepatitis B virus related cryoglobulinemic vasculitis: a multicentre open label study from the Gruppo Italiano di Studio delle Crioglobulinemie - GISC. Dig Liver Dis 2016;48(7):780–4.
16. Franzin F, Efremov DG, Pozzato G, et al. Clonal B-cell expansions in peripheral blood of HCV-infected patients. Br J Haematol 1995;90(3):548–52.
17. Brass V, Moradpour D, Blum HE. Molecular virology of hepatitis C virus (HCV): 2006 update. Int J Med Sci 2006;3:29–34.
18. Reed KE, Rice CM. Overview of hepatitis C virus genome structure, polyprotein processing, and protein properties. Curr Top Microbiol Immunol 2000;242:55–84.

19. Martell M, Esteban JI, Quer J, et al. Dynamic behavior of hepatitis C virus quasispecies in patients undergoing orthotopic liver transplantation. J Virol 1994;68: 3425–36.
20. Simmonds P, Bukh J, Combet C, et al. Consensus proposals for a unified system of nomenclature of hepatitis C virus genotypes. Hepatology 2005;42:962–73.
21. Zignego AL, Macchia D, Monti M, et al. Infection of peripheral mononuclear blood cells by hepatitis C virus. J Hepatol 1992;15:382–6.
22. Pileri P, Uematsu Y, Campagnoli S, et al. Binding of hepatitis C virus to CD81. Science 1998;282:938–41.
23. Petracca R, Falugi F, Galli G, et al. Structure-function analysis of hepatitis C virus envelope-CD81 binding. J Virol 2000;74(10):4824–30.
24. Rosa D, Saletti G, Pozzato G, et al. HCV can activate B cells via CD81 engagement: a molecular mechanism for B cell autoreactivity and crioglobulinemia in HCV. Infect Hepatol 2001;34(4):252.
25. Rosa D, Saletti G, Valiante N, et al. HCV activates naive B cells via CD81 engagement: a pathogenethic mechanism for B cell disturbances in HCV infection. Proceedings of 9th International Symposium on Hepatitis C Virus & Related Viruses. San Diego, luglio 7–11, 2002.
26. Rosa D, Saletti G, De Gregorio E, et al. Activation of naïve B lymphocytes via CD81, a pathogenetic mechanism for hepatitis C virus-associated B lymphocyte disorders. Proc Natl Acad Sci U S A 2005;102(51):18544–9.
27. Ferri C, Monti M, La Civita L, et al. Infection of peripheral blood mononuclear cells by hepatitis C virus in mixed cryoglobulinemia. Blood 1993;82:3701–4.
28. Crovatto M, Pozzato G, Zorat F, et al. Peripheral blood neutrophils from hepatitis C virus-infected patients are replication sites of the virus. Haematologica 2000; 85:356–61.
29. Sansonno D, Lotesoriere C, Cornacchiulo V, et al. Hepatitis C virus infection involves CD34(+) hematopoietic progenitor cells in hepatitis C virus chronic carriers. Blood 1998;92(9):3328–37.
30. Lanford RE, Chavez D, Chisari FV, et al. Lack of detection of negative-strand hepatitis C virus RNA in peripheral blood mononuclear cells and other extrahepatic tissues by the highly strand-specific rTth reverse transcriptase PCR. J Virol 1995;69(12):8079–83.
31. Sung VM, Shimodaira S, Doughty AL, et al. Establishment of B-cell lymphoma cell lines persistently infected with hepatitis C virus in vivo and in vitro: the apoptotic effects of virus infection. J Virol 2003;77(3):2134–46.
32. Ishikawa T, Shibuya K, Yasui K, et al. Expression of hepatitis C virus core protein associated with malignant lymphoma in transgenic mice. Comp Immunol Microbiol Infect Dis 2003;26(2):115–24.
33. Ambinder RF. Gammaherpesviruses and "Hit-and-Run" oncogenesis. Am J Pathol 2000;156(1):1–3.
34. Srinivas SK, Sample JT, Sixbey JW. Spontaneous loss of viral episomes accompanying Epstein-Barr virus reactivation in a Burkitt's lymphoma cell line. J Infect Dis 1998;177:1705–9.
35. Shiramizu B, Barriga F, Neequaye J, et al. Patterns of chromosomal breakpoint locations in Burkitt's lymphoma: relevance to geography and Epstein-Barr virus association. Blood 1991;77:1516–26.
36. Cesarman E, Nador RG, Aozasa K, et al. Kaposi's sarcoma-associated herpes virus in non-AIDS related lymphomas occurring in body cavities. Am J Pathol 1996;149:53–7.

37. Soulier J, Grollet L, Oksenhendler E, et al. Kaposi's sarcoma-associated herpes-virus-like DNA sequences in multicentric Castleman's disease. Blood 1995;86:1276–80.

38. Machida K, Cheng TN, Sung M-H, et al. Somatic hypermutation and mRNA expression levels of the BCL-6 gene in patients with hepatitis C virus-associated lymphoproliferative diseases. J Viral Hepat 2007;14:484–91.

39. Hofmann WP, Fernandez B, Herrmann E, et al. Somatic hypermutation and mRNA expression levels of the BCL-6 gene in patients with hepatitis C virus-associated lymphoproliferative diseases. J Viral Hepat 2007;14(7):484–91.

40. Tucci FA, Broering R, Johansson P, et al. B cells in chronically hepatitis C virus-infected individuals lack a virus-induced mutation signature in the TP53, CTNNB1, and BCL6 genes. J Virol 2013;87(5):2956–62.

41. Wotherspoon AC, Doglioni C, Isaacson PG. Low-grade gastric B-cell lymphoma of mucosa-associated lymphoid tissue (MALT): a multifocal disease. Histopathology 1992;20:29–34.

42. Roggero E, Zucca E, Pinotti G, et al. Eradication of Helicobacter pylori infection in primary low-grade gastric lymphoma of mucosa-associated lymphoid tissue. Ann Intern Med 1995;122:767–9.

43. Mazzaro C, Franzin F, Tulissi P, et al. Regression of monoclonal B-cell expansion in patients affected by mixed cryoglobulinemia responsive to alpha-interferon therapy. Cancer 1996;77(12):2604–13.

44. Mazzaro C, Little D, Pozzato G. Regression of splenic lymphoma after treatment of hepatitis C virus infection. N Engl J Med 2002;347(26):2168–70.

45. Ivanovski M, Silvestri F, Pozzato G, et al. Somatic hypermutation, clonal diversity, and preferential expression of the VH 51p1/VL kv325 immunoglobulin gene combination in hepatitis C virus-associated immunocytomas. Blood 1998;91:2433–42.

46. Marasca R, Vaccari P, Luppi M, et al. Immunoglobulin gene mutations and frequent use of VH1-69 and VH4-34 segments in hepatitis C virus-positive and hepatitis C virus-negative nodal marginal zone B-cell lymphoma. Am J Pathol 2001;159(1):253–61.

47. De Re V, De Vita S, Gasparotto D, et al. Salivary gland B cell lymphoproliferative disorders in Sjögren's syndrome present a restricted use of antigen receptor gene segments similar to those used by hepatitis C virus-associated non-Hodg-kins's lymphomas. Eur J Immunol 2002;32(3):903–10.

48. Quinn ER, Chan CH, Hadlock KG, et al. The B-cell receptor of a hepatitis C virus (HCV)-associated non-Hodgkin lymphoma binds the viral E2 envelope protein, implicating HCV in lymphomagenesis. Blood 2001;98(13):3745–9.

49. Bigot-Corbel E, Gassin M, Corre I, et al. Hepatitis C virus (HCV) infection, mono-clonal immunoglobulin specific for HCV core protein, and plasma-cell malig-nancy. Blood 2008;112(10):4357–8.

50. Pereira MI. Medeiros JA.Role of Helicobacter pylori in gastric mucosa-associated lymphoid tissue lymphomas. World J Gastroenterol 2014;20(3):684–98.

51. Feldmann G, Nischalke HD, Nattermann J, et al. Induction of interleukin-6 by hepatitis C virus core protein in hepatitis C-associated mixed cryoglobulinemia and B-cell non-Hodgkin's lymphoma. Clin Cancer Res 2006;12(15):4491–8.

52. Tanaka T, Kishimoto T. The biology and medical implications of interleukin-6. Cancer Immunol Res 2014;2(4):288–94.

53. Fabris M, Quartuccio L, Sacco S, et al. B-Lymphocyte stimulator (BLyS) up-regulation in mixed cryoglobulinaemia syndrome and hepatitis-C virus infection. Rheumatology (Oxford) 2007;46(1):37–43.
54. Sène D, Limal N, Ghillani-Dalbin P, et al. Hepatitis C virus-associated B-cell pro-liferation–the role of serum B lymphocyte stimulator (BLyS/BAFF). Rheumatology (Oxford) 2007;46(1):65–9.
55. Stadanlick JE, Kaileh M, Karnell FG, et al. Tonic B cell antigen receptor signals supply an NF-kappaB substrate for prosurvival BLyS signaling. Nat Immunol 2008;9(12):1379–87.
56. Yamada T, Lizhong S, Takahashi N, et al. Poly(I: C) induces BLyS-expression of airway fibroblasts through phosphatidylinositol 3-kinase. Cytokine 2010;50(2): 163–9.
57. Zignego AL, Ferri C, Giannelli F, et al. Prevalence of bcl-2 rearrangement in pa-tients with hepatitis C virus-related mixed cryoglobulinemia with or without B-cell lymphomas. Ann Intern Med 2002;137:571–80.
58. Zuckerman E, Zuckerman T, Sahar D, et al. bcl-2 and immunoglobulin gene re-arrangement in patients with hepatitis C virus infection. Br J Haematol 2001;112: 364–9.
59. Gu K, Chan WC, Hawley RC. Practical detection of t(14;18)(IgH/BCL2) in follic-ular lymphoma. Arch Pathol Lab Med 2008;132(8):1355–61.
60. Zignego AL, Giannelli F, Marrocchi ME, et al. T(14; 18) translocation in chronic hepatitis C virus infection. Hepatology 2000;31:474–9.
61. Landgren O, Tageja N. MYD88 and beyond: novel opportunities for diagnosis, prognosis and treatment in Waldenström's Macroglobulinemia. Leukemia 2014;28(9):1799–803.
62. Rossi D. Role of MYD88 in lymphoplasmacytic lymphoma diagnosis and path-ogenesis. Hematol Am Soc Hematol Educ Program 2014;1:113–8.
63. Santini GF, Crovatto M, Modolo ML, et al. Waldenström macroglobulinemia: a role of HCV infection? Blood 1993;82:29–32.
64. Silvestri F, Barillari G, Fanin R, et al. Risk of hepatitis C virus infection, Walden-ström's macroglobulinemia, and monoclonal gammopathies. Blood 1996;88: 1125–6.
65. Neri S, Pulvirenti D, Mauceri B, et al. A case of progression from type II cryoglo-bulinaemia to Waldenstrom's macroglobulinaemia in a patient with chronic hep-atitis C. Clin Exp Med 2005;5(1):40–2.
66. Yang G, Zhou Y, Liu X, et al. A mutation in MYD88 (L265P) supports the survival of lymphoplasmacytic cells by activation of Bruton tyrosine kinase in Walden-ström macroglobulinemia. Blood 2013;122(7):1222–32.
67. Castillo JJ, Treon SP, Davids MS. Inhibition of the Bruton tyrosine kinase pathway in B-Cell lymphoproliferative disorders. Cancer J 2016;22(1):34–9.
68. Castillo JJ, Palomba ML, Advani R, et al. Ibrutinib in Waldenström macroglobu-linemia: latest evidence and clinical experience. Ther Adv Hematol 2016;7(4): 179–86.
69. Ferri C, La Civita L, Longombardo G, et al. Hepatitis C virus and mixed cryoglo-bulinaemia. Br J Rheumatol 1994;33:301.
70. Pozzato G, Mazzaro C, Crovatto M, et al. Low-grade malignant lymphoma, hep-atitis C virus infection, and mixed cryoglobulinemia. Blood 1994;84:3047–53.
71. Gorevic PD, Kassab HJ, Levo Y, et al. Mixed cryoglobulinemia: clinical aspects and long-term follow-up of 40 patients. Am J Med 1980;69:287–308.
72. Silvestri F, Pipan C, Barillari G, et al. Prevalence of hepatitis C virus infection in patients with lymphoproliferative disorders. Blood 1996;87:4296–301.

73. Mazzaro C, Zagonel V, Monfardini S, et al. Hepatitis C virus and non-Hodgkin's lymphomas. Br J Haematol 1996;94:544–50.

74. Osella AR, Misciagna G, Guerra VM, et al. Hepatitis C virus (HCV) infection and liver-related mortality: a population-based cohort study in southern Italy. The Association for the Study of Liver Disease in Puglia. Int J Epidemiol 2000;29(5): 922–7.

75. Maio G, d'Argenio P, Stroffolini T, et al. Hepatitis C virus infection and alanine transaminase levels in the general population: a survey in a southern Italian town. J Hepatol 2000;33(1):116–20.

76. Hanley J, Jarvis L, Simmonds P, et al. HCV and non-Hodgkin lymphoma. Lancet 1996;347(9011):13–39.

77. Thalen DJ, Raemaekers J, Galama J, et al. Absence of hepatitis C virus infection in non-Hodgkin's lymphoma. Br J Haematol 1997;96:880–1.

78. McColl MD, Singer IO, Tait RC, et al. The role of hepatitis C virus in the aetiology of non-Hodgkins lymphoma–a regional association? Leuk Lymphoma 1997; 26(1–2):127–30.

79. Negri E, Little D, Boiocchi M, et al. B-cell non-Hodgkin's lymphoma and hepatitis C virus infection: a systematic review. Int J Cancer 2004;111:1–8.

80. Matsuo K, Kusano A, Sugumar A, et al. Effect of hepatitis C virus infection on the risk of nonHodgkin's lymphoma: a meta-analysis of epidemiological studies. Cancer Sci 2004;95:745–52.

81. Dal Maso L, Franceschi S. Hepatitis C virus and risk of lymphoma and other lymphoid neoplasms: a meta-analysis of epidemiologic studies. Cancer Epidemiol Biomarkers Prev 2006;15:2078–85.

82. Andriani A, Bibas M, di Giacomo C. Liver involvement during HCV infection in chronic lymphoproliferative diseases. Haematologica 1996;81:589–90.

83. Musolino C, Campo S, Pollicino T, et al. Evaluation of hepatitis B and C virus infections in patients with non-Hodgkin's lymphoma and without disease. Hematol 1996;81:162–4.

84. Pioltelli P, Zehender G, Monti G, et al. HCV and non-Hodgkin's lymphoma [letter]. Lancet 1996;347:624–5.

85. Pivetti S, Novarino A, Merico Bertero MT, et al. High prevalence of autoimmune phenomena in hepatitis C virus antibody positive patients with lymphoproliferative and connective tissue disorders. Br J Haematol 1996;95:204–11.

86. Catassi C, Fabiani E, Coppa GV, et al. High prevalence of hepatitis C virus infection in patients with non-Hodgkin's lymphoma at the onset. Preliminary results of an Italian multicenter study. Recenti Prog Med 1998;89(2):63–7.

87. Luppi M, Longo G, Ferrari MG, et al. Clinico-pathological characterization of hepatitis C virus-related B-cell non-Hodgkin's lymphoma without symptomatic cryoglobulinemia. Ann Oncol 1998;106:495–8.

88. Prati D, Zanella A, De Mattei C, et al. Chronic hepatitis C virus infection and primary cutaneous B-cell lymphoma. Br J Haematol 1999;105:841.

89. Vallisa D, Bertè R, Rocca A, et al. Association between hepatitis C virus and non-Hodgkin's lymphoma, and effects of viral infection on histological subtype and clinical course. Am J Med 1999;106:556–60.

90. Pioltelli P, Gargantini L, Cassi E, et al. Hepatitis C virus in non-Hodgkin's lymphoma. A reappraisal after a prospective case-control study of 300 patients. Am J Hematol 2000;64:95–100.

91. Montella M, Crispo A, Frigeri F, et al. HCV and tumors correlated with immune system: a case-control study in area of hyperendemicity. Leuk Res 2001;25: 775–81.

92. Nicolosi Guidicelli S, Lopez-Guillermo A, Falcone U, et al. Hepatitis C virus and GBV-C virus prevalence among patients with B-cell lymphoma in different European regions: a case-control study of the International Extranodal Lymphoma Study Group. Hematol Oncol 2012;30(3):137–42.

93. Schöllkopf C, Smedby KE, Hjalgrim H, et al. Hepatitis C infection and risk of malignant lymphoma. Int J Cancer 2008;122(8):1885–90.

94. Shariff S, Yoshida EM, Gascoyne RD, et al. Hepatitis C infection and B-cell non-Hodgkin's lymphoma in British Columbia: a cross-sectional analysis. Ann Oncol 1999;10(8):961–4.

95. Collier JD, Zanke B, Moore M, et al. No association between hepatitis C and B-cell lymphoma. Hepatology 1999;29(4):1259–61.

96. Zuckerman E, Zuckerman T, Levine AM, et al. Hepatitis C virus infection in patients with B-cell non-Hodgkin's lymphoma. Ann Intern Med 1997;127(6):423–8.

97. Kashyap A, Nademanee A. Molina a hepatitis C and B-cell lymphoma. Ann Intern Med 1998;128(8):695.

98. Izumi T, Sasaki R, Miura Y, et al. Primary hepatosplenic lymphoma: association with hepatitis C virus infection. Blood 1996;87(12):5380–1.

99. Izumi T, Sasaki R, Tsunoda S, et al. B-cell malignancy and hepatitis C. Virus Infect Leuk 1997;11(Suppl 3):516–8.

100. Yoshikawa M, Imazu H, Ueda S, et al. Prevalence of hepatitis C virus infection in patients with non-Hodgkin's lymphoma and multiple myeloma: a report from Japan. J Clin Gastroenterol 1997;25:713–4.

101. Ogino H, Satomura Y, Unoura M, et al. Oguri H Hepatitis B, C and G virus infection in patients with lymphoproliferative disorders. Hepatol Res 1999;14:187–94.

102. Kuniyoshi M, Nakamuta M, Sakai H, et al. Prevalence of hepatitis B or C virus infections in patients with non-Hodgkin's lymphoma. J Gastroenterol Hepatol 2001;16(2):215–9.

103. Imai Y, Ohsawa M, Tanaka H, et al. High prevalence of HCV infection in patients with B-cell non-Hodgkin's lymphoma: comparison with birth cohort- and sex-matched blood donors in a Japanese population. Hepatology 2002;35(4): 974–6.

104. Takeshita M, Sakai H, Okamura S, et al. Prevalence of hepatitis C virus infection in cases of B-cell lymphoma in Japan. Histopathology 2006;48(2):189–98.

105. Pozzato G, Burrone O, Baba K, et al. Ethnic difference in the prevalence of monoclonal B-cell proliferation in patients affected by hepatitis C virus chronic liver disease. J Hepatol 1999;30(6):990–4.

106. Xiong WJ, Li H, Liu HM, et al. Divergence analysis of hepatitis virus infection between aggressive and indolent B cell non-Hodgkin's lymphoma. Zhongguo Shi Yan Xue Ye Xue Za Zhi 2016;24(6):1754–8.

107. Bennett H, Waser N, Johnston K, et al. A review of the burden of hepatitis C virus infection in China, Japan, South Korea and Taiwan. Hepatol Int 2015;9(3): 378–90.

108. Cui Y, Jia J. Update on epidemiology of hepatitis B and C in China. J Gastroenterol Hepatol 2013;28 Suppl(1):7–10.

109. Zhao L-J, Chen F, Li J-G, et al. Hepatitis C virus-related mixed cryoglobulinemia endocapillary proliferative glomerulonephritis and B-cell non-Hodgkin lymphoma: a case report and literature review. Eur Pharmacol Sci 2015;19(16): 3050–5.

110. Pozzato G, Mazzaro C, Dal Maso L, et al. Hepatitis C virus and non-Hodgkin's lymphomas: meta-analysis of epidemiology data and therapy options. World J Hepatol 2016;8(2):107–16.

111. de Sanjose S, Benavente Y, Vajdic CM, et al. Hepatitis C and non-Hodgkin lymphoma among 4784 cases and 6269 controls from the International Lymphoma Epidemiology Consortium. Clin Gastroenterol Hepatol 2008;6(4):451–8.

112. Ferri C, Cacoub P, Mazzaro C, et al. Treatment with rituximab in patients with mixed cryoglobulinemia syndrome: results of multicenter cohort study and review of the literature. Autoimmun Rev 2011;11:48–55.

113. Stasi C, Triboli E, Arena U, et al. Assessment of liver stiffness in patients with HCV and mixed cryoglobulinemia undergoing rituximab treatment. J Transl Med 2014;12:21.

114. Faggioli P, De Paschale M, Tocci A, et al. Acute hepatic toxicity during cyclic chemotherapy in non Hodgkin's lymphoma. Haematologica 1997;82:38–42.

115. Takai S, Tsurumi H, Ando K, et al. Prevalence of hepatitis B and C virus infection in haematological malignancies and liver injury following chemotherapy. Eur J Haematol 2005;74:158–65.

116. Visco C, Arcaini L, Brusamolino E, et al. Distinctive natural history in hepatitis C virus positive diffuse large B-cell lymphoma: analysis of 156 patients from northern Italy. Ann Oncol 2006;17:1434–40.

117. Tursi A, Brandimarte G, Torello M. Disappearance of gastric mucosa-associated lymphoid tissue in hepatitis C virus-positive patients after anti-hepatitis C virus therapy. J Clin Gastroenterol 2004;38:360–3.

118. Saadoun D, Suarez F, Lefrere F, et al. Splenic lymphoma with villous lymphocytes, associated with type II cryoglobulinemia and HCV infection: a new entity? Blood 2005;105:74–6.

119. Mazzaro C, De Re V, Spina M, et al. Pegylated-interferon plus ribavirin for HCVpositive indolent non-Hodgkin lymphomas. Br J Haematol 2009;145:255–7.

120. Vallisa D, Bernuzzi P, Arcaini L, et al. Role of anti-hepatitis C virus (HCV) treatment in HCV-related, low-grade, B-cell, non-Hodgkin's lymphoma: a multicenter Italian experience. J Clin Oncol 2005;23:468–73.

121. European Association for the Study of the Liver. EASL recommendations on treatment of hepatitis C. J Hepatol 2015;63(1):199–236.

122. Koga T, Kawashiri SY, Nakao K, et al. Successful ledipasvir + sofosbuvir treatment of active synovitis in a rheumatoid arthritis patient with hepatitis C virus-related mixed cryoglobulinemia. Mod Rheumatol 2016. [Epub ahead of print].

123. Rossotti R, Travi G, Pazzi A, et al. Rapid clearance of HCV-related splenic marginal zone lymphoma under an interferon-free, NS3/NS4A inhibitor-based treatment. A case report. J Hepatol 2015;62(1):234–7.

124. Sultanik P, Klotz C, Brault P, et al. Regression of an HCV-associated disseminated marginal zone lymphoma under IFN-free antiviral treatment. Blood 2015;125(15):2446–7.

125. Gragnani L, Visentini M, Fognani E, et al. Prospective study of guideline-tailored therapy with direct-acting antivirals for hepatitis C virus-associated mixed cryoglobulinemia. Hepatology 2016;64(5):1473–82.

126. Saadoun D, Thibault V, Si Nafa S-A, et al. Sofosbuvir plus ribavirin for hepatitis C virus-associated cryoglobulaemia vasculitis: VASCUVALDIC study. Ann Rheum Dis 2016;75(10):1777–82.

127. Sise ME, Bloom AK, Wisocky J, et al. Treatment of hepatitis C virus-associated mixed cryoglobulinemia with direct-acting antiviral agents. Hepatology 2016;63(2):408–17.

128. Zignego AL, Gragnani L, Visentini M, et al. The possible persistence of mixed cryoglobulinemia stigmata in spite of viral eradication: insufficient or too late antiviral treatment? Hepatology 2017;65(5):1771–2.

129. Sollima S, Milazzo L, Peri AM, et al. Persistent mixed cryoglobulinaemia vasculitis despite hepatitis C virus eradication after interferon-free antiviral therapy. Rheumatology (Oxford) 2016;55(11):2084–5.
130. Arcaini L, Besson C, Frigeni M, et al. Interferon-free antiviral treatment in B-cell lymphoproliferative disorders associated with hepatitis C virus infection. Blood 2016;128(21):2527–32.

Chronic Hepatitis C Virus Infection and Depression

Luigi Elio Adinolfi, MD*, Riccardo Nevola, MD, Luca Rinaldi, MD, Ciro Romano, MD, Mauro Giordano, MD

KEYWORDS

- HCV • Depression • Quality of life

KEY POINTS

- Depression is an extrahepatic manifestation of chronic hepatitis C virus (HCV) infection reported in one-third of patients.
- The prevalence of depression in patients with HCV has been estimated to be 1.5 to 4.0 times higher than that observed in the general population.
- Direct HCV neuro-invasion, induction of local and systemic inflammation, neurotransmission, and metabolic derangements are the hypothesized pathogenic mechanisms of depression.
- Depression considerably impacts health-related quality of life of HCV-positive patients.
- Clearance of HCV by antiviral treatments is associated with an improvement of both depression and quality of life.

INTRODUCTION

Chronic hepatitis C virus (HCV) infection poses a remarkable burden on the health care system worldwide because of an estimated prevalence of about 3%[1] and association with significant hepatic and extrahepatic manifestations, which are still responsible for significant morbidity and mortality globally.[2]

Indeed, besides liver involvement (chronic hepatitis, cirrhosis, hepatocellular carcinoma), chronic HCV infection is known to be associated with a wide variety of extrahepatic manifestations,[3,4] such as lymphoproliferative disorders (non-Hodgkin lymphoma and mixed cryoglobulinemia),[5] cardiovascular disease (ischemic heart disease, atherosclerosis, ischemic stroke), metabolic derangements (insulin resistance and type 2 diabetes mellitus), renal involvement (membranoproliferative glomerulonephritis), autoimmune diseases (thyroiditis, sicca syndrome), and dermatologic and neuropsychiatric manifestations.[6–16]

Disclosure Statement: The authors have nothing to disclose.
Department of Medicine, Surgery, Neurology, Metabolism, and Aging Sciences, University of Study of Campania "Luigi Vanvitelli", Piazza Miraglia, Naples 80100, Italy
* Corresponding author.
E-mail address: luigelio.adinolfi@unicampania.it

The mechanisms by which HCV induces systemic diseases seem to be multifactorial, correlated to its ability to penetrate and replicate within cells of the main body systems[17] and to induce local and systemic inflammation, metabolic alterations, and immune-mediated phenomena.[18,19]

HCV can target the central nervous system (CNS) causing a wide range of neurologic and psychiatric manifestations; indeed, more than 50% of infected individuals have been reported to have neurologic and psychiatric disorders.[15,20] HCV-associated CNS conditions include cerebrovascular events (atherosclerosis, ischemic stroke),[8,21,22] encephalic and meningeal inflammation (leukoencephalitis, transverse myelitis),[23,24] vascular inflammation (vasculitis),[25] cognitive dysfunction (inadequate concentration, physical and mental fatigue, decreased memory and psychomotor velocity),[15,26] and psychiatric disorders.[27] Among these psychiatric disorders, irrespective of antiviral treatments and alcohol and/or drug abuse, depression is the most frequent and disabling disorder, which has been reported in approximately one-third of HCV-positive patients.[28] The prevalence of depressive disorders seems to be significantly higher among HCV-infected patients compared with that observed in the general population using the criteria of the *Diagnostic and Statistical Manual for Mental Disorders*, (Fourth Edition) (*DSM-IV*). According to the *DSM-IV*, a major depressive disorder is characterized by a period of depressed mood or anhedonia (eg, inability to experience pleasure from normally pleasurable life events, such as eating, exercise, social or sexual interaction) occurring for at least 2 consecutive weeks. Depressed mood or anhedonia must also be accompanied by at least 4 of the following: (1) overwhelming sadness or emptiness; (2) lack of interest or pleasure in daily activities; (3) appetite or weight changes; (4) disturbed sleep patterns; (5) changes in psychomotor activity; (6) fatigue or loss of energy; (7) feelings of guilt or worthlessness; (8) difficulty focusing, concentrating, or making decisions; and (9) recurrent thoughts of death or suicidal ideation.

A direct or indirect effect of HCV on brain function has been hypothesized from the more pronounce metabolic cerebral alterations observed in patients with mild chronic hepatitis C as compared with healthy subjects or patients with chronic hepatitis B.[26,29] Support for this hypothesis has come from the demonstration of replicative forms of HCV in the brain, implying the possibility of CNS as a favorable site for viral replication.[30] Moreover, in chronic HCV infection, alterations in the blood-brain barrier (BBB) so as to allow the passage of circulating proinflammatory cytokines (eg, tumor necrosis factor α [TNFα], interleukin [IL]-1, IL-6),[31] changes in neuronal metabolic pathways,[26,32] and/or ischemia and vasculitis due to cryoglobulinemia[19] all may contribute to the pathogenesis of neuropsychiatric disorders. However, it is important to underline that the mere knowledge of being HCV seropositive can reduce the sense of well-being because the fear of contagion and uncertain prognosis, social marginalization, hopelessness, and depression.[33]

The aim of this review is to analyze the current knowledge about the relation between chronic HCV infection and depression and the possible pathogenic mechanisms as well as the effects of pharmacologic viral clearance on patients' psychiatric features.

HEPATITIS C VIRUS AND DEPRESSION

Several psycho-diagnostic tests have been used in order to assess depression. None of these tests has been shown to possess a high diagnostic performance; however, the Beck Depression Inventory has been widely used because of superior sensibility and specificity when compared with the Hospital Anxiety and Depression Scale.[34,35]

Overall, the prevalence of depression in patients with HCV has been estimated to be 1.5 to 4.0 times higher than that observed in the general population.[16,36] Depressive disorders are generally associated with an impaired quality of life, a limited access to diagnostic workup and therapeutic evaluation, and a reduced adherence to treatment and follow-up.[37]

Both depression prevalence rates and impact on quality of life seem to be unrelated to liver disease severity, preexistent psychological conditions, comorbidities, and interferon (IFN) treatment[38]; however, because concomitant disorders and patient sociocultural background have been reported to be crucial factors or cofactors in the development of depression by some investigators,[39–41] the exact role of these players is still being debated. However, the results of these later reports are controversial because of the presence of confounding bias and the small number of patients examined.

EPIDEMIOLOGY OF DEPRESSION IN CHRONIC HEPATITIS C VIRUS–POSITIVE PATIENTS

The earliest evidence of the role of HCV in the development of depression was provided in 1998 by Johnson and colleagues[42] who reported a significantly higher prevalence of depressive disorders among drug users belonging to the subgroup of HCV-positive patients (57.2%) compared with HCV-negative patients (48.2%).

Using the diagnostic criteria of the *DSM-IV* for major depressive disorder, Carta and colleagues[43] demonstrated a prevalence of 32.6%, among HCV-positive patients, a significantly higher figure when compared with that observed in healthy individuals (12.8%) and hepatitis B virus (HBV)-positive patients (15.1%). These data were, thus, suggestive for a specific role for HCV in inducing depression. Moreover, the same authors showed a significantly higher rate of recurrent brief depression (15.5%) compared with the healthy controls (6.3%).[44] Navines and colleagues[45] reported depressive disorders in 18.2% of HCV positive-patients, with features of a major depressive disorder in 6.4% of patients with HCV. In a group of 90 HCV-positive patients, Golden and colleagues[46] reported a prevalence of 28% of depressive disorders with a strict correlation with psychosocial factors, such as lower acceptance of the disease and social marginalization. Similar rates of depression were reported by Dwight and colleagues,[37] Kraus and colleagues,[47] and Fábregas and colleagues[48] in their patients with HCV. Recently, a large survey of US patients with HCV by Boscarino and colleagues[49] demonstrated a prevalence of depression in 29.7% of cases. A German study[34] showed a prevalence of depression of 25.9%. Interestingly, genotype 3a–infected patients were shown to be at higher risk of depression than those infected by genotype 1.[38] However, because genotype 3a is known to often be associated with drug users, caution should be exercised when interpreting this finding.

Several studies emphasized the observation of significantly higher depression rates in HCV-positive (32.6%) individuals when compared with HBV-positive (15.1%) patients,[38,43,50,51] possibly pointing to a specific role for HCV in the pathogenesis of depression.

In a recent meta-analysis including 130,000 patients with HCV, Younossi and colleagues[16] reported depression rates of 24.5% and 17.2% in patients with HCV and healthy controls, respectively. Patients with HCV were found to have twice the risk of developing depressive symptoms as compared with healthy subjects. Furthermore, the risk seemed to be higher among women and to increase with age. This meta-analysis[16] also ranked depression as the most prevalent extrahepatic manifestation of HCV chronic infection, with health care costs estimated to be around $430 million per year. Indirect costs due to lower work productivity, as highlighted by a 1.5 to 1.85 higher-than-average rate of absenteeism[52] should also be added.

Despite consistent literature on the association between HCV and depression, the true prevalence of depressive disorders in HCV-positive patients remains an unsolved issue. Presently, the prevalence rates of depression seem to be underestimated because of several considerations: (1) screening of psychological profiles of patients with HCV is not performed routinely and often disregarded and (2) many of the afore-mentioned studies reported referred to tertiary center, which may limit the applicability of the data on a broad scale. In this context, Lee and colleagues[53] evaluated a popu-lation of about 10,000 patients with chronic HCV, HBV or alcoholic hepatitis, or nonal-coholic fatty liver disease (NAFLD) sorted from the national surveillance registers of the Centers for Disease Control and Prevention. A strong correlation with depressive dis-orders was shown to exist only for HCV-infected subjects, thus, confirming this asso-ciation on a population level as well. Nonetheless, an increased prevalence of depression was observed in patients with chronic HBV, alcoholic hepatitis, or NAFLD; however, none of these associations could be verified at the population level, unveiling a potential bias for studies including only patients referred to tertiary centers. Although the exact prevalence of depression in patients with HCV remains to be defined, most studies showed a strict association between the two conditions. The main data are re-ported in **Table 1**.

DEPRESSION AND IMPACT ON QUALITY OF LIFE AND CLINICAL MANAGEMENT OF PATIENTS WITH HEPATITIS C VIRUS

Social marginalization with difficult interpersonal relations with both familiars and non-familiars has been observed in patients with HCV with associated depression. More-over, patients with HCV-related depression, in addition to low mood, showed loss of interest in daily activities, low self-esteem, fatigue, and a decreased capability to ideate and focus. Anxiety, insomnia, compulsivity, hypochondria, and phobias may also be present[28]; in some cases, anger, hostility, aggressiveness, and suicidal idea-tion have been reported.[34] HCV-related depression has also been associated with a lower disease acceptance, reduced working capabilities, and a high rate of somatiza-tion.[46] In addition, patients with HCV have been found to exhibit some degree of cognitive impairment in many cases. Using the P300 evoked potential, Kramer and others[54] showed cognitive impairment in about 17% of patients with HCV. Several studies suggest that cognitive damage may already take place in the early phases of HCV disease.[32] Finally, when considering that patients at high risk for psychiatric disorders, such as injecting drug users, are often involved, the association between HCV chronic infection and depression gains further relevance.

Depression and associated conditions considerably impact on health-related qual-ity of life (HRQL) of HCV-positive patients.[16,55,56]

In a recent study on blood donors, HCV-positive subjects (at first diagnosis) were found to display lower HRQL scores than HBV-positive, human T-lymphotropic vi-rus–positive, and healthy individuals[57]; interestingly, scores from HBV-positive donors were shown to overlap those from healthy controls. Similar results emerged from other studies,[58,59] all pointing to a possible direct role of HCV in such disorders.

Depression and HCV-related fatigue have been demonstrated to be the main deter-minants of a low HRQL.[60] The presence of depressive disorders was associated with a remarkable deterioration of HRQL scores and all cognitive domains.[59,61] Kramer and colleagues[62] and Hauser and colleagues[63] provided evidence that HRQL was not influenced by liver disease severity, with the exception of decompensated cirrhosis; conversely, HRQL could be affected by the presence of a comorbidity (eg, internal and psychiatric), age, and severity of fatigue. Finally, onset of psychological disorders

Table 1
Prevalence of depression in chronic hepatitis C virus–infected patients

Author, Year	Country	Study	HCV Patients (n)	Depression Prevalence in HCV (%)	Control Group	Control Patients (n)	Depression Prevalence in Controls (%)
Johnson et al,[42] 1998	United States (Alaska)	Observational	163	57.2	Drug users HCV−	147	48.2
Dwight et al,[37] 2000	United States (California)	Observational	50	28.0	None		
Kraus et al,[47] 2000	Germany	Cross-sectional	113	22.4	None		
Golden et al,[46] 2005	Ireland	Observational	90	28.1	None		
Carta et al,[43] 2007	Italy	Observational	135	32.6	CHB Healthy control	76 540	15.1 12.8
Nelligan et al,[36] 2008	United States	Observational	783	34.0	None		
Erim et al,[34] 2010	Germany	Observational	81	25.9	None		
Karaivazoglou et al,[39] 2010	Greece	Observational	39	—	CHB	45	—
Fábregas et al,[48] 2012	Brazil	Observational	75	28.0	None		
Navinés et al,[45] 2012	Spain	Observational	500	18.2	None		
Lee et al,[53] 2013	United States (Virginia)	Observational	178	54.6	CHB ALD NAFLD Healthy control	46 378 497 9178	26.5 34.7 29.7 27.2
Boscarino et al,[49] 2015	United States (Pennsylvania)	Observational	4781	29.7	None		
Younossi et al,[16] 2016	NA	Meta-analysis	130,039 24,210	29.6 24.5	None HCV−	127,506	17.2

Abbreviations: ALD, alcoholic liver disease; CHB, chronic hepatitis B; NA, not applicable.

and a negative impact on patient quality of life were noted to merely result from a diagnosis of HCV infection as well.[64]

On the other hand, early diagnosis and treatment of depression were shown to have a positive impact on HRQL.[65] Moreover, antiviral treatment-induced HCV eradication was associated with an improvement in quality of life,[66] further supporting a pathogenic role for HCV.

The presence of depression has long been regarded as a substantial barrier to treatment adherence in cases of IFN-based regimens.[67,68] A history of depression is indeed a significant risk factor for new development of depression during IFN treatment.[69] Specifically, moderate to severe depressive symptoms have been described as side effects of IFN-based regimens in about 40% of HCV-infected patients.[70]

MECHANISMS INVOLVED IN HEPATITIS C VIRUS–ASSOCIATED DEPRESSION

The mechanisms by which HCV could be involved in the development of depression and other neuropsychiatric conditions are as yet unclear. Although psychosocial factors (eg, intravenous drug use, alcohol, female gender) may be significantly involved, hint at a possible role of HCV have emerged from several studies. Direct HCV neuroinvasion, induction of local and systemic inflammation, neurotransmission, and metabolic derangements are among the pathogenic mechanisms thus far hypothesized.

A direct effect of HCV on the CNS was proposed more than 15 years ago as a mechanism for the neurocognitive impairment reported in this infection.[26] Apart from the known ability to replicate in different anatomic sites (eg, lymphoid organs, bone marrow, pancreas, thyroid, spleen) and cells (T cells, B cells, macrophages, endothelial cells),[17,71–73] HCV has also been deemed to have a permissive site for replication in the CNS,[23,74–78] owing to the detection of a negative-strand of HCV RNA sequences, that is, intermediate replicative forms of viral genome, in the brain.[74,79]

With regard to mechanisms of viral entry in the CNS, HCV has been theorized to access the brain via the cerebrospinal fluid or, more likely, endowed in infected monocytes/macrophages, thereby crossing the BBB by means of a so-called Trojan horse mechanism.[75] Once in the brain, the colonization of resident microglial cells may take place; their subsequent activation would involve several metabolic changes.[32] Indeed, findings from studies with proton magnetic resonance spectroscopy (MRS), which provides information on cerebral metabolism, pointed to microglial cells as HCV host cells in the brain.[26,32] Regardless of hepatic encephalopathy and substance abuse, an increase in the choline/creatine ratio[26] and a reduction in the levels of N-acetyl aspartate[80] were observed in the white matter and in the basal ganglia of HCV-positive patients as compared with either HBV-positive individuals or healthy controls. Using PET, activation of microglial cells in HCV-affected patients has been recently demonstrated, with a positive correlation with viremia and alterations in cerebral metabolism.[81] Assessment of activation in macrophagic/microglial cells in HCV-positive patients was carried out by Wilkinson and colleagues,[82] who documented increased gene transcription for the proinflammatory cytokines TNFα, IL-1β, and IL-6. As previously shown for human immunodeficiency virus (HIV),[83] TNFα is known to exert a direct neurotoxic effect, whereas IL-1β neurotoxic effects are mediated by the inducible nitric oxide synthase into the astrocytes.[84] Moreover, an altered BBB integrity and efficiency may favor the access of cytokines, pathogens, or immune cells in the CNS, which all may contribute to the genesis of neuropsychiatric manifestations during chronic HCV infection.[85] Fletcher and colleagues[77] have recently located the access site of HCV in the CNS in the BBB endothelial cells. Accordingly, these cells have been found to express the main viral receptors, such as low-density lipoprotein receptor, tetraspanin CD81, scavenger receptor BI, and tight junction proteins claudin-1 and occludin.[86,87] Besides, neuroepithelioma-derived cell lines have been demonstrated to express functional receptors allowing HCV entry, thus, supporting the notion of HCV infecting CNS cells in vivo.[88]

Different HCV strains have been speculated to display a different cellular tropism on discovery of different HCV strains in diverse anatomic sites in the same subject.[74] Forton and colleagues[76] hypothesized that polymorphisms in the internal ribosomal entry site regions of the HCV genome may lead to a decreased synthesis of viral proteins in microglial cells, thus, reducing the chances of immune-mediated recognition and elimination of infected cells. As a result, HCV may persist in the brain; this mechanism would explain its neurotropism.

Besides neuro-invasion, HCV-induced chronic inflammation state may contribute to explain the pathogenesis of neurologic damage.[31] A crosstalk between inflammatory pathways and neuro-circuits in the brain has been determined to underlie behavior response, particularly development of depression.[89] As mentioned earlier, proinflammatory cytokines (TNFα, IL-1, IL-6) produced in situ by cerebral microglial cells or landed into the CNS through a BBB made permeable by the virus have been shown to exert a neurotoxic effect and to modulate cerebral activity. Huckans and colleagues[90] expanded this concept by stressing the role of systemic inflammation, in addition to cerebral inflammation, in the development of neuropsychiatric disorders. Indeed, they reported elevated inflammatory signatures in HCV-positive patients, significantly related to the severity of depression and mood disorders. Likewise, Loftis and colleagues[91] detected higher TNFα plasma levels in HCV-positive patients with respect to seronegative controls; moreover, a direct correlation between depressive symptoms and levels of TNFα and IL-1β was observed, thus, stressing the tight correlation between the severity of depression and the expression of proinflammatory cytokines in patients with HCV.

Several conditions whose hallmark is a strong immune activation has been associated with depressive disorders.[92] In these settings, the chances for mood disorders to manifest would depend on the extent of the contrasting effects on serotoninergic activity exerted by immune activation.[93] Based on these observations, some investigators link the genesis of depressive symptoms in patients with HCV to the virus' ability to generate a state of immune hyperactivation, as opposed to what is commonly observed in HBV infection, which is associated with less psychological deterioration.[43]

Evidence is accumulating that cytokines can interfere with dopaminergic pathways, resulting in a state of decreased motivation or anhedonia, a core symptom of depression.[89] Actually, by means of single-photon emission computerized tomography, alterations in dopaminergic and serotoninergic neurotransmission have been observed in 50% and 60% of patients with HCV, respectively.[94] Of note, these alterations have been found to correlate with cognitive impairment. Consistently, Heeren and colleagues[95] reported significantly reduced levels of striatal and mesencephalic dopamine and glucose metabolism in the limbic area in a cohort of patients with HCV with cognition and mood alterations, thus, supporting the notion that metabolism and cerebral neurotransmission changes may underline neuropsychiatric manifestations in patients with HCV. Moreover, a strict relation between reduced serum levels of tryptophan (precursor of serotonin) and the incidence of depression and anxiety in patients with HCV has been observed[96]; on the contrary, patients with HBV and healthy volunteers failed to display such an association. The development of depression may be aided by an increased platelet serotonin transporter activity, which results in reduced serotonin levels in the intersynaptic space.[97]

Recently, perfusion-weighted MRI allowed to detect concomitant hypoperfusion of several cortical systems (particularly, frontal and temporoparietal cortex) as opposed to hyperperfusion, due to hypermetabolism, in the basal ganglia of patients with HCV.[98] These findings were interpreted as possible signs of inflammation in the early stages of cerebral damage during the course of viral neuro-invasion.[99]

Novel molecular pathways, potentially involved in the pathogenesis of depressive disorders, are being characterized. A possible role for brain-derived neurotrophic factor, a growth factor involved in neural development and regeneration, has been proposed,[51] because of remarkably low levels of this molecule in patients with HCV as opposed to patients with HBV. However, study limitations due to the small number of patients and the presence of confounding factors preclude drawing definitive conclusions.

Sheridan and colleagues[100] focused on the role of apolipoprotein E for its role in maintaining BBB integrity and correct neuronal signaling. Patients with HCV with depression were shown to exhibit lower levels of apolipoprotein E and cholesterol than patients with no psychiatric symptoms. Hence, the investigators suggested that apolipoprotein E deficiency might alter BBB permeability by weakening the tight junctions among adjacent endothelial cells, thus, favoring HCV entry in the CNS.[101] Furthermore, apolipoprotein E receptors were found to interact with N-methyl-D-aspartate receptors, which are involved in brain dopaminergic pathways.[102] This finding provides further evidence of the role of apolipoprotein E in the pathogenesis of HCV-related psychiatric disorders.[100]

Many patients with HCV have been found to have reduced levels of adiponectin.[103] There is evidence on a possible role of low serum adiponectin levels in the pathogenesis of psychiatric disorders.[104,105] Consequently, adiponectin has been suggested to exert a protective role in the development of depression in HCV infection.[106]

In the past, an additional role was also played by IFN-based treatments, which were known to be able to induce depression, suicidal ideation, and several psychiatric symptoms. The incidence of depression during IFN treatment ranged between 17% and 44%, depending on which study is being taken into account.[107,108] History of psychiatric disorders, female sex, patient sociocultural level, drug dosage, and treatment duration were identified as predictive factors for the development of depression during IFN therapy. Other than impairing quality of life, adherence to treatment itself was negatively affected, with a resulting limitation of its efficacy.[108,109] Potentially involved pathogenic mechanisms included neuroendocrine and neurotransmitter alterations, particularly within serotoninergic circuits, as IFN was known to lead to reduced synaptic concentrations of serotonin.[110] Further pathogenic mechanisms of IFN-induced depression have been linked to excessive responses from the hypothalamus-hypophysis-adrenergic axis and alterations in brain cytokine pathways.[111] In this regard, significant TGFβ1 downregulation and secondary changes in the balance of Th1/Th2 cytokines have been shown to correlate with IFN-induced depression.[112]

THERAPEUTIC APPROACHES

Depression and HCV-related fatigue are the main crucial determiners of a low HRQL.[60] Early and adequate management of HCV-associated depression positively affects patients' quality of life.[60] Because IFN is deemed to induce depression by decreasing synaptic concentrations of serotonin,[110] drugs of choice are, hence, selective serotonin reuptake inhibitors.[107] Citalopram, paroxetine, and sertraline, among others, have proved to be effective with a response rate higher than 75%.[113–115] Moreover, such drugs have been successfully used both for treatment of HCV-related depression and prevention and treatment of IFN-related depression.[116] However, when starting antidepressant therapy, drug-drug interactions, baseline hepatic function, drug potential for hepatotoxicity, and other likely adverse side effects should be thoroughly taken into account. Nevertheless, if we assume that chronic HCV infection plays a role in the development of depression, an etiologic therapy would be regarded as the best therapeutic approach. After being the gold standard of HCV treatment for nearly 25 years, IFN and ribavirin have now been replaced by all-oral IFN-free regimens. Second-generation direct-acting antivirals (DAAs) currently enable a sustained virologic response (SVR) in more than 90% of cases.

Depression was an important limitation to the use of an IFN-based regimen.[55,117–119] Nonetheless, despite the possibility of worsening quality of life and depression during an IFN-based treatment,[120] patients who achieve SVR benefitted from a significant improvement in HRQL score,[117,120,121] perceived well-being, and functional state.[66] Moreover, patients with HCV who responded to treatment displayed a reduced choline/creatine ratio in the basal ganglia[26] on MRS, whereas nonresponders and relapsers consistently exhibited a high ratio.[122] These findings were in line with an improvement in cerebral metabolic pathways following HCV clearance. A recent review confirmed the beneficial effects of SVR on HRQL and mental health outcomes, which remained compromised in those failing an SVR.[123]

In 2011, first-generation DAAs, telaprevir and boceprevir, were added to IFN and ribavirin in the treatment of HCV. SVR rates were increased but at the cost of significant side effects. Again, despite limitations in use and worsening quality of life during treatment, patients achieving an SVR, nonetheless, obtained a significant improvement of HRQL.[124]

In the last years, second-generation DAAs have become available and are now the gold standard of HCV treatment. These drugs have allowed more than 90% SVR, with an excellent safety profile; when compared with IFN-based regimes, second-generation DAAs are less likely to negatively impact on patients' quality of life during the treatment.[125] Because of their recent introduction, data on the effect of new DAAs on depression are scant, even though depressive disorders and quality of life seem to improve following an SVR of the subjects who achieved SVR.[125–135] Regardless of the degree of hepatic fibrosis, patients with HCV who achieve an SVR with ledipasvir/sofosbuvir have been shown to exhibit improved quality of life, working productivity, and fatigue[127,136]; because such improvements occurred early following viral clearance, a pathogenic role for HCV rather than the liver damage was hypothesized. Similar results have been reported for sofosbuvir and ribavirin[127] and for the sofosbuvir and velpatasvir combination.[133] Positive results have also been observed in cirrhotic patients[132] and HIV/HCV-coinfected patients.[129] Overall, these preliminary data seem to suggest that viral eradication, independently of the drug used, is of utmost importance to improve patients' quality of life, although caution is necessary because HRQL might be somehow influenced by patients' awareness of treatment success. In addition, viral clearance results in reduced absenteeism from work and increased productive capacity. Younossi and colleagues[130] estimated an annual social cost of $7.1 billion in the United States in case no patients affected by HCV genotype 1 chronic infection were treated. On the other hand, should all the affected patients be treated, an annual net profit of $2.7 billion (taking only genotype 1 into consideration) would result. This prediction may as well be applicable to Europe[131] and Asia.[134]

SUMMARY AND PERSPECTIVES

Depression is a frequent extrahepatic manifestation of HCV chronic infection,[16] with a significant impact on patients' quality of life. Although HCV seems to play a role in the pathogenesis of depression, as inferred by many studies on this topic, there is still much to be elucidated, in terms of both prevalence rate and pathogenic mechanisms. Diagnosis of depression must be made as soon as possible, because adequate management results in improved quality of life. Etiologic treatment of HCV-associated depression would be desirable; however, data on new DAAs' efficacy are currently lacking and eagerly awaited. Now that safe and effective all-oral IFN-free regimens have become available, the relationship between HCV infection and neuropsychiatric conditions can be better investigated; a quick improvement in psychiatric symptoms would be expected if, as correctly hypothesized, they are attributable to HCV itself. The current high cost of the new all-oral regimen allows access to treatment only for a restricted number of HCV-infected patients; at present, many countries have chosen to treat only patients with advanced liver disease. However, this strategy does not take into account the systemic effects of chronic HCV infection, including such a remarkable manifestation as depression.[137] Moreover, it has been reported that patients with HCV under a watchful waiting strategy, for whom the treatment with DAAs has been delayed, might be at a higher risk of developing depression.[138] Thus, a global effort is urgently needed to grant patients large-scale access to all-oral anti-HCV regimens.[139]

REFERENCES

1. Mohd Hanafiah K, Groeger J, Flaxman AD, et al. Global epidemiology of hepatitis C virus infection: new estimates of age-specific antibody to HCV seroprevalence. Hepatology 2013;57:1333–42.

2. El-Kamary SS, Jhaveri R, Shardell MD. All-cause, liver-related, and non-liver-related mortality among HCV-infected individuals in the general US population. Clin Infect Dis 2011;53:150–7.

3. Craxì A, Laffi G, Zignego AL. Hepatitis C virus (HCV) infection: a systemic disease. Mol Aspects Med 2008;29:85–95.

4. Cacoub P, Gragnani L, Comarmond C, et al. Extrahepatic manifestations of chronic hepatitis C virus infection. Dig Liver Dis 2014;46(S5):S165–73.

5. Ferri C, Sebastiani M, Giuggioli D, et al. Hepatitis C virus syndrome: a constellation of organ- and non-organ specific autoimmune disorders, B-cell non-Hodgkin's lymphoma, and cancer. World J Hepatol 2015;7:327–43.

6. Zignego AL, Ferri C, Pileri SA, et al. Italian Association of the Study of Liver Commission on Extrahepatic Manifestations of HCV infection. Extrahepatic manifestations of hepatitis C virus infection: a general overview and guidelines for a clinical approach. Dig Liver Dis 2007;39:2–17.

7. Adinolfi LE, Zampino R, Restivo L, et al. Chronic hepatitis C virus infection and atherosclerosis: clinical impact and mechanisms. World J Gastroenterol 2014; 20:3410–7.

8. Adinolfi LE, Restivo L, Guerrera B, et al. Chronic HCV infection is a risk factor of ischemic stroke. Atherosclerosis 2013;231:22–6.

9. Fallahi P, Ferrari SM, Colaci M, et al. Hepatitis C virus infection and type 2 diabetes. Clin Ter 2013;164:e393–404.

10. Adinolfi LE, Restivo L, Zampino R, et al. Metabolic alterations and chronic hepatitis C: treatment strategies. Expert Opin Pharmacother 2011;12:2215–34.

11. Johnson RJ, Gretch DR, Yamabe H, et al. Membranoproliferative glomerulonephritis associated with hepatitis C virus infection. N Engl J Med 1993;328: 465–70.

12. Shen Y, Wang XL, Xie JP, et al. Thyroid disturbance in patients with chronic hepatitis C infection: a systematic review and meta-analysis. J Gastrointestin Liver Dis 2016;25:227–34.

13. Ramos-Casals M, De Vita S, Tzioufas AG. Hepatitis C virus, Sjögren's syndrome and B-cell lymphoma: linking infection, autoimmunity and cancer. Autoimmun Rev 2005;4:8–15.

14. Carrozzo M, Pellicano R. Lichen planus and hepatitis C virus infection: an updated critical review. Minerva Gastroenterol Dietol 2008;54:65–74.

15. Adinolfi LE, Nevola R, Lus G, et al. Chronic hepatitis C virus infection and neurological and psychiatric disorders: an overview. World J Gastroenterol 2015;21: 2269–80.

16. Younossi Z, Park H, Henry L, et al. Extrahepatic manifestations of hepatitis C: a meta-analysis of prevalence, quality of life, and economic burden. Gastroenterology 2016;150:1599–608.

17. Revie D, Salahuddin SZ. Human cell types important for hepatitis C virus replication in vivo and in vitro: old assertions and current evidence. Virol J 2011;8: 346.

18. Zampino R, Marrone A, Restivo L, et al. Chronic HCV infection and inflammation: clinical impact on hepatic and extra-hepatic manifestations. World J Hepatol 2013;5:528–40.

19. Zignego AL, Craxì A. Extrahepatic manifestations of hepatitis C virus infection. Clin Liver Dis 2008;12:611–36.

20. Mathew S, Faheem M, Ibrahim SM, et al. Hepatitis C virus and neurological damage. World J Hepatol 2016;8:545–56.

21. Enger C, Forssen UM, Bennett D, et al. Thromboembolic events among patients with hepatitis C virus infection and cirrhosis: a matched-cohort study. Adv Ther 2014;31:891–903.

22. He Huang, Kang R, Zhao Z. Hepatitis C virus infection and risk of stroke: a systematic review and meta-analysis. PLoS One 2013;8:e81305.

23. Seifert F, Struffert T, Hildebrandt M, et al. In vivo detection of hepatitis C virus (HCV) RNA in the brain in a case of encephalitis: evidence for HCV neuroinvasion. Eur J Neurol 2008;15:214–8.

24. Zandman-Goddard G, Levy Y, Weiss P, et al. Transverse myelitis associated with chronic hepatitis C. Clin Exp Rheumatol 2003;21:111–3.

25. Dawson TM, Starkebaum G. Isolated central nervous system vasculitis associated with hepatitis C infection. J Rheumatol 1999;26:2273–6.

26. Forton DM, Allsop JM, Main J, et al. Evidence for a cerebral effect of the hepatitis C virus. Lancet 2001;358:38–9.

27. Monaco S, Ferrari S, Gajofatto A, et al. HCV-related nervous system disorders. Clin Dev Immunol 2012;2012:236148.

28. Fontana RJ, Hussain KB, Schwartz SM, et al. Emotional distress in chronic hepatitis C patients not receiving antiviral therapy. J Hepatol 2002;36:401–7.

29. Alvarado Esquivel C, Arreola Valenzuela MA, Mercado Suárez MF, et al. Hepatitis B virus infection among inpatients of a psychiatric hospital of Mexico. Clin Pract Epidemiol Ment Health 2005;1:10.

30. Fletcher NF, McKeating JA. Hepatitis C virus and the brain. J Viral Hepat 2012; 19:301–6.

31. Senzolo M, Schiff S, D'Aloiso CM, et al. Neuropsychological alterations in hepatitis C infection: the role of inflammation. World J Gastroenterol 2011;17: 3369–74.

32. Forton DM, Thomas HC, Murphy CA, et al. Hepatitis C and cognitive impairment in a cohort of patients with mild liver disease. Hepatology 2002;35:433–9.

33. Miller ER, McNally S, Wallace J, et al. The ongoing impacts of hepatitis c–a systematic narrative review of the literature. BMC Public Health 2012;12:672.

34. Erim Y, Tagay S, Beckmann M, et al. Depression and protective factors of mental health in people with hepatitis C: a questionnaire survey. Int J Nurs Stud 2010; 47:342–9.

35. Golden J, Conroy RM, O'Dwyer AM. Reliability and validity of the hospital anxiety and depression scale and the Beck depression inventory (full and FastScreen scales) in detecting depression in persons with hepatitis C. J Affect Disord 2007;100:265–9.

36. Nelligan JA, Loftis JM, Matthews AM, et al. Depression comorbidity and antidepressant use in veterans with chronic hepatitis C: results from a retrospective chart review. J Clin Psychiatry 2008;69:810–6.

37. Dwight MM, Kowdley KV, Russo JE, et al. Depression, fatigue, and functional disability in patients with chronic hepatitis C. J Psychosom Res 2000;49:311–7.

38. Ashrafi M, Modabbernia A, Dalir M, et al. Predictors of mental and physical health in non-cirrhotic patients with viral hepatitis: a case control study. J Psychosom Res 2012;73:218–24.

39. Karaivazoglou K, Iconomou G, Triantos C, et al. Fatigue and depressive symptoms associated with chronic viral hepatitis patients. health-related quality of life (HRQOL). Ann Hepatol 2010;9:419–27.

40. Häuser W, Zimmer C, Schiedermaier P, et al. Biopsychosocial predictors of health-related quality of life in patients with chronic hepatitis C. Psychosom Med 2004;66:954–8.

41. Lowry D, Burke T, Galvin Z, et al. Is psychosocial and cognitive dysfunction misattributed to the virus in hepatitis C infection? Select psychosocial contributors identified. J Viral Hepat 2016;23:584–95.

42. Johnson ME, Fisher DG, Fenaughty A, et al. Hepatitis C virus and depression in drug users. Am J Gastroenterol 1998;93:785–9.

43. Carta MG, Hardoy MC, Garofalo A, et al. Association of chronic hepatitis C with major depressive disorders: irrespective of interferon-alpha therapy. Clin Pract Epidemiol Ment Health 2007;3:22.

44. Carta MG, Angst J, Moro MF, et al. Association of chronic hepatitis C with recurrent brief depression. J Affect Disord 2012;141:361–6.

45. Navinés R, Castellví P, Moreno-España J, et al. Depressive and anxiety disorders in chronic hepatitis C patients: reliability and validity of the Patient Health Questionnaire. J Affect Disord 2012;138:343–51.

46. Golden J, O'Dwyer AM, Conroy RM. Depression and anxiety in patients with hepatitis C: prevalence, detection rates and risk factors. Gen Hosp Psychiatry 2005;27:431–8.

47. Kraus MR, Schäfer A, Csef H, et al. Emotional state, coping styles, and somatic variables in patients with chronic hepatitis C. Psychosomatics 2000;41:377–84.

48. Fábregas BC, Vitorino FD, Rocha DM, et al. Screening inventories to detect depression in chronic hepatitis C patients. Gen Hosp Psychiatry 2012;34:40–5.

49. Boscarino JA, Lu M, Moorman AC, et al, Chronic Hepatitis Cohort Study (CHeCS) Investigators. Predictors of poor mental and physical health status among patients with chronic hepatitis C infection: the Chronic Hepatitis Cohort Study (CHeCS). Hepatology 2015;61:802–11.

50. Foster GR, Goldin RD, Thomas HC. Chronic hepatitis C virus infection causes a significant reduction in quality of life in the absence of cirrhosis. Hepatology 1998;27:209–12.
51. Modabbernia A, Ashrafi M, Keyvani H, et al. Brain-derived neurotrophic factor predicts physical health in untreated patients with hepatitis C. Biol Psychiatry 2011;70:e31–2.
52. DiBonaventura MD, Wagner JS, Yuan Y, et al. The impact of hepatitis C on labor force participation, absenteeism, presenteeism and non-work activities. J Med Econ 2011;14:253–61.
53. Lee K, Otgonsuren M, Younoszai Z, et al. Association of chronic liver disease with depression: a population-based study. Psychosomatics 2013;54:52–9.
54. Kramer L, Bauer E, Funk G, et al. Subclinical impairment of brain function in chronic hepatitis C infection. J Hepatol 2002;37:349–54.
55. Younossi Z, Kallman J, Kincaid J. The effects of HCV infection and management on health-related quality of life. Hepatology 2007;45:806–16.
56. Hilsabeck RC, Hassanein TI, Carlson MD, et al. Cognitive functioning and psychiatric symptomatology in patients with chronic hepatitis C. J Int Neuropsychol Soc 2003;9:847–54.
57. Vahidnia F, Stramer SL, Kessler D, et al. Recent viral infection in US blood donors and health-related quality of life (HRQOL). Qual Life Res 2017;26(2):349–57.
58. Tillmann HL, Wiese M, Braun Y, et al. Quality of life in patients with various liver diseases: patients with HCV show greater mental impairment, while patients with PBC have greater physical impairment. J Viral Hepat 2011;18:252–61.
59. Fábregas BC, de Ávila RE, Faria MN, et al. Health related quality of life among patients with chronic hepatitis C: a cross-sectional study of sociodemographic, psychopathological and psychiatric determinants. Braz J Infect Dis 2013;17:633–9.
60. Younossi ZM, Boparai N, Price LL, et al. Health-related quality of life in chronic liver disease: the impact of type and severity of disease. Am J Gastroenterol 2001;96:2199–205.
61. Barboza KC, Salinas LM, Sahebjam F, et al. Impact of depressive symptoms and hepatic encephalopathy on health-related quality of life in cirrhotic hepatitis C patients. Metab Brain Dis 2016;31:869–80.
62. Kramer L, Hofer H, Bauer E, et al. Relative impact of fatigue and subclinical cognitive brain dysfunction on health-related quality of life in chronic hepatitis C infection. AIDS 2005;19(S3):S85–92.
63. Häuser W, Holtmann G, Grandt D. Determinants of health-related quality of life in patients with chronic liver diseases. Clin Gastroenterol Hepatol 2004;2:157–63.
64. Rodger AJ, Jolley D, Thompson SC, et al. The impact of diagnosis of hepatitis C virus on quality of life. Hepatology 1999;30:1299–301.
65. Gallegos-Orozco JF, Fuentes AP, Gerardo Argueta J, et al. Health-related quality of life and depression in patients with chronic hepatitis C. Arch Med Res 2003;34:124–9.
66. Bonkovsky HL, Woolley JM. Reduction of health-related quality of life in chronic hepatitis C and improvement with interferon therapy. The Consensus Interferon Study Group. Hepatology 1999;29:264–70.
67. Zdilar D, Franco-Bronson K, Buchler N, et al. Hepatitis C, interferon alfa, and depression. Hepatology 2000;31:1207–11.

68. Kraus MR, Schäfer A, Csef H, et al. Compliance with therapy in patients with chronic hepatitis C: associations with psychiatric symptoms, interpersonal problems, and mode of acquisition. Dig Dis Sci 2001;46:2060–5.

69. Wu JY, Shadbolt B, Teoh N, et al. Influence of psychiatric diagnosis on treatment uptake and interferon side effects in patients with hepatitis C. J Gastroenterol Hepatol 2014;29:1258–64.

70. Raison CL, Borisov AS, Broadwell SD, et al. Depression during pegylated interferon-alpha plus ribavirin therapy: prevalence and prediction. J Clin Psychiatry 2005;66:41–8.

71. Laskus T, Radkowski M, Piasek A, et al. Hepatitis C virus in lymphoid cells of patients coinfected with human immunodeficiency virus type 1: evidence of active replication in monocytes/macrophages and lymphocytes. J Infect Dis 2000;181:442–8.

72. Negro F, Levrero M. Does the hepatitis C virus replicate in cells of the hematopoietic lineage? Hepatology 1998;28:261–4.

73. Gowans EJ. Distribution of markers of hepatitis C virus infection throughout the body. Semin Liver Dis 2000;20:85–102.

74. Radkowski M, Wilkinson J, Nowicki M, et al. Search for hepatitis C virus negative-strand RNA sequences and analysis of viral sequences in the central nervous system: evidence of replication. J Virol 2002;76:600–8.

75. Laskus T, Radkowski M, Bednarska A, et al. Detection and analysis of hepatitis C virus sequences in cerebrospinal fluid. J Virol 2002;76:10064–8.

76. Forton DM, Karayiannis P, Mahmud N, et al. Identification of unique hepatitis C virus quasispecies in the central nervous system and comparative analysis of internal translational efficiency of brain, liver, and serum variants. J Virol 2004;78:5170–83.

77. Fletcher NF, Wilson GK, Murray J, et al. Hepatitis C virus infects the endothelial cells of the blood-brain barrier. Gastroenterology 2012;142:634–43.

78. Fishman SL, Murray JM, Eng FJ, et al. Molecular and bio informatic evidence of hepatitis C virus evolution in brain. J Infect Dis 2008;197:597–607.

79. Wilkinson J, Radkowski M, Laskus T. Hepatitis C virus neuroinvasion: identification of infected cells. J Virol 2009;83:1312–9.

80. McAndrews MP, Farcnik K, Carlen P, et al. Prevalence and significance of neurocognitive dysfunction in hepatitis C in the absence of correlated risk factors. Hepatology 2005;41:801–8.

81. Grover VP, Pavese N, Koh SB, et al. Cerebral microglial activation in patients with hepatitis C: in vivo evidence of neuroinflammation. J Viral Hepat 2012;19:e89–96.

82. Wilkinson J, Radkowski M, Eschbacher JM, et al. Activation of brain macrophages/microglia cells in hepatitis C infectio. Gut 2010;59:1394–400.

83. Gelbard HA, Dzenko KA, DiLoreto D, et al. Neurotoxic effects of tumor necrosis factor alpha in primary human neuronal cultures are mediated by activation of the glutamate AMPA receptor subtype: implications for AIDS neuropathogenesis. Dev Neurosci 1993;15:417–22.

84. Jana M, Anderson JA, Saha RN, et al. Regulation of inducible nitric oxide synthase in proinflammatory cytokine-stimulated human primary astrocytes. Free Radic Biol Med 2005;38:655–64.

85. Brabers NA, Nottet HS. Role of the pro-inflammatory cytokines TNF-alpha and IL-1beta in HIV-associated dementia. Eur J Clin Invest 2006;36:447–58.

86. Burlone ME, Budkowska A. Hepatitis C virus cell entry: role of lipoproteins and cellular receptors. J Gen Virol 2009;90:1055–70.

87. Ploss A, Evans MJ, Gaysinskaya VA, et al. Human occludin is a hepatitis C virus entry factor required for infection of mouse cells. Nature 2009;457:882–6.
88. Fletcher NF, Yang JP, Farquhar MJ, et al. Hepatitis C virus infection of neuroepithelioma cell lines. Gastroenterology 2010;139:1365–74.
89. Miller AH, Raison CL. The role of inflammation in depression: from evolutionary imperative to modern treatment target. Nat Rev Immunol 2016;16:22–34.
90. Huckans M, Fuller BE, Olavarria H, et al. Multianalyte profile analysis of plasma immune proteins: altered expression of peripheral immune factors is associated with neuropsychiatric symptom severity in adults with and without chronic hepatitis C virus infection. Brain Behav 2014;4:123–42.
91. Loftis JM, Huckans M, Ruimy S, et al. Depressive symptoms in patients with chronic hepatitis C are correlated with elevated plasma levels of interleukin-1beta and tumor necrosis factor-alpha. Neurosci Lett 2008;430:264–8.
92. Hardoy MC, Cadeddu M, Serra A, et al. A pattern of cerebral perfusion anomalies between major depressive disorder and Hashimoto thyroiditis. BMC Psychiatry 2011;11:148.
93. Maes M, Ringel K, Kubera M, et al. Increased autoimmune activity against 5-HT: a key component of depression that is associated with inflammation and activation of cell-mediated immunity, and with severity and staging of depression. J Affect Disord 2012;136:386–92.
94. Weissenborn K, Ennen JC, Bokemeyer M, et al. Monoaminergic neurotransmission is altered in hepatitis C virus infected patients with chronic fatigue and cognitive impairment. Gut 2006;55:1624–30.
95. Heeren M, Weissenborn K, Arvanitis D, et al. Cerebral glucose utilisation in hepatitis C virus infection-associated encephalopathy. J Cereb Blood Flow Metab 2011;31:2199–208.
96. Cozzi A, Zignego AL, Carpendo R, et al. Low serum tryptophan levels, reduced macrophage IDO activity and high frequency of psychopathology in HCV patients. J Viral Hepat 2006;13:402–8.
97. Franke L, Therstappen E, Schlosser B, et al. A preliminary study on the relationship between platelet serotonin transporter functionality, depression, and fatigue in patients with untreated chronic hepatitis C. Depress Res Treat 2014; 2014:82138.
98. Bladowska J, Zimny A, Knysz B, et al. Evaluation of early cerebral metabolic, perfusion and microstructural changes in HCV-positive patients: a pilot study. J Hepatol 2013;59:651–7.
99. Rumboldt Z. Imaging of topographic viral CNS infections. Neuroimaging Clin N Am 2008;18(1):85–92, viii.
100. Sheridan DA, Bridge SH, Crossey MM, et al. Depressive symptoms in chronic hepatitis C are associated with plasma apolipoprotein E deficiency. Metab Brain Dis 2014;29:625–34.
101. Hafezi-Moghadam A, Thomas KL, Wagner DD. ApoE deficiency leads to a progressive age-dependent blood-brain barrier leakage. Am J Physiol Cell Physiol 2007;292:C1256–62.
102. Hoe HS, Pocivavsek A, Chakraborty G, et al. Apolipoprotein E receptor 2 interactions with the N-methyl-D-aspartate receptor. J Biol Chem 2006;281:3425–31.
103. Durante-Mangoni E, Zampino R, Marrone A, et al. Hepatic steatosis and insulin resistance are associated with serum imbalance of adiponectin/tumour necrosis factor-alpha in chronic hepatitis C patients. Aliment Pharmacol Ther 2006;24: 1349–57.

104. Wędrychowicz A, Zając A, Pilecki M, et al. Peptides from adipose tissue in mental disorders. World J Psychiatry 2014;4:103–11.

105. Carvalho AF, Rocha DQ, McIntyre RS, et al. Adipokines as emerging depression biomarkers: a systematic review and meta-analysis. J Psychiatr Res 2014;59:28–37.

106. Fábregas BC, Vieira ÉL, Moura AS, et al. A follow-up study of 50 chronic hepatitis C patients: adiponectin as a resilience biomarker for major depression. Neuroimmunomodulation 2016;23:88–97.

107. Schäfer A, Wittchen HU, Seufert J, et al. Methodological approaches in the assessment of interferon-alfa-induced depression in patients with chronic hepatitis C - a critical review. Int J Methods Psychiatr Res 2007;16:186–201.

108. Martín-Santos R, Díez-Quevedo C, Castellví P, et al. De novo depression and anxiety disorders and influence on adherence during peginterferon-alpha-2a and ribavirin treatment in patients with hepatitis C. Aliment Pharmacol Ther 2008;27:257–65.

109. Lang JP, Melin P, Ouzan D, et al, CheObs Study Group. Pegylated interferon-alpha2b plus ribavirin therapy in patients with hepatitis C and psychiatric disorders: results of a cohort study. Antivir Ther 2010;15:599–606.

110. Morikawa O, Sakai N, Obara H, et al. Effects of interferon-alpha, interferon-gamma and cAMP on the transcriptional regulation of the serotonin transporter. Eur J Pharmacol 1998;349:317–24.

111. Angelino AF, Treisman GJ. Evidence-informed assessment and treatment of depression in HCV and interferon-treated patients. Int Rev Psychiatry 2005;17:471–6.

112. Birerdinc A, Afendy A, Stepanova M, et al. Gene expression profiles associated with depression in patients with chronic hepatitis C (CH-C). Brain Behav 2012;2:525–31.

113. Hauser P, Khosla J, Aurora H, et al. A prospective study of the incidence and open-label treatment of interferon-induced major depressive disorder in patients with hepatitis C. Mol Psychiatry 2002;7:942–7.

114. Maddock C, Baita A, Orrù MG, et al. Psychopharmacological treatment of depression, anxiety, irritability and insomnia in patients receiving interferon-alpha: a prospective case series and a discussion of biological mechanisms. J Psychopharmacol 2004;18:41–6.

115. Schramm TM, Lawford BR, Macdonald GA, et al. Sertraline treatment of interferon-alfa-induced depressive disorder. Med J Aust 2000;173:359–61.

116. Gleason OC, Yates WR, Isbell MD, et al. An open-label trial of citalopram for major depression in patients with hepatitis C. J Clin Psychiatry 2002;6:194–8.

117. Younossi Z, Henry L. Systematic review: patient-reported outcomes in chronic hepatitis C–the impact of liver disease and new treatment regimens. Aliment Pharmacol Ther 2015;41:497–520.

118. Marcellin P, Chousterman M, Fontanges T, et al, CheObs Study Group. Adherence to treatment and quality of life during hepatitis C therapy: a prospective, real-life, observational study. Liver Int 2011;31:516–24.

119. Falasca K, Mancino P, Ucciferri C, et al. Quality of life, depression, and cytokine patterns in patients with chronic hepatitis C treated with antiviral therapy. Clin Invest Med 2009;32:E212–8.

120. Foster GR. Quality of life considerations for patients with chronic hepatitis C. J Viral Hepat 2009;16:605–11.

121. Hollander A, Foster GR, Weiland O. Health-related quality of life before, during and after combination therapy with interferon and ribavirin in unselected Swedish patients with chronic hepatitis C. Scand J Gastroenterol 2006;41:577–85.

122. Byrnes V, Miller A, Lowry D, et al. Effects of anti-viral therapy and HCV clearance on cerebral metabolism and cognition. J Hepatol 2012;56:549–56.

123. Smith-Palmer J, Cerri K, Valentine W. Achieving sustained virologic response in hepatitis C: a systematic review of the clinical, economic and quality of life benefits. BMC Infect Dis 2015;15:19.

124. Vera-Llonch M, Martin M, Aggarwal J, et al. Health-related quality of life in genotype 1 treatment-naïve chronic hepatitis C patients receiving telaprevir combination treatment in the ADVANCE study. Aliment Pharmacol Ther 2013;38:124–33.

125. Younossi ZM, Stepanova M, Henry L, et al. Minimal impact of sofosbuvir and ribavirin on health related quality of life in chronic hepatitis C (CH-C). J Hepatol 2014;60:741–7.

126. Lawitz E, Mangia A, Wyles D, et al. Sofosbuvir for previously untreated chronic hepatitis C infection. N Engl J Med 2013;368:1878–87.

127. Younossi ZM, Stepanova M, Afdhal N, et al. Improvement of health-related quality of life and work productivity in chronic hepatitis C patients with early and advanced fibrosis treated with ledipasvir and sofosbuvir. J Hepatol 2015;63: 337–45.

128. Younossi ZM, Stepanova M, Zeuzem S, et al. Patient-reported outcomes assessment in chronic hepatitis C treated with sofosbuvir and ribavirin: the VALENCE study. J Hepatol 2014;61:228–34.

129. Younossi ZM, Stepanova M, Sulkowski M, et al. Sofosbuvir and ribavirin for treatment of chronic hepatitis C in patients coinfected with hepatitis C Virus and HIV: the impact on patient-reported outcomes. J Infect Dis 2015;212:367–77.

130. Younossi ZM, Jiang Y, Smith NJ, et al. Ledipasvir/sofosbuvir regimens for chronic hepatitis C infection: insights from a work productivity economic model from the United States. Hepatology 2015;61:1471–8.

131. Younossi Z, Brown A, Buti M, et al. Impact of eradicating hepatitis C virus on the work productivity of chronic hepatitis C (CH-C) patients: an economic model from five European countries. J Viral Hepat 2016;23:217–26.

132. Younossi ZM, Stepanova M, Pol S, et al. The impact of ledipasvir/sofosbuvir on patient-reported outcomes in cirrhotic patients with chronic hepatitis C: the SIRIUS study. Liver Int 2016;36:42–8.

133. Younossi ZM, Stepanova M, Feld J, et al. Sofosbuvir and velpatasvir combination improves outcomes reported by patients with HCV infection, without or with compensated or decompensated cirrhosis. Clin Gastroenterol Hepatol 2017;15(3):421–30.e6.

134. Younossi ZM, Tanaka A, Eguchi Y, et al. The impact of hepatitis C virus outside the liver: evidence from Asia. Liver Int 2017;37(2):159–72.

135. Younossi Z, Henry L. The impact of the new antiviral regimens on patient reported outcomes and health economics of patients with chronic hepatitis C. Dig Liver Dis 2014;46(S5):S186–96.

136. Gerber L, Estep M, Stepanova M, et al. Effects of viral eradication with ledipasvir and sofosbuvir, with or without ribavirin, on measures of fatigue in patients with chronic hepatitis C Virus Infection. Clin Gastroenterol Hepatol 2016;14:156–64.

137. Schaefer M, Capuron L, Friebe A, et al. Hepatitis C infection, antiviral treatment and mental health: a European expert consensus statement. J Hepatol 2012;57: 1379–90.

138. Colagreco JP, Bailey DE, Fitzpatrick JJ, et al. Watchful waiting: role of disease progression on uncertainty and depressive symptoms in patients with chronic hepatitis C. J Viral Hepat 2014;21:727–33.

139. Adinolfi LE, Guerrera B. All-oral interferon-free treatments: the end of hepatitis C virus story, the dream and the reality. World J Hepatol 2015;7:2363–8.

Neurologic Manifestations of Hepatitis C Virus Infection

Sentia Iriana, MD, Michael P. Curry, MD, Nezam H. Afdhal, MD, DSc*

KEYWORDS

- Hepatitis C • Fatigue • Neurocognition • MR spectroscopy • Interferon
- Ledipasvir/sofosbuvir • Cerebrovascular disease

KEY POINTS

- The extrahepatic manifestations of hepatitis C virus (HCV) in the brain include neurocognitive dysfunction, which is manifested by subtle changes in memory, attention, and processing speed.
- Neurocognitive defects are independent of the histologic stage of disease and may be induced by a direct effect of HCV on microglial cells or mediated by systemic cytokines crossing the blood-brain barrier.
- Magnetic resonance spectroscopy demonstrates abnormal metabolism in basal ganglia and prefrontal and frontal cortex, which has been associated with fatigue and abnormal neurocognitive testing.
- Interferon and direct-acting antiviral therapy can improve cerebral metabolism and neurocognition if a sustained virologic response is obtained.
- Cerebrovascular events and mortality are increased in patients with HCV and may be through an increased risk of carotid artery disease and plaque formation.

INTRODUCTION

The neurologic manifestations of hepatitis C virus (HCV) include cognitive impairment that can lead to brain fog and fatigue, markedly impair quality of life, and increase risk of cerebrovascular events and stroke. The mechanisms by which HCV results in these neurologic syndromes is not fully elucidated, but evidence exists that these represent true extrahepatic manifestations of chronic HCV infection.

Cognitive Impairment: Pathophysiology

Our understanding of the exact pathophysiology of neurocognitive defects in HCV is not fully elucidated. Initially, impairment in cognition was thought to be related

The authors have nothing to disclose.
Division of Gastroenterology & Hepatology, Beth Israel Deaconess Medical Center, 110 Francis Street, Boston, MA 02125, USA
* Corresponding author.
E-mail address: nafdhal@bidmc.harvard.edu

Clin Liver Dis 21 (2017) 535–542
http://dx.doi.org/10.1016/j.cld.2017.03.008
1089-3261/17/© 2017 Elsevier Inc. All rights reserved.

predominantly to progressive liver disease with the development of cirrhosis and sub-clinical encephalopathy secondary to portal-systemic shunting and increased ammonia and astrocyte swelling. More recently, the recognition that memory impair-ment, fluctuating disorientation, and fatigue were independent of liver fibrosis led to the concept of a direct effect of HCV on cognition.[1,2]

There is evidence that HCV can cross the blood-brain barrier and even replicate in the brain. HCV has been suggested to enter the brain carried by infected monocytes as a Trojan horse and subsequently infect microglial cells, which are essentially mac-rophages derived from a monocyte lineage.[3–6] HCV negative strand virus, suggesting a replicative intermediate has been found in the brain, and HCV can also be detected in the cerebrospinal fluid (CSF). However, there is little correlation of CSF levels of HCV with serum HCV viral load; neurocognitive defects are not clearly associated with overall viral burden or viral replication.

An alternative theory of the effect of HCV on neurocognition suggests that it is a sec-ondary effect of the chronic activation of the immune system and mediated by cyto-kines.[7–9] Chronic HCV infection is associated with elevated systemic cytokine levels including interferon (IFN)-α and tumor necrosis factor α; these have been shown to cross the blood-brain barrier and affect brain functioning[10–12] where they can cause release of secondary messengers from the vascular endothelium, including prosta-glandins and nitric oxide. Cytokines in the CNS can also stimulate neuroendocrine pathways and neurotransmission.

Cognitive impairment: clinical manifestations
The hallmarks of cognitive dysfunction in HCV are a subtle difficulty in concentration and slowed thinking. This is often clinically manifested as difficulty with higher func-tioning particularly with numbers, sustained attention, psychomotor speed, and learning memory. The pattern of impairment suggests involvement of frontal-subcortical pathways. The constellation of symptoms has been described by patients with HCV as a brain fog, which is an excellent description of the impact on individuals. Hilsabeck and colleagues[13] demonstrated, using a battery of neuropsychological tests, the impaired performance particularly in sustained attention (82%) within a cohort of 66 patients with chronic HCV. Patients with chronic HCV performed less well than a control population with other liver diseases, and there was an association of worsening performance both with the presence of comorbidities and with increased fibrosis. Other studies have confirmed these findings and again documented impairment of working memory, sustained attention, and processing speed.[14,15] Inter-estingly, this pattern of neurocognitive abnormalities involving the subcortical neuro-circuitry is similar to that reported for patients with human immunodeficiency virus infection.

Cognitive impairment and comorbidities
The differentiation of cognitive dysfunction secondary to HCV from comorbidities associated with HCV, such as drug and alcohol addiction or psychiatric disease, is complex. Intravenous drug use (IVDU) and alcohol addiction are extremely common comorbidities and seen in up to 70% and 30% of patients with HCV, respectively, and in themselves have well described associations with cognitive impairment.[16–20] Forton and colleagues studied a group of patients with HCV with active infection, a group with risk factors for HCV but RNA negative, and a matched population of pa-tients with HCV who had been successfully treated and cleared the virus but with matching premorbid conditions. The HCV-infected group was impaired on more neu-ropsychological tests than the HCV-cleared group; these finding were independent of

a history of IVDU, which was reported in 50% of the patients. Kramer and colleagues[21] compared a group of patients with HCV with minimal alcohol consumption with a group with moderate to severe alcohol consumption and found no effect of alcohol history on the cognitive impairment associated with HCV.[21,22] These studies provide evidence of an association of cognitive impairment with HCV regardless of a history of premorbid substance abuse.

Psychiatric disease is also common in patients with HCV, with up to 40% of patients with HCV meeting diagnostic criteria for a concurrent active psychiatric disorder, including anxiety, depression, bipolar disorder, posttraumatic stress disorder, or personality disorders.[18–20] These patients frequently manifest fatigue, anxiety, and depression; all of these may impact neurocognition particularly on measures of concentration, attention, and processing speed.[15] In addition, many neuropsychiatric medications may also affect sensory awareness and neurocognition. Although there is little doubt that these psychiatric syndromes can all worsen neurocognition, the impairment of cognition in patients with HCV has been described independently of prior or active psychiatric conditions again suggesting the independent association of HCV and cognitive impairment.

Cognitive impairment: electroencephalogram and imaging studies

Further evidence for impaired neurocognition comes from electroencephalogram (EEG) and imaging studies performed in patients with HCV. Weissenborn and colleagues[15] compared a group of patients with HCV with mild versus moderate fatigue to a matched controlled population using neuropsychiatric testing, EEG, and cerebral proton MRI with spectroscopy (MRS). The patients with HCV had evidence of cognitive impairment; 25% had slowing of their mean dominant frequency on EEG, and this was seen in patients with both mild and moderate fatigue. There was a correlation of the slowing on EEG to performance characteristics on the neuropsychological tests, particularly on verbal performance, Weschler intelligence test, and working memory tasks.

MRS has the ability to examine the ratio of neural metabolites in areas of the central nervous system (CNS) by targeting different regions of the brain. Commonly targeted areas include the basal ganglia, frontal cortex and prefrontal cortex all of which are involved in neurocognitive processes. The metabolites most frequently measured are N-acetyl aspartate (NAA), choline (Cho), and myoinositol (MI); these are expressed as a ratio when compared with the control metabolite creatine (Cr). Cho and MI are putative markers for glial cell inflammation and activation that could be a direct result of HCV replication in microglial cells or as a secondary effect of peripherally derived proinflammatory cytokines, as discussed previously. NAA is a marker of neuronal health and viability and is reduced in diseases whereby there is neuronal loss particularly in the gray matter.

MRS has shown that HCV-infected patients have elevated levels of Cho in certain brain regions (basal ganglia, white matter, occipital gray matter) and reduced levels of NAA compared with uninfected patients, irrespective of the degree of liver damage and unrelated to hepatic encephalopathy.[15,23] More recently HCV-infected patients were shown to have elevated MI/Cr ratios in the white matter that, in one study, were statistically correlated with impairments in working memory.[24,25] These findings strongly suggest that HCV infection causes brain dysfunction.

Cognitive impairment and hepatitis C virus treatment

Perhaps the best evidence of a cause and effect association between HCV and neurocognition is demonstrated by the effect of viral eradication on subsequent cerebral function both using neurocognitive testing and evaluating changes in MRS metabolism.

Interferon treatment

The standard of care for more than 20 years was IFN and ribavirin for HCV. IFN has direct effects on the CNS that are well recognized and include neuropsychiatric problems, such as depression, anxiety, fatigue, cognitive issues, and sleep disorders. Ribavirin is associated with anemia and insomnia with a secondary increase in fatigue. These effects occur both during treatment and, in some cases, up to 6 months after treatment and would obviously mask improvements in HCV-induced cognitive dysfunction. Some studies have demonstrated diffuse slowing on quantitative EEG and reduced performances on a cognitive screening measure early during IFN-α therapy, which reversed after the end of treatment.[26–28]

Studies have also shown that patients with HCV treated with IFN performed significantly worse than the untreated patients on a measure of complex attention and working memory suggesting that frontal-subcortical systems are adversely affected by IFN-α and that the prefrontal lobe functions of working memory may be the most vulnerable.[29–31] Interestingly, 16% of their patients with HCV continued to complain of cognitive problems after completion of IFN.

In the IFN era of treatment, sustained virologic response (SVR) was defined as no evidence of HCV RNA by a sensitive polymerase chain reaction 12 to 24 weeks after stopping all treatment. At this time point, most of the deleterious effects of IFN on cognition have resolved. Byrnes and colleagues[32] evaluated the effect of SVR prospectively in a well-controlled pilot study of 15 patients with mild fibrosis treated with pegylated IFN and ribavarin (RBV) compared with a matched control population of 7 patients with HCV who did not undergo treatment. MRS and neurocognitive testing were performed at baseline before starting, at week 12 on treatment, and at week 12 after treatment. Thirteen of the 15 treated patients completed the IFN treatment; 8 had an SVR, and 5 remained HCV RNA positive at the week 12 posttreatment time point. MRS was performed on a 3T magnet and targeted ratios of NAA, Cho, and MI compared with Cr in the left basal ganglia, left frontal cortex, and the left dorsolateral prefrontal cortex (DLPFC). The entire population had similar MRS findings at baseline, and the control untreated HCV population had no change in MRS findings over the time period showing the stability of the MRS testing. In the IFN-treated patients there was a significant decrease in both Cho/Cr and MI/Cr in the basal ganglia of patients who achieved SVR at week 12 after treatment, which was not seen in the nonresponder/relapser patients. Reductions in Cho/Cr of 24% were also seen in the DLPFC of SVR patients, but this did not reach statistical significance. No significant changes were seen in NAA/Cr at any site or time point. These changes in cerebral MRS had a clinical correlate with neurocognitive testing in patients achieving SVR who had significant improvements in total verbal learning recall, verbal memory recognition, and visuospatial memory.

In such a relatively small but well-controlled study, the findings support a substantial link between HCV and cerebral dysfunction by demonstrating a reduction in spectroscopic cerebral markers of inflammation associated with an improvement in neurocognition only seen in patients who achieved SVR.

Direct-acting antiviral treatment ± ribavirin

Since 2013, most patients have been treated with direct-acting antiviral (DAA) therapy for HCV; thus, the confounding effects of IFN are removed from studying neurocognition. ION 1 was a large randomized controlled study of ledipasvir and sofosbuvir with or without RBV for genotype 1, treatment-naïve patients with HCV.[33] Alsop and colleagues[34] performed a small substudy within ION 1 whereby they examined MRS in 14 noncirrhotic subjects, 7 treated with ledipasvir/sofosbuvir (LDV/SOF) alone and 7 with LDV/SOF + RBV. MRS was performed at baseline before treatment, at week 4 on treatment, and at week 12 after treatment using a similar protocol as described earlier for the Byrnes and colleagues'[32] study. Mental health (MH) and fatigue-related items of patient-reported outcome (PRO) questionnaires (36-Item Short Form Health Survey [SF-36], Functional Assessment of Chronic Illness Therapy–Fatigue, Chronic Liver Disease Questionnaire-HCV [CLDQ-HCV]) were assessed in all subjects at the same time as MRS was performed.

All subjects had normal alanine aminotransferase and undetectable HCV RNA at week 4 and achieved SVR. MRS demonstrated an increase in basal ganglia NAA/Cr at 4 weeks and a highly significant increase at the week 12 SVR time point, which was more profound in those subjects not receiving RBV and indicated an improvement in neuronal health. Statistical comparisons with the changes in PRO and MRS were very limited by the sample size, but some very interesting trends were seen at the week 12 SVR time point. Looking at individual subjects, an improvement in the MH component of SF-36 was observed in 9 subjects, no change in 2, and a decrease noted in 3. Of the 9 subjects for whom the MH scale of SF-36 improved, 8 subjects had a decrease in their basal ganglia Cho/Cr ratio; whereas for the 5 subjects whose MH scale of SF-36 worsened (or did not change), all of them showed an increase in their basal ganglia Cho/Cr.

Similar findings were seen in basal ganglia MI/Cr and the emotional domain (EM) of the CLDQ-HCV. Of individual subjects, 10 had their EM domain scores improved. Of those, 8 had a decrease in their MI/Cr.

Overall these findings again suggested improvements in brain metabolism particularly within the basal ganglia associated with functional improvements on PRO in MH and emotion. What is of interest is the rapidity with which these changes were seen as HCV RNA was suppressed and that they were established as soon as 12 weeks after viral eradication.

Direct-acting antiviral treatment: no ribavirin

More recently, Curry and colleagues,[35] from the same institution using MRS and a full battery of neurocognitive tests, performed a double-blind placebo-controlled study on 40 noncirrhotic patients with HCV, genotype 1. Twenty-six were randomized to 12 weeks LDV/SOF and 14 to placebo, with the placebo patients transferring to open-label LDV/SOF at week 4 after treatment. The primary end point was the week 4 MRS and neurocognitive tests to see what the effect of viral suppression had on cerebral function. Patients were followed with neurocognitive tests to week 24 SVR, and a subset had late week 24 MRS. Although there were some MRS changes, such as significant decline in Cho/Cr ratio in basal ganglia of LDV/SOF-treated patients, there was overall no major significant differences at week 4 in either MRS or neurocognitive testing between the active and placebo arms. The full study has not been published, but the investigators concluded that at an early (week 4 after treatment) time point there was no major benefit on neurocognition or cerebral metabolism when DAA was compared with placebo. However, by week 24 all treated patients had evidence of improved neurocognition, suggesting that the CNS manifestations of HCV are probably not related to active replication within the brain and that the improvements occur slowly over time and require at least 24 weeks after SVR.

Hepatitis C virus and cerebrovascular disease

There has been a reported association between an increase in carotid arterial plaques and HCV using cross-sectional imaging studies,[36–38] and positive strand HCV RNA has been found in studies of carotid plaques.[39] HCV is associated with serum lipoproteins and can induce oxidative stress and localized inflammation, and all of these features can result in an increased risk of carotid plaque formation.

More importantly, multiple studies have now shown the association between HCV and stroke. Liao and colleagues[40] in Taiwan followed 4094 adults with HCV compared with a matched population of 16,376 adults without HCV. Multivariate adjusted hazard ratios (HRs) and 95% confidence intervals (CIs) were estimated for potential associated factors, including HCV infection, age, sex, low-income status, urbanization, cessation of cigarette smoking, alcohol-related illness, obesity, history of chronic diseases, and medication use.

The cumulative risk of stroke for people with hepatitis C and without hepatitis C infections was 2.5% and 1.9%, respectively, with an adjusted HR of stroke of 1.27 (95% CI 1.14–1.41) for people with hepatitis C indicating that HCV is an independent risk factor for stroke. Lee and colleagues,[41] in a second large community cohort study from Taiwan of 23,665 participants, showed an increased risk of cerebrovascular mortality with a risk-adjusted HR of 2.18. Interestingly, the risk-adjusted HR increased as the HCV RNA increased in the population, suggesting a direct effect of HCV on cerebrovascular risk. Finally, in a large meta-analysis by Ambrosino and colleagues,[42] both an increase in cardiovascular risk and cerebrovascular risk was confirmed with an odds ratio of 1.48 for cerebrovascular events. These studies clearly show an independent and significant association between HCV and risk of cerebrovascular disease. Unfortunately, no data exist as to the effect of SVR on subsequent coronary or cerebrovascular risk.

SUMMARY

The neurologic manifestations of HCV are both common and significant with both an increased morbidity and mortality. HCV-induced neurocognitive dysfunction should be considered in patients even with mild disease, and the overall improvements reported in MH and fatigue with eradication of HCV should be considered when making treatment decisions. Patients with HCV are at risk of cerebrovascular events, and studies to evaluate the effect of eradication of HCV on subsequent vascular risk should be undertaken.

REFERENCES

1. Forton DM, Allsop JM, Main J, et al. Evidence for a cerebral effect of the hepatitis C virus. Lancet 2001;358:38–9.
2. Forton DM, Thomas HC, Murphy CA, et al. Hepatitis C and cognitive impairment in a cohort of patients with mild liver disease. Hepatology 2002;35:433–9.
3. Forton DM, Karayiannis P, Mahmud N, et al. Identification of unique hepatitis C virus quasispecies in the central nervous system and comparative analysis of internal translational efficiency of brain, liver, and serum variants. J Virol 2004;78:5170–83.
4. Laskus T, Radkowski M, Bednarska A, et al. Detection and analysis of hepatitis C virus sequences in cerebrospinal fluid. J Virol 2002;76:10064–8.
5. Radkowski M, Wilkinson J, Nowicki M, et al. Search for hepatitis C virus negative-strand RNA sequences and analysis of viral sequences in the central nervous system: evidence of replication. J Virol 2002;76:600–8.
6. Seifert F, Struffert T, Hildebrandt M, et al. In vivo detection of hepatitis C virus (HCV) RNA in the brain in a case of encephalitis: evidence for HCV neuroinvasion. Eur J Neurol 2008;15:214–8.

7. Wilson CJ, Finch CE, Cohen HJ. Cytokines and cognition – the case for a head-to-toe inflammatory paradigm. J Am Geriatr Soc 2002;50:2041–56.
8. Radkowski M, Bednarska A, Horban A, et al. Infection of primary human macrophages with hepatitis C virus in vitro: induction of tumor necrosis factor-alpha and interleukin 8. J Gen Virol 2004;85:47–59.
9. Licinio J, Kling MA, Hauser P. Cytokines and brain function: relevance to interferon-a-induced mood and cognitive changes. Semin Oncol 1998;25:S30–8.
10. Cacciarelli TV, Martinez OM, Gish RG, et al. Immunoregulatory cytokines in chronic hepatitis C virus infection: pre- and posttreatment with interferon alfa. Hepatology 1996;24:6–9.
11. Farkkila M, Iivanainen M, Roine R, et al. Neurotoxic and other side effects of high-dose interferon in amyotrophic lateral sclerosis. Acta Neurol Scand 1984;70:42–6.
12. Shibata M, Blatteis CM. Human recombinant tumor necrosis factor and interferon affect the activity of neuron in the organum vasculosum laminea terminalis. Brain Res 1991;562:323–6.
13. Hilsabeck RC, Perry W, Hassassein TI. Neuropsychological impairment in patients with chronic hepatitis C. Hepatology 2002;35:440–6.
14. Hilsabeck RC, Hassanein TI, Carlson MD, et al. Cognitive functioning and psychiatric symptomatology in patients with chronic hepatitis C. J Int Neuropsychol Soc 2003;9:847–54.
15. Weissenborn K, Krause J, Bokemeyer M, et al. Hepatitis C virus infection affects the brain-evidence from psychometric studies and magnetic resonance spectroscopy. J Hepatol 2004;41:845–51.
16. Rosenbloom MJ, O'Reilly A, Sassoon SA, et al. Persistent cognitive deficits in community treated alcoholic men and women volunteering for research: limited contribution from psychiatric comorbidity. J Stud Alcohol 2005;66:254–65.
17. Loftis JM, Hauser P. Hepatitis C in patients with psychiatric disease and substance abuse: screening strategies and comanagement models of care. Curr Hepat Rep 2003;2:93–100.
18. Dwight MM, Kowdley KV, Russo JE, et al. Depression, fatigue, and functional disability in patients with chronic hepatitis C. J Psychosom Res 2000;49:311–7.
19. Yovtcheva SP, Aly Rifai M, Moles JK, et al. Psychiatric comorbidity among hepatitis C-positive patients. Psychosomatics 2001;42:411–5.
20. El-Serag HB, Kunik M, Richardson P, et al. Psychiatric disorders among veterans with hepatitis C infection. Gastroenterology 2002;123:476–82.
21. Kramer L, Bauer E, Funk G, et al. Subclinical impairment of brain function in chronic hepatitis C infection. J Hepatol 2002;37:349–54.
22. Gualtieri CT, Johnson LG, Benedict KB. Neurocognition in depression: patients on and off medication versus healthy comparison subjects. J Neuropsychiatry Clin Neurosci 2006;18:217–25.
23. Forton DM, Hamilton G, Allsop JM, et al. Cerebral immune activation in chronic hepatitis C infection: a magnetic resonance spectroscopy study. J Hepatol 2008;49:316–22.
24. Bokemeyer M, Ding XQ, Goldbecker A, et al. Evidence for neuroinflammation and neuroprotection in HCV infection- associated encephalopathy. Gut 2011;60:370–7.
25. Kamei S, Tanaka N, Mastuura M, et al. Blinded, prospective, and serial evaluation by quantitative-EEG in interferon-alpha-treated hepatitis-C. Acta Neurol Scand 1999;100:25–33.

26. Kamei S, Sakai T, Matsuura M, et al. Alterations of quantitative EEG and mini-mental state examination in interferon-a-treated hepatitis C. Eur Neurol 2002; 48:102–7.

27. Hilsabeck RC, Hassanein TI, Ziegler EA, et al. Effect of interferon-alpha on cognitive functioning in patients with chronic hepatitis C. J Int Neuropsychol Soc 2005; 11:16–22.

28. Amodio P, De Toni EN, Cavalletto L, et al. Mood, cognition and EEG changes during interferon alpha (alpha-IFN) treatment for chronic hepatitis C. J Affect Disord 2005;84:93–8.

29. Capuron L, Pagnoni G, Demetrashvili M, et al. Anterior cingulate activation and error processing during interferon-alpha treatment. Biol Psychiatry 2005;58: 190–6.

30. Kraus MR, Schafer A, Wissmann S, et al. Neurocognitive changes in patients with hepatitis C receiving interferon alfa-2b and ribavirin. Clin Pharmacol Ther 2005; 77:90–100.

31. Lieb K, Engelbrecht MA, Gut O, et al. Cognitive impairment in patients with chronic hepatitis treated with interferon alpha (IFNa): results from a prospective study. Eur Psychiatry 2006;21:204–10.

32. Byrnes V, Miller A, Lowry D, et al. Effects of antiviral therapy and HCV clearance on cerebral metabolism and cognition. J Hepatol 2012;56:549–56.

33. Afdhal N, Zeuzem S, Kwo P, et al, the ION-1 Investigators. Ledipasvir and sofosbuvir for untreated HCV genotype 1 infection. N Engl J Med 2014;370:1889–98.

34. Alsop D, Younossi Z, Stepanova M, et al. Cerebral MR spectroscopy and patient-reported mental health outcomes in hepatitis C genotype 1 naive patients treated with ledipasvir and sofosbuvir (abstr 48). Hepatology 2014;60:221A.

35. Curry MP, Moczynski NP, Liu H, et al. The effect of sustained virologic response on cerebral metabolism and neurocognition in patients with chronic genotype 1 HCV infection. J Hepatol 2016;62(2):S797.

36. Ishizaka N, Ishizaka Y, Takahashi E, et al. Association between hepatitis C virus seropositivity, carotid-artery plaque, and intima–media thickening. Lancet 2002; 359:133–5.

37. Ishizaka Y, Ishizaka N, Takahashi E, et al. Association between hepatitis C virus core protein and carotid atherosclerosis. Circ J 2003;67:26–30.

38. Bilora F, Rinaldi R, Boccioletti V, et al. Chronic viral hepatitis: a prospective factor against atherosclerosis. A study with echo-color Doppler of the carotid and femoral arteries and the abdominal aorta. Gastroenterol Clin Biol 2002;26: 1001–4.

39. Boddi M, Abbate R, Chellini B, et al. HCV infection facilitates asymptomatic carotid atherosclerosis: preliminary report of HCV RNA localization in human carotid plaques. Dig Liver Dis 2007;39(Suppl 1):S55–60.

40. Liao CC, Su TC, Sung FC, et al. Does hepatitis C virus infection increase risk for stroke? A population-based cohort study. PLoS One 2012;7(2):e31527.

41. Lee M, Yang HI, Wang CH, et al. Hepatitis C virus infection and increased risk of cerebrovascular disease. Stroke 2010;41:2894–900.

42. Ambrosino P, Lupoli R, DiMinno A, et al. The risk of coronary artery disease and cerebrovascular disease in patients with hepatitis C: a systematic review and meta-analysis. Int J Cardiol 2016;221:746–54.

Hepatitis C and Risk of Nonhepatic Malignancies

Maya Balakrishnan, MD, MPH[a],*, Matthew T. Glover, MD[a], Fasiha Kanwal, MD[a,b]

KEYWORDS

- Hepatitis C virus • Cholangiocarcinoma • Pancreatic adenocarcinoma
- Papillary thyroid cancer • Oral squamous cell cancer • Renal/kidney cancer

KEY POINTS

- The association between HCV and intrahepatic CCA is most compelling with supporting epidemiologic and biologic evidence; in contrast, the evidence argues against an association between HCV and extrahepatic CCA.
- The epidemiologic evidence is in favor of an HCV and renal/kidney cancer association; however, the biologic basis is still not fully substantiated.
- Evidence regarding the association between HCV and PAC and OSSC each is mixed, confounded by alcohol and tobacco exposure, and requires further study.
- Based on the available data, HCV is not associated with PTC; epidemiologic studies examining this association are largely negative and there is not a biologically convincing mechanism for the association.

INTRODUCTION

Chronic hepatitis C virus (HCV) is a recognized oncovirus, primarily known for its association with hepatocellular carcinoma (HCC) and non-Hodgkin lymphoma. Epidemiologic studies show an increased risk of mortality among HCV-infected individuals compared with uninfected individuals from hepatic and nonhepatic causes; the latter include several nonhepatic malignancies.[1,2] These and other findings, discussed here, have raised the possibility of a link between HCV and nonhepatic malignancies.

HCV may promote extrahepatic cancers directly or indirectly. HCV has been isolated in extrahepatic tissues and may thus promote carcinogenesis directly through persistent inflammation and oncogenesis of target tissues.[3,4] Alternatively, HCV's effects may be indirect by promoting a proinflammatory systemic state conducive to

The authors have nothing to disclose.

[a] Section of Gastroenterology and Hepatology, Department of Medicine, Baylor College of Medicine, One Baylor Plaza, Houston, TX 77030, USA; [b] Department of Medicine, Houston VA HSR&D Center for Innovations in Quality, Effectiveness and Safety, Michael E. DeBakey Veterans Affairs Medical Center, 2002 Holcombe Boulevard, Houston, TX 77030, USA

* Corresponding author.

E-mail address: maya.balakrishnan@bcm.edu

cancer development. HCV-infected individuals also have a higher prevalence of tobacco and alcohol use than uninfected individuals,.[5] Thus, compared with general populations, HCV-infected persons could be at increased risk of cancer, not only because of the pathogenic effect of the virus but also because of a higher degree of exposure to other known carcinogens.

This article reviews the association between HCV and five of the most frequently studied non-HCC cancers: (1) cholangiocarcinoma (CCA), (2) pancreatic adenocarcinoma (PAC), (3) papillary thyroid cancer (PTC), (4) oral squamous cell cancer (OSCC), and (5) renal/kidney cancer.[6] We examine the putative association between HCV and each included cancer by reviewing the biologic plausibility of HCV in promoting each cancer, the strength of the epidemiologic evidence, and the coherence of the association. Few studies have examined the relationship between HCV and other cancers, such as breast, colon, prostate, and lung cancer, with mixed results; most studies suggest lack of any significant association between these nonhepatic cancers in HCV. Thus, these cancers are not discussed in this review.

CHOLANGIOCARCINOMA

CCA, malignant biliary epithelial tumors arising from anywhere along the biliary tree, are rare but insidious and highly lethal malignancies. They are broadly categorized into two anatomic subtypes: intrahepatic and extrahepatic CCA. Each subtype is different with respect to clinical presentation, biology, and treatment. Intrahepatic CCAs arise in the peripheral bile ducts within the hepatic parenchyma. They originate from biliary epithelial or hepatic progenitor cells and some intrahepatic CCAs are proposed to share features with primary liver cancers.[7-10] Extrahepatic CCAs, however, arise outside of the hepatic parenchyma distal to the bifurcation of the left and right hepatic ducts, and originate from biliary epithelial cells and peribiliary glands.[11]

Chronic biliary inflammation and cholestasis are key factors in CCA pathogenesis. Although most cases are sporadic, established CCA risk factors have been identified and include primary sclerosing cholangitis, chronic hepatobiliary parasitic infection (*Opisthorchis viverrini* and *Clonorchis sinensis*), hepatolithiasis, and biliary duct congenital malformations. HCV emerged as a potential risk factor for CCA based on early observations of CCA cases among HCV-infected patients. Since then a large body of work has been published examining the association between HCV infection and CCA.

Biologic Mechanism

A clear mechanism for how HCV may induce biliary tract carcinogenesis has yet to be delineated. However, several clinical and bench observations suggest a possible role for HCV in inducing bile duct inflammation and cholangiocarcinogenesis. HCV RNA and NS5 protein have been identified in bile duct epithelium among chronically infected patients,[12,13] suggesting that HCV may promote chronic inflammation of the bile duct epithelium. HCV RNA sequences have been demonstrated in extrahepatic CCA tissue, lending support to an etiologic role for HCV.[14-16] Biliary intraepithelial neoplasia has been observed in the large and septal-sized bile ducts of explanted livers from HCV-infected individuals alone and in association with alcohol,[17,18] providing support for an association between HCV and a putative preneoplastic condition.

Bench observations have lent some basis for a mechanistic role of HCV in the pathogenesis of CCA. HCV-transfected normal human biliary epithelial cells have exhibited transformation to show CCA-like features.[19] HCV core proteins were shown to modulate cellular proliferation and apopotosis in CCA tissues.[20] In a separate experiment, HCV core protein was significantly associated with CCA invasion and metastasis.[21] Together, these findings suggest that HCV core proteins can participate in malignant transformation of normal human biliary epithelial cells.

Epidemiologic Observations: Hepatitis C Virus–Cholangiocarcinomas Association

Epidemiologic studies have observed an increased risk of CCA among HCV-infected compared with HCV-uninfected persons with pooled odds ratios (OR) ranging 1.8 (95% confidence interval [CI], 1.4–2.4)[22] to 5.4 (95% CI, 2.7–10.9).[23] The association between HCV and CCA varies by anatomic subtype and by geographic region. For example, studies demonstrate an increased risk of intrahepatic CCA but little or no increased risk of extrahepatic CCA among HCV-infected individuals. In available meta-analyses, HCV was associated with statistically significant increased risk of intrahepatic CCA with pooled OR ranging 3.42 (95% CI, 1.96–5.99)[24] to 4.84 (95% CI, 2.41–9.71).[25] In contrast, HCV was not associated with a statistically significant risk of extrahepatic CCA (pooled OR, 1.75; 95% CI, 1.00–3.05) based on meta-analysis that included all five available case-control studies evaluating the association.[23] Similarly, in a large retrospective cohort study that separately examined extrahepatic and intrahepatic CCAs, El-Serag and coworkers[26] found an increased incidence of intrahepatic CCA (hazard ratio [HR], 2.55; 95% CI, 1.31–4.95) but not extrahepatic CCA (HR, 1.05; 95% CI, 0.60–1.85) among HCV-infected compared with matched HCV-uninfected military veterans (incidence rate of intrahepatic CCA among HCV-infected vs -uninfected: 4/100,000 vs 1.6/100,000).

The association between HCV and intrahepatic CCA is modified by geographic location.[23,25] The HCV-CCA association was stronger in studies including North American populations (pooled OR, 6.48; 95% CI, 4.97–8.46) than studies of Asian populations (pooled OR, 2.01; 95% CI, 1.44–2.79).[23] This variability is explained by a higher prevalence of established CCA risk factors including chronic hepatobiliary parasites, hepatolithiasis, and potentially chronic hepatitis B in Asia.

Summary

Epidemiologic evidence supports an association between HCV and intrahepatic CCA, particularly in geographic areas with low prevalence of other competing CCA risk factors. HCV does not seem to increase the risk of extrahepatic CCA. However, most of the data are based on case-control and one retrospective cohort study. There is a paucity of population-based or prospective cohort studies. Yet, similarities in origin and pathogenesis between subtypes of intrahepatic CCA and HCC along with observed transformations of HCV transfected biliary epithelial cells provide biologic plausibility for the relationship.

PANCREATIC ADENOCARCINOMA

PAC is one of the most aggressive and lethal cancers with an overall 5-year survival rate less than 5%. Established risk factors for PAC include tobacco use and hereditary factors. Other less established, potential risk factors include diabetes, chronic pancreatitis, heavy alcohol consumption, and HCV.

Biologic Mechanism

The anatomic proximity and shared blood supply with the liver make the pancreas potentially susceptible to the inflammatory complications of HCV. Indeed, data show that HCV can infect, replicate in, and chronically inflame exocrine pancreatic tissue. HCV antigens, HCV RNA, and HCV replicative intermediates have been identified in the pancreatic acinar cells of subjects with HCV.[3] HCV has also been associated with hyperlipasemia[27,28] and acute pancreatitis[28–30] Given these observations, it is plausible that HCV might be a risk factor for PAC.

Epidemiologic Observations: Hepatitis C Virus–Pancreatic Cancer Association

Several studies have examined the association between HCV and PAC over the past decade. These include six cohort studies,[2,26,31–34] two case control studies,[35,36] and three meta-analyses.[4,37,38] Three cohort studies, none of which adjusted for alcohol or tobacco exposure, demonstrated an increased incidence of PAC among HCV-infected persons compared with general population with a standardized incidence ratio ranging from 2.5 (95% CI, 1.6–3.2) to 3.95 (95% CI, 1.07–10.11).[2,33,34] In contrast, studies that adjusted for exposure to tobacco and alcohol failed to detect a significant association between HCV and PAC. Similar findings were reported from two separate hospital-based case-control studies conducted in the United States[36] and Taiwan[35]; there was no association between HCV and PAC after adjusting for tobacco and alcohol use (OR, 0.9 and 95% CI, 0.3–2.8; OR, 1.36 and 95% CI, 0.8–2.31, respectively).

Meta-analyses of these observational studies have yielded mixed results, likely because of heterogeneity in the study populations and inconsistent adjustment of coexisting risk factors. For example, Fiorino and colleagues[4] did not find a statistically significant association between anti-HCV positivity and PAC in a meta-analysis of studies that adjusted for alcohol and tobacco exposure (relative risk [RR], 1.16; 95% CI, 0.99–1.3). In contrast, Xu and colleagues[37] found a small increased risk for PAC among HCV-infected persons in the meta-analysis of four studies that adjusted for smoking (OR, 1.32; 95% CI, 1.08–1.56) and three studies that adjusted for alcohol use (OR, 1.51; 95% CI, 1.17–1.85).

Summary

Isolation of HCV from pancreatic exocrine tissue and evidence of HCV-induced pancreatic inflammation has raised the possibility that HCV infection may play a role in the development of PAC. However, epidemiologic studies that accounted for established risk factors for PAC (tobacco and alcohol) do not support the association between HCV and PAC.

PAPILLARY THYROID CANCER

Thyroid cancer has tripled in incidence since 1975. PTC, which arises from the follicular cells of the thyroid and has several subtypes, accounts for 85% of thyroid cancers.[39] Part of the observed increase in thyroid cancer incidence is thought to be a function of better imaging techniques and greater vigilance leading to overdetection of subclinical disease. However, there is general agreement that there has been a "real" rise in thyroid cancer potentially because of greater exposure to acquired risk factors.[40] Established nonmodifiable risk factors for PTC are female gender, older age, and family history. The most established environmental risk factor for PTC is exposure to ionizing radiation. Other possible less-established risk factors include obesity and dietary factors. Recent studies have examined an association between HCV and PTC, with mixed results.

Biologic Mechanism

Autoimmune thyroid disease is a recognized extrahepatic manifestation of HCV: Graves disease, Hashimoto thyroiditis, and isolated increases in antithyroid antibodies are frequent among chronically HCV-infected persons.[41–44] HCV-infected persons have a greater risk of autoimmune thyroid disease compared with hepatitis B virus–infected (pooled OR, 3.3; 95% CI, 2.4–4.6) and healthy control subjects (pooled OR, 1.3; 95% CI, 1.1–1.7).[41] Studies have postulated that HCV may exert an indirect oncogenic effect on thyroid by inducing autoimmune thyroiditis.[45] However, this notion remains controversial. Indeed, the relationship between autoimmune thyroiditis and PTC is still not firmly established in the general endocrine literature. HCV has been isolated from thyroid tissue[46]; however, a direct oncogenic effect of HCV on thyroid is unlikely.

Epidemiologic Evidence: Hepatitis C Virus–Papillary Thyroid Cancer

A total of 10 observational studies have examined the association between HCV infection and thyroid cancer. Antonelli and colleagues[47] reported a significantly higher prevalence of PTC among 139 HCV-infected persons compared with 839 HCV-negative controls in Italy (2.2% vs 0%; $P = .004$). Later, the same group confirmed these findings in a larger study where a significantly higher prevalence of PTC was observed among 308 HCV-infected persons compared with 616 age- and gender-matched HCV-negative control subjects from iodine-deficient and 616 matched HCV-negative control subjects from iodine-sufficient regions (1.9% vs 0% vs 0.2%; $P = .001$).[48] They also reported a higher prevalence of PTC among 94 HCV-infected patients with mixed cryoglobulinemia compared with 470 control subjects from the general population (2.1% vs 0%; $P<.01$).[49] Subsequently, in a case control study, Montella and colleagues[50] found that the odds of PTC was 3.3 times greater among HCV-infected than HCV-uninfected persons (OR, 3.3; 95% CI, 1.5–7.4; $P = .003$). The association between HCV and PTC was similar among women (OR, 3.3; 95% CI, 1.4–8.1; $P = .008$) and men (OR, 3.3; 95% CI, 0.8–13.4; $P = .1$), although the latter did not reach statistical significance.[50] All studies took place in Italy, potentially reflecting the moderately high HCV infection prevalence in the region,[51] thus limiting their generalizability to other regions.

Indeed, six retrospective cohort studies from geographically diverse regions with relatively lower HCV prevalence rates (United States,[2,52] Australia,[32,33] Sweden,[53] and Denmark[34]) were unable to replicate the findings from the Italian centers. These cohort studies compared the observed incidence of thyroid cancer among HCV-infected persons with the expected incidence in the general population. In contrast to the previous case-control and cross-sectional studies that specifically identified PTC based on histology or cytology, thyroid cancer was ascertained by international classification diagnostic codes. It is possible that the use of international classification diagnostic codes for thyroid cancer in general, rather than histology specifically for PTC, might have attenuated the associations between HCV and thyroid cancer. However, the cohort study design is superior to case-control and cross-sectional designs for determination of causality, in this case the role of HCV in thyroid cancer incidence. Further strengths of the available cohort studies include use of nationally representative samples with large sample sizes from geographically diverse populations.

Summary

The association of HCV with thyroid cancer is not clear, because studies have differing conclusions and there is a paucity of prospective cohort studies that used standardized and histologic criteria for thyroid cancer diagnosis.

ORAL SQUAMOUS CELL CANCER

OSCC is the most common type of oral malignant tumors. Established risk factors include tobacco, alcohol, betel leaf, and areca nut use. In addition, the human papilloma virus is a recognized viral cause of OSCC. Oral lichen planus, leukoplakia, and oral dysplasia are premalignant oral lesions that can transform into OSCC. HCV can proliferate in the oral mucosa and has been detected directly in tissue from oral lichen planus, oral cancer, and salivary glands.[54,55] The HCV predilection for oral tissue has thus generated interest in its potential role as an infectious risk factor for OSCC.

Biologic Mechanism

The main putative pathogenic link between HCV and oral cancer is via oral lichen planus. Oral lichen planus is the oral phenotype of lichen planus, which is an inflammatory mucocutaneous condition and an established extrahepatic manifestation of HCV. Compared with HCV-uninfected persons, HCV-infected persons have a twofold greater risk for lichen planus.[56] The association between chronic HCV infection and oral lichen planus is even stronger, with estimated OR ranging 4.6 (95% CI, 3.0–7.7) to 5.6 (95% CI, 3.5–8.8) in separate meta-analyses.[57,58] HCV most likely promotes oral lichen planus indirectly by stimulating an immune response rather than through a direct viral effect.[57] The role of oral lichen planus as an OSCC premalignant lesion[59,60] suggests that HCV may also be a potential risk factor for OSCC.

Epidemiologic Evidence: Hepatitis C Virus–Oral Squamous Cell Cancer Association

Case reports published in the late-1990s documented the progression of oral lichen planus to OSCC in HCV-infected patients.[61,62] These clinical observations raised the possibility of HCV as a novel infectious risk factor for OSCC. Since then three cross-sectional and five retrospective cohort studies have examined the relationship between HCV and OSCC, with inconsistent results. A Veterans Affairs–based study in the United States reported a significantly higher prevalence of HCV among patients with OSCC (21%) compared with the general population (9.9%).[63] In contrast, a study from Japan found that HCV prevalence was not different among patients with OSCC compared with those with impacted teeth (OR, 0.44; $P<.05$).[64] Eftekharian and colleagues[65] observed a very low HCV prevalence (0.9%) among consecutive patients with squamous cell head and neck cancers in a multicenter study from Iran.

Cohort studies have also reported conflicted results. Using data from the Taiwanese national insurance database, Su and colleagues[66] found that HCV was associated with an increased risk for OSCC (HR, 1.92; 95% CI, 1.21–3.04). In a multicenter hepatitis C cohort, Allison and colleagues[2] did not find a significantly increased incidence of OSCC (Standardized Rate Ratio (SRR), 2.5; 95% CI, 0.9–4.1) but reported significantly increased OSCC-related mortality risk (RR, 5.2; 95% CI, 5.1–5.4) among HCV-infected persons compared with the general population. Findings of three other cohort studies from Denmark and Australia did not support an association between HCV and risk of oral cancer.[32–34] Notably, none of these studies adjusted for tobacco exposure, although Su and colleagues[66] attempted to account for smoking by excluding participants who ever developed a smoking-related cancer.

Summary

The association between HCV and OSCC is plausible yet remains unproven. The biologic basis for the association between HCV and OSCC via oral lichen planus, a recognized premalignant condition and established HCV complication, is compelling. However, the available epidemiologic evidence is inconsistent and therefore insufficient to support the association at this time.

RENAL CELL CARCINOMA/KIDNEY CANCER

Renal cell carcinoma (RCC) consists of malignancies arising from the renal cortex and accounts for 90% of kidney cancers. RCC incidence has increased over the past two decades, particularly among men and African-Americans.[67] Established risk factors for RCC include tobacco, obesity, dialysis, and hereditary factors. HCV has been implicated in RCC because of its association with chronic kidney disease. Early case reports of RCC in HCV-positive patients suggested a pathogenic link between the two.

Biologic Mechanism

Kidney disease is a well-recognized complication of chronic HCV infection. Compared with HCV-uninfected, HCV-infected persons have an increased risk of developing chronic kidney disease and end-stage renal disease (pooled RR, 1.23; 95% CI, 1.12–1.34).[56] The most frequent HCV-associated renal disease is glomerulonephritis, typically the consequence of cryoglobulin glomerular deposition. Other HCV glomerular diseases include membranous nephropathy, rapidly progressive glomerulonephritis, and fibrillary and immunotactoid glomerulonephritis.[68]

The mechanism by which HCV could promote RCC is not entirely understood. The HCV-chronic kidney disease association is probably not a sufficient biologic mechanism. Instead, three main hypotheses have been put forth to explain the possible association between HCV and RCC. One hypothesis implicates a role for HCV in RCC pathogenesis via the NY-REN-54 protein, an altered ubiquitin-related protein that may promote oncogenesis.[69] A second postulated mechanism is HCV-induced increased expression of serine protease inhibor Kazal (SPIK), a protein that inhibits serine protease-related apoptosis.[70] The third hypothesis implicates HCV inhibition of cytotoxic T-cell dependent apoptosis, which disturbs host immunity and normal tissue and leads to renal oncogenesis.[71]

Epidemiologic Evidence: Hepatitis C Virus–Renal/Kidney Cancer Association

A total of 10 studies have examined the association between HCV and RCC. These include four cross-sectional[72–75] and six cohort studies.[2,32–34,76,77] In addition, one meta-analysis has been conducted that included all but three of the available studies.[78]

Most cross-sectional studies have found a positive association between RCC and HCV infection. A recent case-control study using Taiwanese national health insurance data found a 24% increased odds of RCC among HCV-infected compared with uninfected persons after adjusting for chronic disease, age, and socioeconomic status[67]; notably this study did not adjust for known RCC risk factors including tobacco or family history. In a separate case-control study based in a single-center, Gonzalez and colleagues[73] noted a significantly higher odds of HCV infection among patients with RCC compared with patients with colon cancer (OR, 24; 95% CI, 2.4–999; P = .042) after adjustment for several variables including smoking. Similar findings were reported by Malaguarnera and colleagues[75] who found an significantly higher HCV infection prevalence among elderly patients with RCC compared with elderly healthy control subjects in an single Italian center (53% vs 10%; P<.05). In contrast, Budakoglu and colleagues[72] did not find a significant association between RCC and HCV infection in a multicenter case-control study.

The findings of cohort studies have been mixed. Using a multicenter cohort of HCV infected persons, Allison and colleagues[2] found that HCV-infected persons had higher incidence of RCC compared with the general population (SRR, 1.6; 95% CI, 1.1–2.2).

Gordon and colleagues[77] also found an increased RCC incidence among HCV-infected persons in a single center study (HR, 2.02; 95% CI, 1.01–4.06). In contrast, four separate cohort studies from Denmark,[34] Australia,[32,33] and Sweden[76] did not find a statistically increased incidence of RCC among HCV-infected persons compared with the general population.

The meta-analysis found that the pooled risk for RCC was 1.86 times greater among HCV-infected compared with HCV-uninfected persons. Furthermore HCV-infected persons developed RCC at a significantly younger age than HCV-uninfected persons.[78]

Summary

Available epidemiologic evidence supports the association between HCV and RCC but the findings are not entirely consistent. However, proposed biologic mechanisms for the association are still hypothetical and need to be elucidated in future studies.

OVERALL SUMMARY

The association between HCV and intrahepatic CCA is most compelling with supporting epidemiologic and biologic evidence; in contrast, the evidence argues against an association between HCV and extrahepatic CCA. The epidemiologic evidence is in favor of an HCV and renal/kidney cancer association; however, the biologic basis is still not fully substantiated. Evidence regarding the association between HCV and PAC and OSSC each is mixed, confounded by alcohol and tobacco exposure, and requires further study. Based on the available data, HCV is not associated with PTC; epidemiologic studies examining this association are largely negative and there is not a biologically convincing mechanism for the association.

REFERENCES

1. Lee MH, Yang HI, Lu SN, et al. Chronic hepatitis C virus infection increases mortality from hepatic and extrahepatic diseases: a community-based long-term prospective study. J Infect Dis 2012;206:469–77.
2. Allison RD, Tong X, Moorman AC, et al. Increased incidence of cancer and cancer-related mortality among persons with chronic hepatitis C infection, 2006-2010. J Hepatol 2015;63:822–8.
3. Yan FM, Chen AS, Hao F, et al. Hepatitis C virus may infect extrahepatic tissues in patients with hepatitis C. World J Gastroenterol 2000;6:805–11.
4. Fiorino S, Chili E, Bacchi-Reggiani L, et al. Association between hepatitis B or hepatitis C virus infection and risk of pancreatic adenocarcinoma development: a systematic review and meta-analysis. Pancreatology 2013;13:147–60.
5. Simon D, Michita RT, Beria JU, et al. Alcohol misuse and illicit drug use are associated with HCV/HIV co-infection. Epidemiol Infect 2014;142:2616–23.
6. Fiorino S, Bacchi-Reggiani L, de Biase D, et al. Possible association between hepatitis C virus and malignancies different from hepatocellular carcinoma: a systematic review. World J Gastroenterol 2015;21:12896–953.
7. Banales JM, Cardinale V, Carpino G, et al. Expert consensus document: cholangiocarcinoma: current knowledge and future perspectives consensus statement from the European Network for the Study of Cholangiocarcinoma (ENS-CCA). Nat Rev Gastroenterol Hepatol 2016;13:261–80.
8. Fan B, Malato Y, Calvisi DF, et al. Cholangiocarcinomas can originate from hepatocytes in mice. J Clin Invest 2012;122:2911–5.

9. Sekiya S, Suzuki A. Intrahepatic cholangiocarcinoma can arise from Notch-mediated conversion of hepatocytes. J Clin Invest 2012;122:3914–8.
10. Sempoux C, Jibara G, Ward SC, et al. Intrahepatic cholangiocarcinoma: new insights in pathology. Semin Liver Dis 2011;31:49–60.
11. Rizvi S, Gores GJ. Pathogenesis, diagnosis, and management of cholangiocarcinoma. Gastroenterology 2013;145:1215–29.
12. Fillipowicz EA, Xiao S, Sower LE, et al. Detection of HCV in bile duct epithelium by laser capture microdissection (LCM). In Vivo 2005;19:737–9.
13. Haruna Y, Kanda T, Honda M, et al. Detection of hepatitis C virus in the bile and bile duct epithelial cells of hepatitis C virus-infected patients. Hepatology 2001; 33:977–80.
14. Lu H, Ye MQ, Thung SN, et al. Detection of hepatitis C virus RNA sequences in cholangiocarcinomas in Chinese and American patients. Chin Med J (Engl) 2000;113:1138–41.
15. Perumal V, Wang J, Thuluvath P, et al. Hepatitis C and hepatitis B nucleic acids are present in intrahepatic cholangiocarcinomas from the United States. Hum Pathol 2006;37:1211–6.
16. Yin F, Chen B. Detection of hepatitis C virus RNA sequences in hepatic portal cholangiocarcinoma tissue by reverse transcription polymerase chain reaction. Chin Med J (Engl) 1998;111:1068–70.
17. Torbenson M, Yeh MM, Abraham SC. Bile duct dysplasia in the setting of chronic hepatitis C and alcohol cirrhosis. Am J Surg Pathol 2007;31:1410–3.
18. Wu TT, Levy M, Correa AM, et al. Biliary intraepithelial neoplasia in patients without chronic biliary disease: analysis of liver explants with alcoholic cirrhosis, hepatitis C infection, and noncirrhotic liver diseases. Cancer 2009;115:4564–75.
19. Chen RF, Li ZH, Liu RY, et al. Malignant transformation of the cultured human normal biliary tract epithelial cells induced by hepatitis C virus core protein. Oncol Rep 2007;17:105–10.
20. Chen RF, Li ZH, Zou SQ, et al. Effect of hepatitis C virus core protein on modulation of cellular proliferation and apoptosis in hilar cholangiocarcinoma. Hepatobiliary Pancreat Dis Int 2005;4:71–4.
21. Li T, Li D, Cheng L, et al. Epithelial-mesenchymal transition induced by hepatitis C virus core protein in cholangiocarcinoma. Ann Surg Oncol 2010;17:1937–44.
22. Shin HR, Oh JK, Masuyer E, et al. Epidemiology of cholangiocarcinoma: an update focusing on risk factors. Cancer Sci 2010;101:579–85.
23. Li H, Hu B, Zhou ZQ, et al. Hepatitis C virus infection and the risk of intrahepatic cholangiocarcinoma and extrahepatic cholangiocarcinoma: evidence from a systematic review and meta-analysis of 16 case-control studies. World J Surg Oncol 2015;13:161.
24. Zhou Y, Zhao Y, Li B, et al. Hepatitis viruses infection and risk of intrahepatic cholangiocarcinoma: evidence from a meta-analysis. BMC Cancer 2012;12:289.
25. Palmer WC, Patel T. Are common factors involved in the pathogenesis of primary liver cancers? A meta-analysis of risk factors for intrahepatic cholangiocarcinoma. J Hepatol 2012;57:69–76.
26. El-Serag HB, Engels EA, Landgren O, et al. Risk of hepatobiliary and pancreatic cancers after hepatitis C virus infection: a population-based study of U.S. veterans. Hepatology 2009;49:116–23.
27. Yoffe B, Bagri AS, Tran T, et al. Hyperlipasemia associated with hepatitis C virus. Dig Dis Sci 2003;48:1648–53.
28. Katakura Y, Yotsuyanagi H, Hashizume K, et al. Pancreatic involvement in chronic viral hepatitis. World J Gastroenterol 2005;11:3508–13.

29. Alvares-Da-Silva MR, Francisconi CF, Waechter FL. Acute hepatitis C complicated by pancreatitis: another extrahepatic manifestation of hepatitis C virus? J Viral Hepat 2000;7:84–6.

30. Taranto D, Carrato A, Romano M, et al. Mild pancreatic damage in acute viral hepatitis. Digestion 1989;42:93–7.

31. Huang J, Magnusson M, Torner A, et al. Risk of pancreatic cancer among individuals with hepatitis C or hepatitis B virus infection: a nationwide study in Sweden. Br J Cancer 2013;109:2917–23.

32. Amin J, Dore GJ, O'Connell DL, et al. Cancer incidence in people with hepatitis B or C infection: a large community-based linkage study. J Hepatol 2006;45: 197–203.

33. Swart A, Burns L, Mao L, et al. The importance of blood-borne viruses in elevated cancer risk among opioid-dependent people: a population-based cohort study. BMJ Open 2012;2. [pii:e001755].

34. Omland LH, Farkas DK, Jepsen P, et al. Hepatitis C virus infection and risk of cancer: a population-based cohort study. Clin Epidemiol 2010;2:179–86.

35. Chang MC, Chen CH, Liang JD, et al. Hepatitis B and C viruses are not risks for pancreatic adenocarcinoma. World J Gastroenterol 2014;20:5060–5.

36. Hassan MM, Li D, El-Deeb AS, et al. Association between hepatitis B virus and pancreatic cancer. J Clin Oncol 2008;26:4557–62.

37. Xu JH, Fu JJ, Wang XL, et al. Hepatitis B or C viral infection and risk of pancreatic cancer: a meta-analysis of observational studies. World J Gastroenterol 2013;19: 4234–41.

38. Xing S, Li ZW, Tian YF, et al. Chronic hepatitis virus infection increases the risk of pancreatic cancer: a meta-analysis. Hepatobiliary Pancreat Dis Int 2013;12: 575–83.

39. Fagin JA, Wells SA Jr. Biologic and clinical perspectives on thyroid cancer. N Engl J Med 2016;375:1054–67.

40. Wiltshire JJ, Drake TM, Uttley L, et al. Systematic review of trends in the incidence rates of thyroid cancer. Thyroid 2016;26:1541–52.

41. Antonelli A, Ferri C, Fallahi P, et al. Thyroid disorders in chronic hepatitis C virus infection. Thyroid 2006;16:563–72.

42. Antonelli A, Ferri C, Fallahi P, et al. Thyroid involvement in patients with overt HCV-related mixed cryoglobulinaemia. QJM 2004;97:499–506.

43. Quaranta JF, Tran A, Regnier D, et al. High prevalence of antibodies to hepatitis C virus (HCV) in patients with anti-thyroid autoantibodies. J Hepatol 1993;18:136–8.

44. Antonelli A, Ferri C, Pampana A, et al. Thyroid disorders in chronic hepatitis C. Am J Med 2004;117:10–3.

45. Okayasu I, Fujiwara M, Hara Y, et al. Association of chronic lymphocytic thyroiditis and thyroid papillary carcinoma. A study of surgical cases among Japanese, and white and African Americans. Cancer 1995;76:2312–8.

46. Bartolome J, Rodriguez-Inigo E, Quadros P, et al. Detection of hepatitis C virus in thyroid tissue from patients with chronic HCV infection. J Med Virol 2008;80: 1588–94.

47. Antonelli A, Ferri C, Fallahi P. Thyroid cancer in patients with hepatitis C infection. Jama 1999;281:1588.

48. Antonelli A, Ferri C, Fallahi P, et al. Thyroid cancer in HCV-related chronic hepatitis patients: a case-control study. Thyroid 2007;17:447–51.

49. Antonelli A, Ferri C, Fallahi P, et al. Thyroid cancer in HCV-related mixed cryoglobulinemia patients. Clin Exp Rheumatol 2002;20:693–6.

50. Montella M, Pezzullo L, Crispo A, et al. Risk of thyroid cancer and high prevalence of hepatitis C virus. Oncol Rep 2003;10:133–6.
51. Thrift AP, El-Serag HB, Kanwal F. Global epidemiology and burden of HCV infection and HCV-related disease. Nat Rev Gastroenterol Hepatol 2016;14:122–32.
52. Giordano TP, Henderson L, Landgren O, et al. Risk of non-Hodgkin lymphoma and lymphoproliferative precursor diseases in US veterans with hepatitis C virus. JAMA 2007;297:2010–7.
53. Duberg AS, Nordstrom M, Torner A, et al. Non-Hodgkin's lymphoma and other nonhepatic malignancies in Swedish patients with hepatitis C virus infection. Hepatology 2005;41:652–9.
54. Nagao Y, Sata M, Noguchi S, et al. Detection of hepatitis C virus RNA in oral lichen planus and oral cancer tissues. J Oral Pathol Med 2000;29:259–66.
55. Arrieta JJ, Rodriguez-Inigo E, Casqueiro M, et al. Detection of hepatitis C virus replication by in situ hybridization in epithelial cells of anti-hepatitis C virus-positive patients with and without oral lichen planus. Hepatology 2000;32:97–103.
56. Younossi Z, Park H, Henry L, et al. Extrahepatic manifestations of hepatitis C: a meta-analysis of prevalence, quality of life, and economic burden. Gastroenterology 2016;150:1599–608.
57. Lodi G, Pellicano R, Carrozzo M. Hepatitis C virus infection and lichen planus: a systematic review with meta-analysis. Oral Dis 2010;16:601–12.
58. Petti S, Rabiei M, De Luca M, et al. The magnitude of the association between hepatitis C virus infection and oral lichen planus: meta-analysis and case control study. Odontology 2011;99:168–78.
59. Silverman S Jr. Oral lichen planus: a potentially premalignant lesion. J Oral Maxillofac Surg 2000;58:1286–8.
60. Gandolfo S, Richiardi L, Carrozzo M, et al. Risk of oral squamous cell carcinoma in 402 patients with oral lichen planus: a follow-up study in an Italian population. Oral Oncol 2004;40:77–83.
61. Porter SR, Lodi G, Chandler K, et al. Development of squamous cell carcinoma in hepatitis C virus-associated lichen planus. Oral Oncol 1997;33:58–9.
62. Carrozzo M, Carbone M, Gandolfo S, et al. An atypical verrucous carcinoma of the tongue arising in a patient with oral lichen planus associated with hepatitis C virus infection. Oral Oncol 1997;33:220–5.
63. Nobles J, Wold C, Fazekas-May M, et al. Prevalence and epidemiology of hepatitis C virus in patients with squamous cell carcinoma of the head and neck. Laryngoscope 2004;114:2119–22.
64. Takata Y, Takahashi T, Fukuda J. Prevalence of hepatitis virus infection in association with oral diseases requiring surgery. Oral Dis 2002;8:95–9.
65. Eftekharian A, Khajavi M, Shokoofi S, et al. Hepatitis C virus in patients with squamous cell carcinoma of the head and neck in Iran: is there any relation? Eur Arch Otorhinolaryngol 2012;269:2571–3.
66. Su FH, Chang SN, Chen PC, et al. Positive association between hepatitis C infection and oral cavity cancer: a nationwide population-based cohort study in Taiwan. PLoS One 2012;7:e48109.
67. Znaor A, Lortet-Tieulent J, Laversanne M, et al. International variations and trends in renal cell carcinoma incidence and mortality. Eur Urol 2015;67:519–30.
68. Ferri C, Sebastiani M, Giuggioli D, et al. Hepatitis C virus syndrome: a constellation of organ- and non-organ specific autoimmune disorders, B-cell non-Hodgkin's lymphoma, and cancer. World J Hepatol 2015;7:327–43.
69. Wiwanitkit V. Renal cell carcinoma and hepatitis C virus infection: is there any cause-outcome relationship? J Cancer Res Ther 2011;7:226–7.

70. Lukkonen A, Lintula S, von Boguslawski K, et al. Tumor-associated trypsin inhibitor in normal and malignant renal tissue and in serum of renal-cell carcinoma patients. Int J Cancer 1999;83:486–90.

71. Chisari FV. Cytotoxic T cells and viral hepatitis. J Clin Invest 1997;99:1472–7.

72. Budakoglu B, Aksoy S, Arslan C, et al. Frequency of HCV infection in renal cell carcinoma patients. Med Oncol 2012;29:1892–5.

73. Gonzalez HC, Lamerato L, Rogers CG, et al. Chronic hepatitis C infection as a risk factor for renal cell carcinoma. Dig Dis Sci 2015;60:1820–4.

74. Lin YS, Yeh CC, Lin YC, et al. Kidney cancer linked to chronic hepatitis in the Asia-Pacific: a population-based analysis. Am J Nephrol 2016;45:22–31.

75. Malaguarnera M, Gargante MP, Risino C, et al. Hepatitis C virus in elderly cancer patients. Eur J Intern Med 2006;17:325–9.

76. Hofmann JN, Torner A, Chow WH, et al. Risk of kidney cancer and chronic kidney disease in relation to hepatitis C virus infection: a nationwide register-based cohort study in Sweden. Eur J Cancer Prev 2011;20:326–30.

77. Gordon SC, Moonka D, Brown KA, et al. Risk for renal cell carcinoma in chronic hepatitis C infection. Cancer Epidemiol Biomarkers Prev 2010;19:1066–73.

78. Wijarnpreecha K, Nissaisorakarn P, Sornprom S, et al. Hepatitis C infection and renal cell carcinoma: a systematic review and meta-analysis. World J Gastrointest Pathophysiol 2016;7:314–9.

Dermatologic Manifestations of Chronic Hepatitis C Infection

Mehmet Sayiner, MD[a,b], Pegah Golabi, MD[a], Freba Farhat, MD[b], Zobair M. Younossi, MD, MPH[a,b],*

KEYWORDS

- Hepatitis C • Extrahepatic manifestation • Dermatologic manifestation
- Cryoglobulinemia • Porphyria • Lichen planus

KEY POINTS

- HCV infection is associated with several dermatologic diseases, such as symptomatic mixed cryoglobulinemia, lichen planus, porphyria cutanea tarda, and necrolytic acral erythema.
- Most of the dermatologic manifestations may be caused by immune complexes.
- In the interferon and ribavirin era, treatment was associated with dermatologic side effects.
- The new generation of interferon-free and ribavirin-free anti-HCV regimens is devoid of dermatologic side effects.

INTRODUCTION

Chronic hepatitis C virus (HCV) infection is a global health problem and causes significant liver disease among infected patients. It is estimated that millions of people worldwide carry HCV antibodies with higher prevalence in Asia, the Middle East, and North Africa.[1] In the United States, the estimated prevalence of HCV infection is around 1.3% in the general population, but the rate is 3.2% in individuals who are born between 1945 and 1965.[2] HCV is a multifaceted disease and associated with not only liver disease, but also with multiple extrahepatic manifestations, including

Disclosure Statement: The authors have nothing to disclose.
[a] Betty and Guy Beatty Center for Integrated Research, Inova Health System, Inova Fairfax Hospital, Claude Moore Health Education and Research Building, 3rd Floor, 3300 Gallows Road, Falls Church, VA 22042, USA; [b] Department of Medicine, Center for Liver Disease, Inova Fairfax Hospital, Claude Moore Health Education and Research Building, 3rd Floor, 3300 Gallows Road, Falls Church, VA 22042, USA
* Corresponding author. Betty and Guy Beatty Center for Integrated Research, Claude Moore Health Education and Research Building, 3300 Gallows Road, Falls Church, VA 22042.
E-mail address: Zobair.Younossi@inova.org

Clin Liver Dis 21 (2017) 555–564
http://dx.doi.org/10.1016/j.cld.2017.03.010
1089-3261/17/© 2017 Elsevier Inc. All rights reserved.

kidney, eyes, musculoskeletal system, skin, nervous system, and immune system involvement.[3]

Chronic HCV infection has been linked to multiple dermatologic conditions, such as mixed cryoglobulinemia (MC), porphyria cutanea tarda (PCT), lichen planus (LP), and necrolytic acral erythema.[4,5] Also, there are some anecdotal associations with psoriasis and prurigo.[5] This article provides the reader the basic mechanisms and clinical features of these clinical conditions, and the management of these dermatologic manifestations.

MIXED CRYOGLOBULINEMIA

MC is one of the common extrahepatic manifestations of chronic HCV infection. In addition to its association with rheumatologic diseases and lymphoma, MC can cause dermatologic manifestation manifested by a rash, usually in the lower extremities. In this context, MC is responsible for small vessel vasculitis caused by the precipitation and deposition of immune complexes in the small vessels at temperatures lower than 37°C.[6]

Based on the composition of the precipitated immune complex, three different immunochemical types of cryoglobulins have been described. Type 1 cryoglobulins consist of pure monoclonal components and are most often caused by underlying multiple myeloma or Waldenström macroglobulinemia.[7] Type 2 is a mixture of monoclonal IgM and polyclonal IgG, and is most often seen in patients with chronic HCV infection, although infection with hepatitis B virus and Epstein-Barr virus were also implicated in some cases. Type 3, in which both IgG an IgM rheumatoid factor are polyclonal, is usually seen in some patients with HCV infection and chronic autoimmune diseases, such as systemic lupus erythematosus.[8] In patients with HCV with MC, type 2 cryoglobulins with rheumatoid factor activity are involved in more than half of the cases, whereas type 3 cryoglobulins account for nearly 40% of MC, and these cryoprecipitates are rich in HCV-RNA.[9,10]

Among all causes of MC, HCV infection accounts for 95% of all cases.[11] However, among patients with chronic HCV infection, the rate of detectable cryoglobulins is around 25% to 50%, albeit the rate of symptomatic patients is lower at 10% to 30%.[12,13] In fact, the gap in these ratios may be attributed to the varying degree of underlying liver disease, the differences in the rates of fibrosis, and the duration of the infection.[14] It has also been shown that the risk of significant cryoglobulinemia increases with the severity of underlying liver disease.[15]

The three most common symptoms of patients with MC are palpable purpura, arthralgia, and weakness, which were named as the core symptoms of cryoglobulinemia by Meltzer and Franklin in 1966.[16,17] The intravascular precipitation of immunoglobulins in lower temperatures causes reversible mechanical obstruction primarily in the small vessels of skin, kidneys, liver, and peripheral nerves and lead to Raynaud phenomenon and immune-complex mediated vasculitis. Among these patients, skin is the most frequently affected organ and palpable purpura is the most common symptom, although chronic ulcers may also occur.[18] The obstructive immune complexes may also cause pruritus, urticaria, and leukocytoclastic vasculitis.[19]

MC is typically diagnosed with history, clinical manifestations, and detecting hypocomplementemia, especially low C4, and cryoglobulins in the laboratory.[20] HCV seropositivity also supports the diagnosis of MC. Rheumatoid factor is almost always positive in patients with MC. Other markers of chronic inflammation can also be present, including elevated erythrocyte sedimentation rate, C-reactive protein, or normocytic anemia.[21] Furthermore, the purpuric skin lesion can be biopsied and pathologic diagnosis of leukocytoclastic vasculitis can be made. In the affected small blood vessels, cryoglobulins, and immune complexes are shown in the vessel walls.[22]

In summary, MC is an immune-complex mediated small vessel disease affecting mostly skin, but also kidneys, liver, and nervous system, and manifests with palpable purpura, weakness, and arthralgia. Treatment of underlying HCV can suppress the manifestations of vasculitis but immunosuppressive treatment with rituximab may be required, and plasma exchange in some patients.[23–25]

LICHEN PLANUS

LP is an uncommon disease of the stratified squamous epithelium, and may affect various body parts involving skin, oral cavity, genitalia, scalp, and even nails and esophagus.[26] The classic LP lesions are usually pruritic, polygonal, purple papules or plaques.[4] The size of the violaceous, flat-topped lesions may vary from pinpoint to larger than a centimeter.[27]

LP often develops between the ages of 30 and 60 and is seen in less than 1% of the general population.[28,29] The disease does not show any preference for sex and there is no strong racial predilection.[28,30] LP lesions are most commonly seen on the flexor aspects of wrists, forearms, and extensor aspects of hands, ankles, shins, and also genital area.[5] There are more than a dozen different clinical variants of LP; annular LP is common in the genital area; inverse type is usually seen in the intertriginous sites, such as axilla and inframammary area; and atrophic LP is often seen in the legs.[31] New lesions may develop in previously unaffected areas after scratching and trauma, which is known as Koebner phenomenon, also seen in patients with psoriasis. Although LP lesions rarely scars and they are usually self-limited, oral LP lesions more frequently become chronic and considered as premalignant lesions.[32]

The cause of LP is not known; however, it has been proposed that an immune mechanism directed by activated $CD8^+$ T cells against basal keratinocytes plays a major role in the pathophysiology of the disease.[33] Certain types of cytokines, such as tumor necrosis factor-α, interferon-γ, and interleukin-6 and -8, may also play a role in the pathogenesis of LP in patients with HCV infection.[34] During the era of interferon, several studies reported development or worsening of LP lesions during treatment with interferon.[35]

Although the cause and effect relationship has not been clearly shown for HCV infection and LP, previous studies evidently found statistically significant associations between chronic HCV infection and LP.[36–38] A meta-analysis by Shengyuan and colleagues[27] with 70 studies from five continents revealed that the presence of HCV may be used as a predictive marker for certain types of LP, because there was a significant risk for development of LP in patients with HCV infection. This meta-analysis also reported that compared with control subjects, patients with LP had higher HCV prevalence rates with an odds ratio of 5.4. Furthermore, a systematic review by Lodi and colleagues[37] found that compared with control group, the prevalence of LP was 4.8 times higher in patients with HCV. It is estimated that among patients with LP, the prevalence of HCV ranges from 4% in Europe to 24% in the Middle East and it is hypothesized that the difference in these rates was caused by genetic factors, such as different human leukocyte antigen types and the difference in most common HCV genotype in those geographic areas.[39,40] Although there is no definitive screening recommendations for HCV in patients with LP, likely because of the variability in the prevalence of HCV in different parts of the world, screening is an option where the association between two entities is stronger.[41]

The diagnosis of LP mostly relies on the combination of history and physical examination findings. The entire cutaneous surface should be examined, including external genitalia and oral cavity. However, in case of uncertainty, a punch or shave biopsy reaching to mid-dermis level is useful for diagnosis.[42] The characteristic histopathologic finding of LP is saw-tooth pattern of epidermal hyperplasia; thickening of the granular cell layer; vacuolization of the basal layer; apoptotic keratinocytes called Civatte bodies; and an intense infiltration of dermal-epidermal junction, mainly with T cells.[42]

Cutaneous LP is mostly self-limited and may resolve spontaneously. In cases where treatment is required, high-potency corticosteroids are usually the first line of treatment.[42–44]

In patients with HCV, the response of the LP lesion to interferon treatment is controversial, because there are studies reporting both improvement and exacerbation of symptoms with interferon treatment.[45] Similarly, a meta-analysis by Petti and colleagues[46] showed that treatment of HCV infection with anti-HCV medications does not necessarily lead to regression of LP lesions. Interferon-free direct-acting antiviral treatment is a new standard treatment of HCV, albeit the data about the effectiveness of these regimens in patients with HCV and LP are not available.

In conclusion, LP is a disease of the stratified squamous epithelium involving the skin and orogenital mucosa with unknown cause and can be seen in subjects with chronic HCV infection. It is characterized by pruritic, purple, plaques and papules and is diagnosed clinically or with a biopsy. Treatment of LP with interferon-based regimens did not show satisfactory results; however, newly developed direct-acting antivirals are an option for HCV-associated LP.

PORPHYRIA CUTANEA TARDA

The porphyrias are inherited or acquired metabolic disorders caused by reduced activity of enzymes in heme and porphyrin synthesis.[47] PCT, which is also called symptomatic porphyria, is the most common form of these disorders and caused by significant deficiency of hepatic uroporphyrinogen decarboxylase (UROD).[48,49] It is a rare disease of adults and the prevalence of PCT in the United States is estimated to be 1 in 25,000. Although both sexes are equally susceptible to the disease, because of the risk factors, such as alcohol abuse and HCV infection, PCT is seen more commonly in men.[50,51]

There are different types of PCT; type 1 is also called the sporadic form and accounts for nearly 80% of all PCT cases. There is no UROD mutation in this type and enzymatic deficiency is limited to liver. Type 2 is a familial form and UROD mutation is inherited in an autosomal-dominant fashion. Type 2 accounts for nearly 20% of all PCT cases and there is decreased enzymatic activity in all tissues.[52]

The enzymatic deficiency lies in the core of the pathogenesis of PCT. UROD is the fifth enzyme in the heme synthetic pathway and catalyzes the decarboxylation of uroporphyrinogen to coproporphyrinogen.[53] Clinical manifestations of PCT are seen when hepatic UROD activity goes lower than 20% of normal. Accumulation of porphyrinogens leads to formation of uroporphyrin and hepatocarboxyl porphyrins, and the conversion continues with the help of different enzymes and modifications by intestinal bacteria. Finally, porphyrins are transported from liver to skin and lead to phototoxicity.[54] When exposed to light with 400-nm wavelength, these phototoxic porphyrins release photons and cause production of reactive oxygen species, which damage membranes, lipids, and proteins.[55]

The association between HCV and PCT is strong and a meta-analysis by Gisbert and colleagues[56] revealed about 50% of patients with PCT have HCV and this rate goes up to greater than 70% in southern Europe. In the United States, HCV prevalence in patients with PCT was estimated to be around 66%.[5] Although the exact mechanism through which HCV unmasks the enzymatic deficiency has not been clearly shown, the possible mechanism may include HCV-induced production of reactive oxygen species, which down-regulates hepcidin and cause hepatic iron overload, rather than a direct effect on the enzymatic pathway.[57,58]

The clinical manifestations of PCT are variable and include blistering skin lesions, subepidermal bullae, erosions, milia, hypertrichosis, alopecia, onycholysis, and hypopigmentation.[59] The sun-exposed areas, such as back of the hand, forearm, face, neck, and feet, are more prone to photo damage. Skin lesions may be painful and scarring of the lesions may progress to contractions and calcifications that resemble systemic scleroderma.[60] Because two most common risk factors for PCT are HCV infection and alcohol abuse, hepatocyte injury and transaminase elevations are common in PCT.[61,62] It was also reported that patients with PCT have increased risk for developing cirrhosis and hepatocellular carcinoma.[63]

The diagnosis of PCT is typically suspected on clinical grounds and relies on laboratory testing to detect elevated levels of porphyrins. The first step for diagnosis in a patients with symptomatic PCT is to check total plasma, serum, or spot urine porphyrins.[54] Patients with symptomatic PCT have markedly elevated urinary uroporphyrin and hepatocarboxyl porphyrin. Another useful tool for diagnosis is the plasma porphyrin fluorescent assay, which has a characteristic peak at 620 nm.[54] In subjects with PCT, screening for HCV is important.

The standard treatment of PCT consists of phlebotomy and/or low-dose hydroxychloroquine.[5] It is also important to minimize the risk factors, such as alcohol consumption, estrogen use, iron supplementation, and smoking.[64,65] Additionally, controlling the sun exposure is recommended, with customization of clothing. In familial inheritance cases, genetic counseling is exceptionally important. In patients with HCV, presence of PCT is an indication for treatment of HCV. Historically, treatment with interferon regimens was associated with low response and PCT was reported to be independently associated with insufficient viral response to interferon treatment.[66] In contrast, combining interferon therapy with iron reduction was more beneficial treatment in patients with HCV infection.[67] Finally, despite scarcity of data, treatment of PCT with direct-acting antivirals seems to be more effective than interferon-based regimens.[68]

In summary, PCT is a disease of heme and porphyrin metabolism, caused by decreased activity of UROD enzyme, and manifests with blistering skin lesions. HCV is highly associated with PCT and should be screened when the diagnosis of PCT is made. Although interferon-based treatment regimens show unpredictable response, new direct-acting antivirals have much more promising results in the treatment of HCV-associated PCT.

OTHER DERMATOLOGIC ENTITIES
Psoriasis

Psoriasis is a common, chronic, immune-mediated skin disorder that manifests itself with well-demarcated erythematous plaques with silver scale. Psoriasis is associated with an up-regulated systemic inflammation and overproduction of inflammatory markers, such as tumor necrosis factor-α, interferon-γ, or interleukin-17.[69] The disease does not have a gender predilection and global prevalence ranges between 1% and 8%.[70]

A few hospital-based clinical studies and observational studies have reported an association between HCV infection and psoriasis. Two relatively old studies from Japan revealed an increased prevalence of anti-HCV antibody among patients with psoriasis compared with the general population.[71,72] A new study by Chun and colleagues[73] reported that HCV infection may up-regulate the inflammatory cytokines and may increase susceptibility to developing psoriasis. However, based on a population-based database study by Kanada and colleagues[74] psoriasis does not seem to be associated with an increased risk of HCV. Additional prospective studies are needed to support the role of HCV in the pathogenesis of psoriasis and whether psoriasis is a true dermatologic manifestation of HCV infection. Nevertheless, in patients with psoriasis, screening for HCV is performed before starting systemic immunosuppressive treatment.[75]

Necrolytic Acral Erythema

Necrolytic acral erythema is a rare, psoriasis-like dermatologic disorder characterized by pruritic, sharply marginated, erythematous to hypopigmented plaques with variable scale on the lower extremities.[76] The histopathologic appearance resembles psoriasis because keratinocyte necrosis, papillomatosis, and psoriasiform changes are usually detected. In a study by Abdallah and colleagues[77] in Egypt, among 30 patients with necrolytic acral erythema, all of them were found to be positive for HCV. There are other studies and case-reports linking this rare dermatologic disease to HCV, and to zinc deficiency.[78] Topical and systemic corticosteroids have been used as the first-line treatment. Additionally, sustained HCV viral eradication seems to improve the skin lesions.[79]

Pruritus

Rather than a dermatologic disease, pruritus is a common symptom in some patients with HCV infection and may be caused in part from cholestasis.[40,57] Nearly 15% of all patients with chronic HCV suffer from pruritus, making it one of their most common dermatologic complaints. Patients with chronic HCV may present either with generalized pruritus on apparently normal skin, or with pruritus with secondary skin findings, such as excoriations and lichenification. The latter is typical for prurigo nodularis and lichen simplex chronicus, both of which are associated with higher HCV prevalence.[80]

Pruritus should be carefully evaluated during HCV treatment, because it may either be secondary to treatment, or to one of the previously mentioned dermatologic manifestations. Interferon and ribavirin regimens were associated with new onset of significant pruritus in more than 10% of patients.[4] In this context, ribavirin was the most important culprit responsible for rash and pruritus. However, the rate of pruritus and rash became much more frequent with first-generation protease inhibitors, between 40% and 60%.[81] In fact, a small number of these patients developed rashes resembling Stevens-Johnson syndrome and was one of the reasons for discontinuation of these regimens. With the advent of new anti-HCV regimens free of interferon and ribavirin, rash and pruritus are no longer important complications of HCV treatment.

SUMMARY

Chronic HCV infection is a systemic disease and associated with various types of extrahepatic manifestations, one of which is dermatologic involvement. Although a myriad of dermatologic diseases have been linked to chronic HCV infection, the evidence is weak except for the association of HCV with MC, LP, PCT, and necrolytic acral erythema. Although the efficacy of interferon-based treatment was low and interferon and ribavirin caused dermatologic complications, viral eradication with the new regimens seems to be high and these regimens are well tolerated. Nevertheless, more data are needed to establish the efficacy of these regimens in the context of dermatologic manifestation of HCV.

REFERENCES

1. Mohd Hanafiah K, Groeger J, Flaxman AD, et al. Global epidemiology of hepatitis C virus infection: new estimates of age-specific antibody to HCV seroprevalence. Hepatology 2013;57:1333–42.
2. Sayiner M, Wymer M, Golabi P, et al. Presence of hepatitis C (HCV) infection in baby boomers with Medicare is independently associated with mortality and resource utilisation. Aliment Pharmacol Ther 2016;43:1060–8.
3. Vigano M, Colombo M. Extrahepatic manifestations of hepatitis C virus. Gastroenterol Clin North Am 2015;44:775–91.
4. Berk DR, Mallory SB, Keeffe EB, et al. Dermatologic disorders associated with chronic hepatitis C: effect of interferon therapy. Clin Gastroenterol Hepatol 2007;5:142–51.
5. Dedania B, Wu GY. Dermatologic extrahepatic manifestations of hepatitis C. J Clin Transl Hepatol 2015;3:127–33.
6. Ferri C, Giuggioli D, Cazzato M, et al. HCV-related cryoglobulinemic vasculitis: an update on its etiopathogenesis and therapeutic strategies. Clin Exp Rheumatol 2003;21:S78–84.
7. Paueksakon P, Revelo MP, Horn RG, et al. Monoclonal gammopathy: significance and possible causality in renal disease. Am J Kidney Dis 2003;42:87–95.
8. Brouet JC, Clauvel JP, Danon F, et al. Biologic and clinical significance of cryoglobulins. A report of 86 cases. Am J Med 1974;57:775–88.
9. Saadoun D, Asselah T, Resche-Rigon M, et al. Cryoglobulinemia is associated with steatosis and fibrosis in chronic hepatitis C. Hepatology 2006;43:1337–45.
10. Agnello V, Chung RT, Kaplan LM. A role for hepatitis C virus infection in type II cryoglobulinemia. N Engl J Med 1992;327:1490–5.
11. Misiani R, Bellavita P, Fenili D, et al. Hepatitis C virus infection in patients with essential mixed cryoglobulinemia. Ann Intern Med 1992;117:573–7.
12. Matignon M, Cacoub P, Colombat M, et al. Clinical and morphologic spectrum of renal involvement in patients with mixed cryoglobulinemia without evidence of hepatitis C virus infection. Medicine (Baltimore) 2009;88:341–8.
13. Donada C, Crucitti A, Donadon V, et al. Systemic manifestations and liver disease in patients with chronic hepatitis C and type II or III mixed cryoglobulinaemia. J Viral Hepat 1998;5:179–85.
14. Ramos-Casals M, Stone JH, Cid MC, et al. The cryoglobulinaemias. Lancet 2012;379:348–60.
15. Stefanova-Petrova DV, Tzvetanska AH, Naumova EJ, et al. Chronic hepatitis C virus infection: prevalence of extrahepatic manifestations and association with cryoglobulinemia in Bulgarian patients. World J Gastroenterol 2007;13:6518–28.
16. Sene D, Limal N, Cacoub P. Hepatitis C virus-associated extrahepatic manifestations: a review. Metab Brain Dis 2004;19:357–81.
17. Ferri C, Sebastiani M, Giuggioli D, et al. Mixed cryoglobulinemia: demographic, clinical, and serologic features and survival in 231 patients. Semin Arthritis Rheum 2004;33:355–74.
18. Cacoub P, Gragnani L, Comarmond C, et al. Extrahepatic manifestations of chronic hepatitis C virus infection. Dig Liver Dis 2014;46(Suppl 5):S165–73.

19. Dupin N, Chosidow O, Lunel F, et al. Essential mixed cryoglobulinemia. A comparative study of dermatologic manifestations in patients infected or noninfected with hepatitis C virus. Arch Dermatol 1995;131:1124–7.

20. Sene D, Ghillani-Dalbin P, Thibault V, et al. Longterm course of mixed cryoglobulinemia in patients infected with hepatitis C virus. J Rheumatol 2004;31:2199–206.

21. Frankel AH, Singer DR, Winearls CG, et al. Type II essential mixed cryoglobulinaemia: presentation, treatment and outcome in 13 patients. Q J Med 1992;82:101–24.

22. Rongioletti F, Patterson JW, Rebora A. The histological and pathogenetic spectrum of cutaneous disease in monoclonal gammopathies. J Cutan Pathol 2008;35:705–21.

23. Pietrogrande M, De Vita S, Zignego AL, et al. Recommendations for the management of mixed cryoglobulinemia syndrome in hepatitis C virus-infected patients. Autoimmun Rev 2011;10:444–54.

24. Saadoun D, Resche-Rigon M, Thibault V, et al. Antiviral therapy for hepatitis C virus–associated mixed cryoglobulinemia vasculitis: a long-term followup study. Arthritis Rheum 2006;54:3696–706.

25. Visentini M, Tinelli C, Colantuono S, et al. Efficacy of low-dose rituximab for the treatment of mixed cryoglobulinemia vasculitis: phase II clinical trial and systematic review. Autoimmun Rev 2015;14:889–96.

26. Lodi G, Pellicano R, Carrozzo M. Hepatitis C virus infection and lichen planus: a systematic review with meta-analysis. Oral Dis 2010;16:601–12.

27. Shengyuan L, Songpo Y, Wen W, et al. Hepatitis C virus and lichen planus: a reciprocal association determined by a meta-analysis. Arch Dermatol 2009;145:1040–7.

28. Le Cleach L, Chosidow O. Clinical practice. Lichen planus. N Engl J Med 2012;366:723–32.

29. Eisen D, Carrozzo M, Bagan Sebastian JV, et al. Number V oral lichen planus: clinical features and management. Oral Dis 2005;11:338–49.

30. Wagner G, Rose C, Sachse MM. Clinical variants of lichen planus. J Dtsch Dermatol Ges 2013;11:309–19.

31. Gorouhi F, Davari P, Fazel N. Cutaneous and mucosal lichen planus: a comprehensive review of clinical subtypes, risk factors, diagnosis, and prognosis. ScientificWorldJournal 2014;2014:742826.

32. Eisen D. The clinical manifestations and treatment of oral lichen planus. Dermatol Clin 2003;21:79–89.

33. Lehman JS, Tollefson MM, Gibson LE. Lichen planus. Int J Dermatol 2009;48:682–94.

34. Farhi D, Dupin N. Pathophysiology, etiologic factors, and clinical management of oral lichen planus, part I: facts and controversies. Clin Dermatol 2010;28:100–8.

35. Nagao Y, Kawaguchi T, Ide T, et al. Exacerbation of oral erosive lichen planus by combination of interferon and ribavirin therapy for chronic hepatitis C. Int J Mol Med 2005;15:237–41.

36. Carrozzo M, Gandolfo S. Oral diseases possibly associated with hepatitis C virus. Crit Rev Oral Biol Med 2003;14:115–27.

37. Lodi G, Giuliani M, Majorana A, et al. Lichen planus and hepatitis C virus: a multicentre study of patients with oral lesions and a systematic review. Br J Dermatol 2004;151:1172–81.

38. Gumber SC, Chopra S. Hepatitis C: a multifaceted disease. Review of extrahepatic manifestations. Ann Intern Med 1995;123:615–20.

39. Bigby M. The relationship between lichen planus and hepatitis C clarified. Arch Dermatol 2009;145:1048–50.
40. Jadali Z. Dermatologic manifestations of hepatitis C infection and the effect of interferon therapy: a literature review. Arch Iran Med 2012;15:43–8.
41. Harman M, Akdeniz S, Dursun M, et al. Lichen planus and hepatitis C virus infection: an epidemiologic study. Int J Clin Pract 2004;58:1118–9.
42. Usatine RP, Tinitigan M. Diagnosis and treatment of lichen planus. Am Fam Physician 2011;84:53–60.
43. Carbone M, Arduino PG, Carrozzo M, et al. Topical clobetasol in the treatment of atrophic-erosive oral lichen planus: a randomized controlled trial to compare two preparations with different concentrations. J Oral Pathol Med 2009;38:227–33.
44. Jensen JT, Bird M, Leclair CM. Patient satisfaction after the treatment of vulvovaginal erosive lichen planus with topical clobetasol and tacrolimus: a survey study. Am J Obstet Gynecol 2004;190:1759–63 [discussion: 1763–5].
45. Mayo MJ. Extrahepatic manifestations of hepatitis C infection. Am J Med Sci 2003;325:135–48.
46. Petti S, Rabiei M, De Luca M, et al. The magnitude of the association between hepatitis C virus infection and oral lichen planus: meta-analysis and case control study. Odontology 2011;99:168–78.
47. Deybach JC, Badminton M, Puy H, et al. European porphyria initiative (EPI): a platform to develop a common approach to the management of porphyrias and to promote research in the field. Physiol Res 2006;55(Suppl 2):S67–73.
48. Alla V, Bonkovsky HL. Iron in nonhemochromatotic liver disorders. Semin Liver Dis 2005;25:461–72.
49. Elder GH, Worwood M. Mutations in the hemochromatosis gene, porphyria cutanea tarda, and iron overload. Hepatology 1998;27:289–91.
50. Elder GH. Porphyria cutanea tarda. Semin Liver Dis 1998;18:67–75.
51. Siegesmund M, van Tuyll van Serooskerken AM, Poblete-Gutierrez P, et al. The acute hepatic porphyrias: current status and future challenges. Best Pract Res Clin Gastroenterol 2010;24:593–605.
52. Frank J, Poblete-Gutierrez P. Porphyria cutanea tarda: when skin meets liver. Best Pract Res Clin Gastroenterol 2010;24:735–45.
53. Sams H, Kiripolsky MG, Bhat L, et al. Porphyria cutanea tarda, hepatitis C, alcoholism, and hemochromatosis: a case report and review of the literature. Cutis 2004;73:188–90.
54. Szlendak U, Bykowska K, Lipniacka A. Clinical, biochemical and molecular characteristics of the main types of porphyria. Adv Clin Exp Med 2016;25:361–8.
55. Magnus IA. Cutaneous porphyria. Clin Haematol 1980;9:273–302.
56. Gisbert JP, Garcia-Buey L, Pajares JM, et al. Prevalence of hepatitis C virus infection in porphyria cutanea tarda: systematic review and meta-analysis. J Hepatol 2003;39:620–7.
57. Garcovich S, Garcovich M, Capizzi R, et al. Cutaneous manifestations of hepatitis C in the era of new antiviral agents. World J Hepatol 2015;7:2740–8.
58. Nishina S, Hino K, Korenaga M, et al. Hepatitis C virus-induced reactive oxygen species raise hepatic iron level in mice by reducing hepcidin transcription. Gastroenterology 2008;134:226–38.
59. Sarkany RP. The management of porphyria cutanea tarda. Clin Exp Dermatol 2001;26:225–32.
60. Khayat R, Dupuy A, Panse I, et al. Sclerodermatous changes in porphyria cutanea tarda: six cases. Ann Dermatol Venereol 2013;140:589–97 [in French].
61. Puy H, Gouya L, Deybach JC. Porphyrias. Lancet 2010;375:924–37.

62. Schulenburg-Brand D, Katugampola R, Anstey AV, et al. The cutaneous porphyrias. Dermatol Clin 2014;32:369–84, ix.

63. Linet MS, Gridley G, Nyren O, et al. Primary liver cancer, other malignancies, and mortality risks following porphyria: a cohort study in Denmark and Sweden. Am J Epidemiol 1999;149:1010–5.

64. Maynard B, Peters MS. Histologic and immunofluorescence study of cutaneous porphyrias. J Cutan Pathol 1992;19:40–7.

65. Balwani M, Desnick RJ. The porphyrias: advances in diagnosis and treatment. Hematology Am Soc Hematol Educ Program 2012;2012:19–27.

66. Fernandez I, Castellano G, de Salamanca RE, et al. Porphyria cutanea tarda as a predictor of poor response to interferon alfa therapy in chronic hepatitis C. Scand J Gastroenterol 2003;38:314–9.

67. Desai TK, Jamil LH, Balasubramaniam M, et al. Phlebotomy improves therapeutic response to interferon in patients with chronic hepatitis C: a meta-analysis of six prospective randomized controlled trials. Dig Dis Sci 2008;53:815–22.

68. Aguilera P, Laguno M, To-Figueras J. Treatment of chronic hepatitis with boceprevir leads to remission of porphyria cutanea tarda. Br J Dermatol 2014;171: 1595–6.

69. Boehncke WH, Schon MP. Psoriasis. Lancet 2015;386:983–94.

70. Parisi R, Symmons DP, Griffiths CE, et al. Global epidemiology of psoriasis: a systematic review of incidence and prevalence. J Invest Dermatol 2013;133:377–85.

71. Kanazawa K, Aikawa T, Tsuda F, et al. Hepatitis C virus infection in patients with psoriasis. Arch Dermatol 1996;132:1391–2.

72. Yamamoto T, Katayama I, Nishioka K. Psoriasis and hepatitis C virus. Acta Derm Venereol 1995;75:482–3.

73. Chun K, Afshar M, Audish D, et al. Hepatitis C may enhance key amplifiers of psoriasis. J Eur Acad Dermatol Venereol 2016. [Epub ahead of print].

74. Kanada KN, Schupp CW, Armstrong AW. Association between psoriasis and viral infections in the United States: focusing on hepatitis B, hepatitis C and human immunodeficiency virus. J Eur Acad Dermatol Venereol 2013;27:1312–6.

75. Frankel AJ, Van Voorhees AS, Hsu S, et al. Treatment of psoriasis in patients with hepatitis C: from the medical board of the National psoriasis foundation. J Am Acad Dermatol 2009;61:1044–55.

76. Raphael BA, Dorey-Stein ZL, Lott J, et al. Low prevalence of necrolytic acral erythema in patients with chronic hepatitis C virus infection. J Am Acad Dermatol 2012;67:962–8.

77. Abdallah MA, Ghozzi MY, Monib HA, et al. Necrolytic acral erythema: a cutaneous sign of hepatitis C virus infection. J Am Acad Dermatol 2005;53:247–51.

78. Iyengar S, Chang S, Ho B, et al. Necrolytic acral erythema masquerading as cellulitis. Dermatol Online J 2014;20:3.

79. Hivnor CM, Yan AC, Junkins-Hopkins JM, et al. Necrolytic acral erythema: response to combination therapy with interferon and ribavirin. J Am Acad Dermatol 2004;50:S121–4.

80. Soylu S, Gul U, Kilic A. Cutaneous manifestations in patients positive for anti-hepatitis C virus antibodies. Acta Derm Venereol 2007;87:49–53.

81. Roujeau JC, Mockenhaupt M, Tahan SR, et al. Telaprevir-related dermatitis. JAMA Dermatol 2013;149:152–8.

Patient-Reported Outcomes and Fatigue in Patients with Chronic Hepatitis C Infection

Pegah Golabi, MD[a], Mehmet Sayiner, MD[a,b], Haley Bush, MSPH[a], Lynn H. Gerber, MD[a,b], Zobair M. Younossi, MD, MPH[a,b,*]

KEYWORDS

- Hepatitis C • Fatigue • Patient-reported outcome

KEY POINTS

- Fatigue is the most common, the most under-reported and undertreated symptom of chronic hepatitis C.
- Degree of fatigue varies among patients and often does not correlate with disease severity.
- Fatigue differs from and should be distinguished from other common conditions including depression, sleepiness, drowsiness, and weakness.
- There are 2 types of fatigue, central and peripheral; the former is associated with disturbances of mood and motivation, and the latter, physical fatigue, is associated with weakness and decreased level of physical performance.
- The diagnosis of fatigue is challenging, and it can be assisted by performing a thorough medical evaluation to identify comorbidities.

INTRODUCTION

Hepatitis C virus (HCV) infection causes a systemic infection associated with significant chronic liver disease. In addition to the impact on the liver, HCV infection is often associated with extrahepatic manifestations. These include but are not limited to

Disclosure Statement: The authors have nothing to disclose.
[a] Betty and Guy Beatty Center for Integrated Research, Inova Health system, Claude Moore Health Education and Research Building, 3rd floor, 300 Gallows Road, Falls Church, VA 22042, USA; [b] Center for Liver Disease, Department of Medicine, Inova Fairfax Hospital, Claude Moore Health Education and Research Building, 3rd floor, 3300 Gallows Road, Falls Church, VA 22042, USA
* Corresponding author. Betty and Guy Beatty Center for Integrated Research, Claude Moore Health Education and Research Building, 3rd floor, 3300 Gallows Road, Falls Church, VA 22042.
E-mail address: zobair.younossi@inova.org

involvement of the cardiovascular, respiratory, endocrine, and connective tissue systems. There is report of metabolic changes including glucose and lipid metabolism, as well as musculoskeletal and central nervous systems (CNS) function.[1] In addition to organ system involvement, symptoms such as fatigue, somnolence, and mood/affect change may be part of the clinical picture.

In addition to its clinical impact, HCV negatively affects patient-reported outcomes (PROs). PROs are the measurements based on reports that come directly from patients about their health condition, without an interpretation by a clinician or anyone else. PRO is an umbrella term that includes quality of life, including those captured by self-reports for health-relate quality of life (HRQL) and fatigue. Given that fatigue is such a prominent driver of PROs in patients with HCV, this article will initially focus on fatigue and then discuss HRQL concepts in HCV.

Definition of Fatigue

Fatigue is one of the most common symptoms affecting patients with chronic liver diseases. It negatively impacts their quality of life and daily activities.[2] Fatigue is a complex phenomenon for which definition and contributors continue to be explored.

Daniel Defoe first described fatigue in his novel about the life of Robinson Crusoe in 1719, as it was the reason for the mutineers to be defeated. Oxford English Dictionary describes fatigue as "lassitude or weariness resulting from either bodily or mental exertion" or "a condition of muscles, organs or cells characterized by a temporary reduction in power or sensitivity following a period of prolonged activity or stimulation."[3,4] Even this definition does not take into account fatigue that is not temporally related to exertion.

HOW COMMON IS FATIGUE?

In the general population, fatigue is reported in 5% to 40% of patients attending physician visits, but fatigue lasting more than 6 months is reported only in 2% to 10% of patients.[5] On the other hand, the picture is quite different in patients with chronic HCV infection, in whom fatigue has been regarded as the most frequent extrahepatic manifestation.[6] Although most studies report that more than 50% of patients with HCV experience fatigue, some reports claim that the prevalence of fatigue in HCV infected patients can be as high as 80%.[7–9] This fatigue is often distressing, not easily treated, and not likely to respond to sleep or rest. Interestingly it does not correlate with markers of liver disease severity or level of viremia.[10–12] Further, fatigue is frequently misreported as depression or sleepiness. In fact, because of significant differences in diagnosis and treatment, it is important to differentiate fatigue from other diagnoses as well as determine how fatigue is accurately measured and clinically managed.

MANIFESTATIONS OF FATIGUE

Patients with chronic HCV infection describe their fatigue in a variety of different ways. One goal of this article is to alert clinicians to the types of descriptors that are used to describe fatigue. Patients with chronic HCV may define fatigue as lethargy, lack of energy, malaise, motivation loss, exhaustion, or lassitude. Additionally, attention deficit, word finding difficulty, depression, headache, and even sleep disturbance are the other common complaints patients use to describe their fatigue.[13] It is important to note that there are some associations between fatigue and these complaints, but, it must be emphasized that fatigue should not be used as a synonym for any of these symptoms. As an example, there are bidirectional associations. Fatigue is not depression, although depressed patients have higher prevalence of fatigue and vice versa. In this context, a recent meta-analysis revealed that the prevalence of depression among patients with HCV was 24.5%, and the risk for developing depression in patients with HCV was more than 2 times greater than patients without HCV.[14] In patients with depressive disorders, the prevalence of fatigue can be as high as 90%, and it is not easy to clearly discriminate the 2 disorders most of the time.[15–17]

Another strong association is described between fatigue and excessive daytime sleepiness.[18] Nevertheless, different than fatigue, excessive daytime sleepiness has been linked to some pathologic conditions like narcolepsy, sleep apnea–hypopnea syndrome, periodic limb movement disorder, idiopathic hypersomnia, or sleep deprivation.[19] The definition and semiological distinction of both concepts remain difficult, but, there are also some tools like Epworth Sleepiness Scale (ESS), Fatigue Severity Scale (FSS), and Empirical Fatigue and Sleepiness Scales, for the assessment of fatigue and sleepiness.[20]

Fatigue in patients with chronic HCV infection can also be caused by several nonvirus-related pathologic conditions such as anemia and cirrhosis. In patients with chronic HCV infection, anemia can be secondary to acute gastrointestinal bleeding, iron deficiency, or chronic disease. Interestingly, treating anemia does not always alleviate HCV-related fatigue, which indeed supports the fact that these 2 conditions are distinct from each other.[21]

There are also numerous other metabolic and clinical entities that go hand in hand with fatigue. For example, fatigue can accompany some pulmonary diseases. A recent study showed that both sarcoidosis and idiopathic pulmonary fibrosis patients suffer from fatigue, and sarcoidosis patients tend to report more severe fatigue scores.[22] Similarly, multiple endocrinopathies, including but not limited to diabetes, thyroid disorders, adrenal insufficiency, Cushing syndrome, gonadal dysfunction, and many metabolic abnormalities, such as hyper or hypoglycemia and dyslipidemia, can contribute to fatigue.[23] Among clinical conditions, autoimmune and rheumatological diseases may be the most carefully studied and typically include multiple sclerosis, rheumatoid arthritis, systemic lupus erythematosus, myasthenia, and CNS disorders.[24–26] Given the coexistence of these diseases in HCV patients, it is important be aware of these associations in the clinical practice.

CLASSIFICATION OF FATIGUE

The classification of fatigue depends on an agreed upon construct. This is not yet widely accepted, but there are investigators and clinicians who have begun to use the concept of peripheral and central fatigue. This approach helps distinguish between fatigue typically associated with activity and that not necessarily induced by either physical or mental activity.

Depending on the duration, fatigue can be divided into acute or chronic fatigue. This is based on duration of symptom: acute, if the duration is less than 6 months, and chronic, if the duration is longer than 6 months.[5] The main classification, however, is according to underlying mechanism, in which fatigue is categorized as central or peripheral. Old nomenclature frequently used pathological or nonpathological. The former refers to fatigue that is persistent, often difficult to treat, and without an underlying pathology. The latter usually is attributable to an identifiable cause (eg, respiratory infection, influenza, or extreme exertion, and thought to be self-limited or responsive to treating the underlying disease). In this article, the term central fatigue is used interchangeably with mental fatigue, and the term peripheral fatigue is used for physical fatigue.

PERIPHERAL FATIGUE

One of the important contributors to fatigue is the peripheral component, which is also regarded as the physical fatigue. Two historical studies have described physical fatigue as "the inability to maintain the required or expected force or power output" of muscle or "any decline in muscle performance associated with muscle activity at the original intensity."[27,28] This type of fatigue is, therefore, usually associated with physical activity and usually resolves with rest.

Although physical fatigue is a common symptom during sport and exercise activities, it can also be observed secondary to many chronic diseases and health conditions. In fact, mechanisms of peripheral fatigue can be attributable to some neuromuscular conditions. Examples of neuronal conditions can be axonal loss, demyelination, and conduction block, whereas muscular conditions can include loss of electrical conduction on the muscle membrane to the T-tubule system, impaired release of calcium ions from the sarcoplasmic reticulum in the myocyte, dysfunctions between actin and myosin filaments, or impaired oxidative phosphorylation or glycolysis.[29] Classically, myositis and neuromuscular diseases, including upper and lower motor neuron diseases, polyradiculitis, polyneuropathies, neuromuscular transmission diseases, myopathies, and rhabdomyolysis, are associated with muscle weakness and poor peak muscle performance or sustained activity. In many chronic disease conditions, inactivity causes physical deconditioning, which further results in reductions in total body muscle mass and strength, as well as increased fatigability due to changes in muscle metabolism.[30] Other significant contributors include cardiac and pulmonary dysfunction, altered metabolism, and sedentary lifestyle.[31–33]

CENTRAL FATIGUE

Central fatigue, sometimes referred to as mental fatigue, is different from physical fatigue and is not attributable to physical effort. This type of fatigue is a result of the unwillingness or inability to continue to engage in muscular activity, despite not reaching the level of muscle exhaustion. It can also be defined as the perception of mental fatigue after performing cognitive activities that involve concentration, attention, alertness or endurance.[5] Mental fatigue may be experienced as change in mood such as depressive symptoms, lack of motivation and anxiety, decreased motivation, or neurocognitive performance, (eg, slowing of thought processes, distraction, memory deficits).[34] Other conditions such as major depression or brain fog are used by the patients to describe their fatigue.[35]

Several explanations for the mechanisms of central fatigue imply a role for serotonin (5-hydroxytryptamine [5-HT]), dopamine, and acetylcholine. There is evidence that elevations of 5-HT activity during prolonged exercise hasten fatigue. Approaches designed to attenuate brain 5-HT synthesis during prolonged exercise improve endurance performance.[36] Cytokines and ammonia have been shown to associate with reduced exercise tolerance, in particular with acute viral and bacterial infection. Also, the changes in midbrain serotoninergic and dopaminergic pathways were related to increased levels of fatigue, anxiety, and depression in patients with chronic HCV infection.[37,38] Indeed, it was not only the change in the level of hormones; there was also decreased binding capacity of these transporters in midbrain and striatal regions of the CNS. As a supportive finding, it was also shown that usage of ondansetron, which is a serotonin type-3 receptor antagonist, might ameliorate HCV-associated fatigue.[39] Decreased levels of tryptophan, which is the precursor of serotonin, was also found to be associated with fatigue.[40]

It is noteworthy that although central and peripheral fatigue can coexist, fatigue in chronic HCV patients has been thought to be central fatigue. Studies in specific patient groups, such as patients with Parkinson disease or cancer, revealed that the severity of central fatigue did not correlate with that of physical fatigue, and concluded that physical and mental fatigue were independent symptoms and should be assessed separately.[41,42] These reports suggest that the 2 symptoms may have different etiologies and may require different treatments.

DIAGNOSTICS FOR FATIGUE

Fatigue rarely is an isolated symptom. Significant literature relates fatigue with pain, insomnia, depression, distress, and anxiety.[43] It has also been associated with perceived neurocognitive dysfunction, but not always with poor performance.[44] The clinician should routinely assess for these associated symptoms, with an awareness that often depressive symptoms and fatigue are difficult to distinguish. Instrumentation designed to measure each should be sought. Additionally, other illnesses may be characterized by fatigue, as mentioned previously, and should be included in the differential and appropriate tests done.

To rule out possible secondary causes of fatigue, a good clinical history is the first step. Although there are no globally accepted routine blood works for fatigue,[45] the initial laboratory tests include, but are not limited to, complete blood count, serum glucose, electrolytes, urea and creatinine, liver function tests, erythrocyte sedimentation rate, C reactive protein level, thyroid stimulant hormone, and iron level.[45] In some cases, the biochemical investigation can be even more detailed, with checking serum levels of glucocorticoids and catecholamines. In order to assess physical fatigue, muscle-specific markers like serum lactate and ammonia can be helpful, as well as some inflammatory markers like tumor necrosis factor alpha and interleukin 6.[46]

Measurement is critical for assessing fatigue, and because it may have physical and mental (CNS) contributors, both objective and self-reports may be needed. The subjective nature of fatigue makes it difficult to define, measure, quantify, and treat, which may lead hepatologists to overlook or minimize the patients' reports.

In distinguishing peripheral and central fatigue, there has been concern over which metrics to use and for what purpose. The former is frequently measured using objective measures of peak muscle strength, muscle endurance, and aerobic capacity. Physical activity level can be measured using self-reports or sensors, an objective, quantitative measure of activity. Additionally, some evaluations rely on biochemical tests (hemoglobin, thyroid), neuromuscular function employing nerve conduction studies, electromyography and magnetic resonance-based imaging modalities, exercise stress testing, and cardiac echoes.

When the clinician suspects physical fatigue and decides to assess muscle function, there are a variety of options the clinician can choose. Peripheral muscle fatigue can be shown as a decline in maximal voluntary contraction readings during isometric contraction phase. Also, as Finsterer and Mahjoub[5] described, various electromyography parameters may be changed when fatigue is caused by impaired firing of the alpha motor neurons. These parameters include spectral frequency, reduced amplitude, or density of interference pattern, and nerve conduction studies may be helpful to determine the muscle twitch force.[29] Additionally, creatine phosphokinase, aldolase, alanine, aspartate amino transferase, and measures of inflammation such as erythrocyte sedimentation rate may be helpful.

MRI is able to detect key muscle abnormalities like size, shape, and signal intensity changes. During exercise, there is increased production of lactate in myocytes, which generate an acidic environment and cause an increase in the amount of hydrogen ions. The increased production of these hydrogen ions, which are also protons, results in an enhancement with contrast medium on T2 MRI. In fact, this enhancement is directly correlated with the amount of acidosis.[47] Also, magnetic resonance spectroscopy serves as a complementary tool to MRI, and can provide objective measurements of muscle energy metabolism and cytosolic pH at rest, during activity, and after the exercise is completed.[48]

It is helpful to couple these objective measures with patient self-reports that can help determine the patient's level of activity, his or her experience of the amount of effort expended and whether he or she is able to carry out necessary and desired daily routines.

Central fatigue is usually measured through self-reports or neuropsychological testing if there is a question about cognitive impairment. Neurocognitive testing usually focuses on recall, memory, reaction time, and executive functioning. In the past, there has been some difficulty accepting the self-reports as reliable and sensitive, but it is worth noting that in some situations, the only tool the clinician has in hand may be the self-reports from the patients. The data collected from self-reports is extremely valuable.

There are many instruments that have been designed to measure fatigue. Depending on the number of properties the scales evaluate, they can be unidimensional or multidimensional. The examples of these dimensions can be the impact of fatigue on patient's function, momentary perception, trait perception, or the severity of fatigue.[49]

Most commonly used fatigue scales in liver disease include the fatigue severity scale (FSS), the fatigue assessment inventory (FAI), functional assessment of chronic illness therapy fatigue scale (FACIT-F), Iowa fatigue scale, and fatigue impact scale (FIS).

A recent publication from members of the authors' group has demonstrated that there may be at least 2 separate factors explaining fatigue scores from commonly used fatigue measures. Physical fatigue and central fatigue seem to be separate factors, as determined by the nature of responses to specific questions on the FSS and the FACT-F.[50]

More specific to HCV, large numbers of HRQL instruments and multidimensional specific fatigue metrics have been used to assess fatigue, energy, and vitality in patients with chronic HCV infection. These instruments include the short form-36 (SF-36), chronic liver disease questionnaire for HCV (CLDQ-HCV), hepatitis quality of life questionnaire, liver disease quality of life index, and sickness impact profile (SIP).[51] Recently, the application of item response theory has been used to select items that can be customized to certain groups, while minimizing the numbers of questions. The PROMIS (The Patient-Reported Outcomes Measurement Information System) network describes this approach.[52]

TREATMENT

As in many medical conditions, treating the underlying disease frequently reduces or eliminates symptoms as the underlying cause of the illness is mitigated. This is true for patients with chronic HCV. The successful treatment of HCV by achieving sustained virologic response (SVR) reduces fatigue in a large majority of people, but this sometimes takes a protracted period of time, and even then, it may persist.[53,54]

From the pharmacologic standpoint, amantadine, acetylsalicylic acid, modafinil, and thiamine were shown to have a beneficial effect on fatigue in patients with cancer diagnoses.[5] Also, as discussed in the central fatigue section, the decrease in serotonin and dopamine in the CNS are associated with increased fatigue perception. Methylphenidate, a medication that increases dopamine levels in the CNS, was also shown to be effective in lowering fatigue perception in those with cancer diagnoses.[49] Nevertheless, in patients with HCV, there is no other established treatment for fatigue. Given the impact of achieving SVR on fatigue and fatigue-related HRQL domains, the authors believe that clinical fatigue must be an indication for treatment of HCV regardless of severity of liver disease.

IMPACT OF TREATMENT OF HEPATITIS C VIRUS

Data suggest that fatigue, decreased quality of life, and depression are exacerbated by treatment with interferon, and fatigue is increased during ribavirin therapy.[54–57] In studies comparing interferon-based treatment with interferon-free direct antiviral therapy, interferon was independently associated with up to −26.0% worsening of the PRO scores, including those measuring some aspect of fatigue. Furthermore, there was a 9% worsening of scores during ribavirin treatment.[58]

Ribavirin is associated with development of anemia that is reversible with discontinuation. Interferon fatigue is associated with treatment and resolves upon discontinuation or completion. Both work independently of viral clearance.[59]

Also noted is that there seems to be a delay in improvement in fatigue levels after achieving sustained virologic response (SVR).[53] Fatigue continues to abate weeks after treatment completion and months after reaching SVR. Some of this may be attributable to the impact of ribavirin and its associated anemia; other possible explanations include that the delay may be needed for physiologic responses to viral clearance. Data suggest that improvement in fatigue reduction continues through 4 weeks after the treatment phase, which will continue with longer follow-up.[53] Some of this may be related to drug washout, while the other portion may be an indication of the benefit of achieving SVR.

Much has been published substantiating the effectiveness of treatment of HCV for reducing fatigue in people with HCV.[2,60–63] Data from published studies also suggest that achieving SVR may reduce the level of insulin resistance and improve physical function.[63] This may serve as a link between metabolic abnormalities associated with HCV, such as insulin resistance and diabetes, and peripheral fatigue.

Nonpharmacological treatment approaches to fatigue can be effective. As in the healthier life style recommendations, any type of exercise, but more specifically aerobic exercise and progressive resistance training, has been shown to be effective.[29] It is critical to prescribe specific exercise recommendations. To support this recommendation, some reports suggest that for cancer survivors, moderate-intensity exercise is effective in fatigue treatment when the exercise prescription is individualized.[64,65] Other methods include adequate sleep and rest, having a healthy and balanced diet, occupational therapies, acupuncture, energy conservative courses, and mindfulness training.[66–68] For patients with HCV, exercise has been shown to be effective in reducing fatigue symptomatology. The combination of exercise and diet is more effective than exercise alone.[69]

HEALTH-RELATED QUALITY OF LIFE

As noted PROs can capture important aspects of health-related quality of life (HRQL) in patients with HCV infection. In fact, HCV infection causes a profound negative effect on HRQL through fatigue, depression, and decreased physical and mental functioning.[70] HRQL surveys have been used to measure the negative effects of the disease on PROs. These PRO measures can be important to evaluate the impact of chronic infection, eligibility and readiness for treatment, and assessment of HRQL during and after treatment.[51,71]

HEALTH-RELATED QUALITY OF LIFE BEFORE, DURING, AND AFTER TREATMENT

The literature clearly shows that patients with chronic HCV infection have lower baseline PRO scores when compared with norms for uninfected people.[51] These include measures of various symptoms (eg, fatigue and lower energy levels) and often poorer sleep and mood.[14,72–74] In fact, patients with chronic HCV infection who do not have advanced liver disease also suffer from HRQL impairments.[75,76] Fatigue, as discussed in length previously, and depression are thought to be the major factors for this baseline impairment. In fact, studies reported that fatigue and depression were the independent predictors of PRO impairment in patients with chronic HCV infection.[61,77,78] Fatigue and impairment in cognitive functioning are the leading extrahepatic manifestations of HCV in patients with early liver disease. The severity of liver disease also effects patients' HRQL, as worsening hepatic dysfunction in patients with cirrhosis (higher MELD [Model For End-Stage Liver Disease] score) and development of complications, such as ascites and hepatic encephalopathy, can cause severe impairment of HRQL.[79,80]

IMPACT OF DIFFERENT TREATMENT OPTIONS ON HEALTH-RELATED QUALITY OF LIFE

As PROs are surrogates for patients' experience, SVR is a surrogate for clinical outcomes. Achieving SVR with HCV treatment was found to be associated with an improvement in HRQL scores.[81]

Nevertheless, patients with HCV can have different experience with different antiviral regimens. During the interferon and ribavirin era, treatment had a negative impact on HRQL, which in turn negatively impacted treatment adherence and effectiveness in clinical practice.[51,58,82] These impairments were mostly driven by the adverse effect profile of interferon-based regimens, which include influenza-like symptoms, fatigue, rash, and depression, excluded many patients from receiving treatment. Furthermore, the presence of certain comorbidities like anemia, renal or cardiac disease, psychiatric issues, and autoimmune conditions, contraindicated the use of interferon, ribavirin, and first-generation direct-acting antivirals.[83] Second-generation agents that were based on a triple combination therapy with pegylated interferon, ribavirin, and a protease inhibitor increased HCV clearance rates but continued to impair HRQL during treatment.[84]

Newly developed interferon-free regimens have been shown to improve HRQL during treatment and after achieving SVR.[53,61,85–87] Some of this improvement during treatment may be due to the rapid clearing of virus. The data from clinical trials have shown that among patients with HCV genotype 1, treatment with interferon and ribavirin-free regimens resulted in early suppression of HCV and simultaneous improvement in PROs, which continued to improve throughout the duration of treatment and after treatment.[88] In fact, PRO improvements were noted as early as 2 weeks after the initiation of treatment, which coincided with complete viral suppression. The same regimen also significantly improves PROs in patients coinfected with HCV and human immunodeficiency virus.[86] Similar PRO improvements were noted with newly approved pan-genotypic regimens.[85,89] One study concluded that patients with HCV infection, and especially the ones with decompensated cirrhosis, had significant increases in their PRO scores during treatment with these regimens and after achieving sustained virologic response. The most prominent improvements were in general health of SF-36, emotional well-being and total FACIT-F, and all domains of CLDQ-HCV.[89]

These and other data are convincing to show that the new anti-HCV regimens have superior PRO profiles during treatment and after achieving SVR.[85-90]

SUMMARY

PROs are important surrogates for patient experience. PROs as captured by HRQL and fatigue instruments show significant impairment in HCV infection. In fact, fatigue is the most common but poorly understood and often underdiagnosed symptom for patients with chronic HCV infection. Even for patients who have achieved SVR, in some patients fatigue may persist and negatively impact HRQL. It is difficult to identify causes for fatigue for many patients, suggesting that it may be secondary to numerous clinical conditions. It may be associated with abnormalities in almost every organ system. It is often the final endpoint for complex human metabolic or inflammatory pathways. Additionally, it may be a reflection of mood and associated with changes in neuropeptides and catecholamines. Regardless of potential cause, the clinician should inquire about fatigue and look for potential contributors when signs are present for all with HCV, even those who have achieved SVR. This is important not only to assess patients' experience with their disease but also to construct a treatment regimen.

In addition to fatigue, other aspects of HRQL are also impaired in patients with HCV infection. Although the older regimens with interferon substantially worsened these HRQL impairments during treatment, newer regimens free of interferon and ribavirin document substantial improvement of PROs during treatment and after achieving SVR, and are durable. These data document the fact that SVR not only leads to improvement of important clinical outcomes but also patients' experience as documented by better PRO scores.

REFERENCES

1. Cacoub P, Gragnani L, Comarmond C, et al. Extrahepatic manifestations of chronic hepatitis C virus infection. Dig Liver Dis 2014;46(Suppl 5):S165–73.
2. Sarkar S, Jiang Z, Evon DM, et al. Fatigue before, during and after antiviral therapy of chronic hepatitis C: results from the Virahep-C study. J Hepatol 2012;57(5): 946–52.
3. Fatigue (Def.1,2) In Oxford English Dictionary Available at: http://public.oed.com. Accessed September 14, 2016.
4. Austin PW, Gerber L, Karrar AK. Fatigue in chronic liver disease: exploring the role of the autonomic nervous system. Liver Int 2015;35(5):1489–91.
5. Finsterer J, Mahjoub SZ. Fatigue in healthy and diseased individuals. Am J Hosp Palliat Care 2014;31(5):562–75.
6. Cacoub P, Poynard T, Ghillani P, et al. Extrahepatic manifestations of chronic hepatitis C. MULTIVIRC Group. Multidepartment Virus C. Arthritis Rheum 1999; 42(10):2204–12.
7. Stefanova-Petrova DV, Tzvetanska AH, Naumova EJ, et al. Chronic hepatitis C virus infection: prevalence of extrahepatic manifestations and association with cryoglobulinemia in Bulgarian patients. World J Gastroenterol 2007;13(48):6518–28.
8. McAndrews MP, Farcnik K, Carlen P, et al. Prevalence and significance of neurocognitive dysfunction in hepatitis C in the absence of correlated risk factors. Hepatology 2005;41(4):801–8.
9. Thames AD, Castellon SA, Singer EJ, et al. Neuroimaging abnormalities, neurocognitive function, and fatigue in patients with hepatitis C. Neurol Neuroimmunol Neuroinflamm 2015;2(1):e59.

10. Swain MG. Fatigue in liver disease: pathophysiology and clinical management. Can J Gastroenterol 2006;20(3):181–8.

11. Goh J, Coughlan B, Quinn J, et al. Fatigue does not correlate with the degree of hepatitis or the presence of autoimmune disorders in chronic hepatitis C infection. Eur J Gastroenterol Hepatol 1999;11(8):833–8.

12. Poynard T, Cacoub P, Ratziu V, et al. Fatigue in patients with chronic hepatitis C. J Viral Hepat 2002;9(4):295–303.

13. Adinolfi LE, Nevola R, Lus G, et al. Chronic hepatitis C virus infection and neurological and psychiatric disorders: an overview. World J Gastroenterol 2015;21(8): 2269–80.

14. Younossi Z, Park H, Henry L, et al. Extrahepatic manifestations of hepatitis C: a meta-analysis of prevalence, quality of life, and economic burden. Gastroenterology 2016;150(7):1599–608.

15. Ferentinos P, Kontaxakis V, Havaki-Kontaxaki B, et al. The fatigue questionnaire: standardization in patients with major depression. Psychiatry Res 2010;177(1–2): 114–9.

16. Targum SD, Fava M. Fatigue as a residual symptom of depression. Innov Clin Neurosci 2011;8(10):40–3.

17. Fava M, Ball S, Nelson JC, et al. Clinical relevance of fatigue as a residual symptom in major depressive disorder. Depress Anxiety 2014;31(3):250–7.

18. Neu D, Hoffmann G, Moutrier R, et al. Are patients with chronic fatigue syndrome just 'tired' or also 'sleepy'? J Sleep Res 2008;17(4):427–31.

19. Young TB. Epidemiology of daytime sleepiness: definitions, symptomatology, and prevalence. J Clin Psychiatry 2004;65(Suppl 16):12–6.

20. Neu D, Mairesse O, Hoffmann G, et al. Do 'sleepy' and 'tired' go together? Rasch analysis of the relationships between sleepiness, fatigue and nonrestorative sleep complaints in a nonclinical population sample. Neuroepidemiology 2010; 35(1):1–11.

21. Bager P. Fatigue and acute/chronic anaemia. Dan Med J 2014;61(4):B4824.

22. Atkins CP, Gilbert D, Brockwell C, et al. Fatigue in sarcoidosis and idiopathic pulmonary fibrosis: differences in character and severity between diseases. Sarcoidosis Vasc Diffuse Lung Dis 2016;33(2):130–8.

23. Kaltsas G, Vgontzas A, Chrousos G. Fatigue, endocrinopathies, and metabolic disorders. PM R 2010;2(5):393–8.

24. Balsamo S, Diniz LR, dos Santos-Neto LL, et al. Exercise and fatigue in rheumatoid arthritis. Isr Med Assoc J 2014;16(1):57–60.

25. Induruwa I, Constantinescu CS, Gran B. Fatigue in multiple sclerosis - a brief review. J Neurol Sci 2012;323(1–2):9–15.

26. Elsais A, Wyller VB, Loge JH, et al. Fatigue in myasthenia gravis: is it more than muscular weakness? BMC Neurol 2013;13:132.

27. Edwards RH. Human muscle function and fatigue. Ciba Found Symp 1981;82: 1–18.

28. Simonson E, Weiser PC. Psychological aspects and physiological correlates of work and fatigue. In: Simonson E, Weiser PC, editors. Psychological aspects and physiological correlates of work and fatigue. Springfield (IL): Charles C. Thomas Pub Ltd; 1976. p. 336–405.

29. Davis MP, Walsh D. Mechanisms of fatigue. J Support Oncol 2010;8(4):164–74.

30. Rimmer JH, Schiller W, Chen MD. Effects of disability-associated low energy expenditure deconditioning syndrome. Exerc Sport Sci Rev 2012;40(1):22–9.

31. Bogdanis GC. Effects of physical activity and inactivity on muscle fatigue. Front Physiol 2012;3:142.

32. D'Mello C, Swain MG. Liver-brain interactions in inflammatory liver diseases: implications for fatigue and mood disorders. Brain Behav Immun 2014;35:9–20.
33. Chaudhuri A, Behan PO. Fatigue in neurological disorders. Lancet 2004; 363(9413):978–88.
34. Smith MR, Marcora SM, Coutts AJ. Mental fatigue impairs intermittent running performance. Med Sci Sports Exerc 2015;47(8):1682–90.
35. Senzolo M, Schiff S, D'Aloiso CM, et al. Neuropsychological alterations in hepatitis C infection: the role of inflammation. World J Gastroenterol 2011;17(29): 3369–74.
36. Davis JM, Bailey SP. Possible mechanisms of central nervous system fatigue during exercise. Med Sci Sports Exerc 1997;29(1):45–57.
37. Weissenborn K, Krause J, Bokemeyer M, et al. Hepatitis C virus infection affects the brain-evidence from psychometric studies and magnetic resonance spectroscopy. J Hepatol 2004;41(5):845–51.
38. Weissenborn K, Ennen JC, Bokemeyer M, et al. Monoaminergic neurotransmission is altered in hepatitis C virus infected patients with chronic fatigue and cognitive impairment. Gut 2006;55(11):1624–30.
39. Piche T, Vanbiervliet G, Cherikh F, et al. Effect of ondansetron, a 5-HT3 receptor antagonist, on fatigue in chronic hepatitis C: a randomised, double blind, placebo controlled study. Gut 2005;54(8):1169–73.
40. Castell LM, Yamamoto T, Phoenix J, et al. The role of tryptophan in fatigue in different conditions of stress. Adv Exp Med Biol 1999;467:697–704.
41. Luo YM, Hart N, Mustfa N, et al. Effect of diaphragm fatigue on neural respiratory drive. J Appl Physiol (1985) 2001;90(5):1691–9.
42. Dimeo F, Stieglitz RD, Novelli-Fischer U, et al. Correlation between physical performance and fatigue in cancer patients. Ann Oncol 1997;8(12):1251–5.
43. Fiorentino L, Rissling M, Liu L, et al. The symptom cluster of sleep, fatigue and depressive symptoms in breast cancer patients: severity of the problem and treatment options. Drug Discov Today Dis Models 2011;8(4):167–73.
44. Millikin CP, Rourke SB, Halman MH, et al. Fatigue in HIV/AIDS is associated with depression and subjective neurocognitive complaints but not neuropsychological functioning. J Clin Exp Neuropsychol 2003;25(2):201–15.
45. Wilson J, Morgan S, Magin PJ, et al. Fatigue–a rational approach to investigation. Aust Fam Physician 2014;43(7):457–61.
46. Finsterer J. Biomarkers of peripheral muscle fatigue during exercise. BMC Musculoskelet Disord 2012;13:218.
47. Bendahan D, Giannesini B, Cozzone PJ. Functional investigations of exercising muscle: a noninvasive magnetic resonance spectroscopy-magnetic resonance imaging approach. Cell Mol Life Sci 2004;61(9):1001–15.
48. Tonon C, Gramegna LL, Lodi R. Magnetic resonance imaging and spectroscopy in the evaluation of neuromuscular disorders and fatigue. Neuromuscul Disord 2012;22(Suppl 3):S187–91.
49. Kluger BM, Krupp LB, Enoka RM. Fatigue and fatigability in neurologic illnesses: proposal for a unified taxonomy. Neurology 2013;80(4):409–16.
50. Weinstein AA, Diao G, Baghi H, et al. Demonstration of two types of fatigue in subjects with chronic liver disease using factor analysis. Qual Life Res 2017. [Epub ahead of print].
51. Younossi Z, Henry L. Systematic review: patient-reported outcomes in chronic hepatitis C–the impact of liver disease and new treatment regimens. Aliment Pharmacol Ther 2015;41(6):497–520.

52. PROMIS. Health measures - PROMIS. Available at: http://www.healthmeasures. net/explore-measurement-systems/promis. Accessed October 4, 2016.

53. Gerber L, Estep M, Stepanova M, et al. Effects of viral eradication with ledipasvir and sofosbuvir, with or without ribavirin, on measures of fatigue in patients with chronic hepatitis C virus infection. Clin Gastroenterol Hepatol 2016;14(1): 156–64.e3.

54. Cacoub P, Ratziu V, Myers RP, et al. Impact of treatment on extra hepatic manifestations in patients with chronic hepatitis C. J Hepatol 2002;36(6):812–8.

55. Koskinas J, Merkouraki P, Manesis E, et al. Assessment of depression in patients with chronic hepatitis: effect of interferon treatment. Dig Dis 2002;20(3–4):284–8.

56. Younossi ZM, Stepanova M, Esteban R, et al. Superiority of interferon-free regimens for chronic hepatitis C: the effect on health-related quality of life and work productivity. Medicine (Baltimore) 2017;96(7):e5914.

57. Kwo P, Gane EJ, Peng CY, et al. Effectiveness of elbasvir and grazoprevir combination, with or without ribavirin, for treatment-experienced patients with chronic hepatitis C infection. Gastroenterology 2017;152(1):164–75.e4.

58. Younossi ZM, Stepanova M, Henry L, et al. An in-depth analysis of patient-reported outcomes in patients with chronic hepatitis C treated with different anti-viral regimens. Am J Gastroenterol 2016;111(6):808–16.

59. Marcellin F, Protopopescu C, Poizot-Martin I, et al. Short article: fatigue in the long term after HCV treatment in HIV-HCV-coinfected patients: functional limitations persist despite viral clearance in patients exposed to peg-interferon/ribavirin-containing regimens (ANRS CO13-HEPAVIH cohort). Eur J Gastroenterol Hepatol 2016;28(9):1003–7.

60. Bonkovsky HL, Snow KK, Malet PF, et al. Health-related quality of life in patients with chronic hepatitis C and advanced fibrosis. J Hepatol 2007;46(3):420–31.

61. Younossi ZM, Stepanova M, Henry L, et al. Effects of sofosbuvir-based treatment, with and without interferon, on outcome and productivity of patients with chronic hepatitis C. Clin Gastroenterol Hepatol 2014;12(8):1349–59.e13.

62. Younossi ZM, Stepanova M, Nader F, et al. The patient's journey with chronic hepatitis C from interferon plus ribavirin to interferon- and ribavirin-free regimens: a study of health-related quality of life. Aliment Pharmacol Ther 2015;42(3):286–95.

63. Negro F, Forton D, Craxi A, et al. Extrahepatic morbidity and mortality of chronic hepatitis C. Gastroenterology 2015;149(6):1345–60.

64. Schneider CM, Hsieh CC, Sprod LK, et al. Effects of supervised exercise training on cardiopulmonary function and fatigue in breast cancer survivors during and after treatment. Cancer 2007;110(4):918–25.

65. Dennett AM, Peiris CL, Shields N, et al. Moderate-intensity exercise reduces fatigue and improves mobility in cancer survivors: a systematic review and meta-regression. J Physiother 2016;62(2):68–82.

66. Sturkenboom IH, Graff MJ, Borm GF, et al. Effectiveness of occupational therapy in Parkinson's disease: study protocol for a randomized controlled trial. Trials 2013;14:34.

67. Deng G, Chan Y, Sjoberg D, et al. Acupuncture for the treatment of post-chemotherapy chronic fatigue: a randomized, blinded, sham-controlled trial. Support Care Cancer 2013;21(6):1735–41.

68. Dalgas U, Stenager E, Jakobsen J, et al. Fatigue, mood and quality of life improve in MS patients after progressive resistance training. Mult Scler 2010;16(4): 480–90.

69. Golabi P, Locklear CT, Austin P, et al. Effectiveness of exercise in hepatic fat mobilization in non-alcoholic fatty liver disease: systematic review. World J Gastroenterol 2016;22(27):6318–27.

70. Foster GR. Quality of life considerations for patients with chronic hepatitis C. J Viral Hepat 2009;16(9):605–11.

71. Armstrong AR, Herrmann SE, Chassany O, et al. The International development of PROQOL-HCV: an instrument to assess the health-related quality of life of patients treated for Hepatitis C virus. BMC Infect Dis 2016;16(1):443.

72. Younossi Z, Stepanova M, Omata M, et al. Health utilities using SF-6D scores in Japanese patients with chronic hepatitis C treated with sofosbuvir-based regimens in clinical trials. Health Qual Life Outcomes 2017;15(1):25.

73. Whiteley D, Elliott L, Cunningham-Burley S, et al. Health-related quality of life for individuals with hepatitis C: a narrative review. Int J Drug Policy 2015;26(10): 936–49.

74. Hsu PC, Federico CA, Krajden M, et al. Health utilities and psychometric quality of life in patients with early- and late-stage hepatitis C virus infection. J Gastroenterol Hepatol 2012;27(1):149–57.

75. Gutteling JJ, de Man RA, van der Plas SM, et al. Determinants of quality of life in chronic liver patients. Aliment Pharmacol Ther 2006;23(11):1629–35.

76. Loria A, Doyle K, Weinstein AA, et al. Multiple factors predict physical performance in people with chronic liver disease. Am J Phys Med Rehabil 2014; 93(6):470–6.

77. Dan AA, Crone C, Wise TN, et al. Anger experiences among hepatitis C patients: relationship to depressive symptoms and health-related quality of life. Psychosomatics 2007;48(3):223–9.

78. Younossi Z, Kallman J, Kincaid J. The effects of HCV infection and management on health-related quality of life. Hepatology 2007;45(3):806–16.

79. van der Plas SM, Hansen BE, de Boer JB, et al. Generic and disease-specific health related quality of life of liver patients with various aetiologies: a survey. Qual Life Res 2007;16(3):375–88.

80. Sanyal A, Younossi ZM, Bass NM, et al. Randomised clinical trial: rifaximin improves health-related quality of life in cirrhotic patients with hepatic encephalopathy - a double-blind placebo-controlled study. Aliment Pharmacol Ther 2011; 34(8):853–61.

81. Tossing G. Treating hepatitis C in HIV-HCV coinfected patients. Infection 2002; 30(5):329–31.

82. Younossi ZM, Stepanova M, Henry L, et al. Adherence to treatment of chronic hepatitis C: from interferon containing regimens to interferon and ribavirin free regimens. Medicine (Baltimore) 2016;95(28):e4151.

83. McGowan CE, Fried MW. Barriers to hepatitis C treatment. Liver Int 2012; 32(Suppl 1):151–6.

84. Trembling PM, Tanwar S, Dusheiko GM. Boceprevir: an oral protease inhibitor for the treatment of chronic HCV infection. Expert Rev Anti Infect Ther 2012;10(3): 269–79.

85. Younossi ZM, Stepanova M, Feld J, et al. Sofosbuvir/velpatasvir improves patient-reported outcomes in HCV patients: results from ASTRAL-1 placebo-controlled trial. J Hepatol 2016;65(1):33–9.

86. Younossi ZM, Stepanova M, Sulkowski M, et al. Sofosbuvir and ledipasvir improve patient-reported outcomes in patients co-infected with hepatitis C and human immunodeficiency virus. J Viral Hepat 2016;23(11):857–65.

87. Younossi ZM, Stepanova M, Pol S, et al. The impact of ledipasvir/sofosbuvir on patient-reported outcomes in cirrhotic patients with chronic hepatitis C: the SIRIUS study. Liver Int 2016;36(1):42–8.

88. Younossi ZM, Stepanova M, Marcellin P, et al. Treatment with ledipasvir and sofosbuvir improves patient-reported outcomes: results from the ION-1, -2, and -3 clinical trials. Hepatology 2015;61(6):1798–808.

89. Younossi ZM, Stepanova M, Feld J, et al. Sofosbuvir and velpatasvir combination improves outcomes reported by patients with HCV infection, without or with compensated or decompensated cirrhosis. Clin Gastroenterol Hepatol 2017; 15(3):421–30.e6.

90. Poordad F, Agarwal K, Younes Z, et al. Low relapse rate leads to high concordance of sustained virologic response (SVR) at 12 weeks with SVR at 24 weeks after treatment with ABT-450/ritonavir, ombitasvir, and dasabuvir plus ribavirin in subjects with chronic hepatitis C virus genotype 1 infection in the AVIATOR study. Clin Infect Dis 2015;60(4):608–10.

Economic Burden of Hepatitis C Infection

Maria Stepanova, PhD[a,b], Zobair M. Younossi, MD[a,b,c],*

KEYWORDS

- Cost of illness • Cost-effectiveness • Cost-utility • Pharmacoeconomic
- Work productivity • Fatigue • Societal perspective • Screening

KEY POINTS

- Chronic hepatitis C virus (HCV) infection places a significant economic burden to societies worldwide.
- Economic burden of HCV includes direct medical costs and indirect costs owing to impaired quality of life and loss of work productivity.
- In addition to chronic liver disease caused by HCV, extrahepatic manifestations of the virus add substantially to the economic burden of the disease.
- Treatment of chronic HCV should be assessed by budgetary cost and by accounting for the benefits of cure including prevented morbidity, mortality, and improved work productivity.

INTRODUCTION

The studies of economic burden of chronic diseases have generally been falling behind similar studies related to their epidemiology, morbidity, and mortality.[1] However, understanding the economic burden of diseases, or the cost of illness, seems to be increasingly valuable given recent evidence that chronic diseases might have significantly detracted from economic growth in developed countries.[1] The economic aspect is also important as a reference for resource allocation, policy development, and for determining the cost-effectiveness of new therapies. Currently, many health policy decisions in Western countries require cost-effectiveness analysis, as one of the most relevant surrogates of total use of resources, in support or denial of intervention decisions.[2]

The authors have nothing to disclose.

[a] Center for Outcomes Research in Liver Diseases, 2411 I Street NW, Washington, DC 20037, USA; [b] Betty and Guy Beatty Center for Integrated Research, Inova Health System, 3300 Gallows Road, Falls Church, VA 22042, USA; [c] Department of Medicine, Center for Liver Diseases, Inova Fairfax Hospital, 3300 Gallows Road, Falls Church, VA 22042, USA

* Corresponding author. Betty and Guy Beatty Center for Integrated Research, Claude Moore Health Education and Research Building, 3300 Gallows Road, Falls Church, VA 22042.
E-mail address: zobair.younossi@inova.org

ECONOMICS OF CHRONIC HEPATITIS C TREATMENT

Recent emergence of direct-acting antivirals (DAAs) for the treatment of chronic hepatitis C virus (HCV) infection has made a substantial push toward examining the disease from the economic point of view. In particular, relatively high cost per pill for the newly developed drugs has highlighted the price controversy, which might have overshadowed their excellent efficacy and safety. In the United States, that controversy and concerns about access to treatment have been discussed at congressional hearings and, at some point, included suggestions of nonvoluntary acquisition of patents based on the principles of eminent domain.[3] Indeed, unprecedented treatment effectiveness for communicable diseases has made price-based rationing of treatment look questionable from an ethical point of view. At the same time, in the scientific literature, the value of a cure with DAAs has been being extensively studied in multiple economic models developed for different clinical populations in a number of countries.[4–14]

There are several different approaches to evaluating the economic impact of a chronic disease and its treatment. The simplest is a budgetary cost analysis where only immediate costs of treatment, such as the costs of the drug, its adverse events, and expected use of health care resources, are considered. This approach, although often relied on by payers, may result in the perception that the most economically beneficial drug is the cheapest one. In contrast, a more comprehensive analysis would rather consider the cost of the treatment weighed against expected outcomes to understand the true net benefit of the intervention. That being the case, the benefit of the treatment would include prevented morbidity and mortality as well as potential changes of other relevant outcomes (such as patient-reported outcomes and workers' productivity) in comparison with alternative treatments or to the natural course of the disease (the no-treatment option).[15]

Self-contained cost–benefit analyses of treatment requires transformation of all studied outcomes to monetary values. For practical purposes, this is often difficult or impossible without additional assumptions. For chronic hepatitis C, a more meaningful economic outcome is the cost of cure (which is sustained virologic response) that can be used in cost-effectiveness analysis.[16] Another outcome, which is often perceived as the most relevant to both patients and the society, is the number of quality-adjusted life-years (QALYs) gained after treatment, which can be fed into a cost-utility analysis, thus producing the cost per QALY. That outcome is then compared with the willingness to pay threshold (WPT), which is the amount the society is believed to be willing to pay for gaining an additional QALY in its member. Historically, in the United States, a WPT threshold of $50,000 per QALY has been used[17]; a similar value in the United Kingdom is £20,000 to £30,000 per QALY,[18] and it varies between €20,000 and €50,000 in other European Union countries.[19] However, many researchers believe that these values might be outdated and, generally, not based on scientific evidence.[20,21] Indeed, the US threshold was originally established in the 1970s based on the Medicare cost of coverage for renal dialysis. More recently, WTP thresholds of $100,000 to 200,000 have been proposed.[20] In fact, the World Health Organization has suggested that that value should be determined within the context of economic reality of each country, and recommends that WPT to not exceed three times the national per-capita gross domestic product.[22]

In this context, despite a high cost per pill, multiple studies have indicated that DAAs could be cost-effective in most patients with chronic hepatitis C. In fact, DAA-based treatments have been evaluated from the economic point of view since their arrival to the market in early 2010s. Pharmacoeconomic analysis of the first-generation

DAAs showed that these drugs were clearly cost-effective only in certain subpopulations (advanced fibrosis, favorable IL28 B genotype).[4] After the arrival of the second-generation DAAs, these regimens were no longer cost-effective and were pulled from the US market.[23,24]

Pharmacoeconomic studies of the second generation DAAs have generally suggested that all-oral interferon-free regimens are cost-effective across a variety of clinical populations in developed countries.[25] One study estimated an incremental cost-effectiveness ratio of such regimens to be approximately US$45,000 per QALY in the 2013 U.S. dollars, minimized in genotype 1 patients.[26] Another study reported the all-oral interferon-free combination of sofosbuvir and ledipasvir (LDV/SOF) to be associated with the lowest 1-year cost per sustained virologic response among all available DAA-based treatments (including interferon-containing regimens) in all patient subcohorts in HCV genotype 1 population owing to both high efficacy and good tolerability. The same regimen was also found to be either dominant or the most cost-effective with regard to the lifetime incremental cost-effectiveness ratio per QALY in the United States, and was also cheaper in the long term than the no-treatment option owing to prevented cases of advanced liver disease.[27] Furthermore, for all interferon-free regimens, treatment initiation at earlier stages of liver fibrosis was predicted to result in improved economic outcomes, albeit projected to incur substantial aggregate costs.[27–29] The regimen of choice, however, does vary between HCV genotypes owing to varying efficacy of the drugs, and this typically affects cost-effectiveness conclusions.[30,31] In particular, for treatment-naïve (but not treatment-experienced) patients with genotypes 2 and 3, the incremental cost-effectiveness ratio of an all-oral DAA-based treatment was close to or exceeded WPT of $100,000, suggesting questionable cost-effectiveness at present.[26,32] However, none of these studies considered the benefit of treatment beyond prevention of liver-related sequelae of the disease. Given that, it is possible that presently inconclusive cost-effectiveness inference may change if the comprehensive benefit of the cure, including prevention and resolution of extrahepatic manifestations (EHMs) of HCV, improvement of fatigue, quality of life, and work productivity, is considered.

The DAA-based regimens have also been studied in certain clinical populations to which findings from the general HCV population might be not directly applicable. In the human immunodeficiency virus–HCV coinfected population, the interferon-free regimen with a combination of ombitasvir/paritaprevir/ritonavir with or without ribavirin was found to be the most effective in preventing excessive adverse clinical outcomes and deaths; that regimen was also found to be more cost-effective in comparison with LDV/SOF in anti-HCV treatment-naïve human immunodeficiency virus–HCV patients.[14] The cost-effectiveness of sofosbuvir-based therapy was also confirmed in incarcerated patients,[11] patients with decompensated cirrhosis,[13] and posttransplant patients.[33] One report from the Netherlands suggested cost-effectiveness of treating patients who inject drugs with DAAs, primarily because curing their infection would reduce HCV epidemics in that population.[34] Notably, preliminary cost-effectiveness results obtained from real-world clinical practices seem to parallel findings reported from clinical trials.[35,36]

Outside the United States, the cost-effectiveness of DAA-based therapy was found to depend on a country-specific WPT.[6] In Europe, the National Institute for Health and Care Excellence recommended interferon- and ribavirin-free LDV/SOF to be used only in patients of genotypes 1 and 4 with a history of failing another HCV treatment and/or cirrhosis, or in patients for whom 8-week-long treatment would be clinically appropriate (treatment-naïve HCV genotype 1 without cirrhosis only).[37] A similar association of cost-effectiveness with treatment duration was reported from Canada.[38] In

Switzerland, treatment of a mixed cohort with sofosbuvir-containing regimens was found to be, on average, cost-effective with a WPT of CHF 100,000, but not so in certain subgroups (genotypes 2 and 3 interferon-eligible treatment-naïve patients without cirrhosis).[12] Similarly, a study from Spain suggested that interferon-free options were not cost-effective at the current price level for patients with HCV genotype 3.[39] Reports from Japan suggested that LDV/SOF was cost-effective in HCV genotype 1 patients, and an interferon-free combination of sofosbuvir and ribavirin was the most cost-effective in genotype 2.[40,41] Another study suggested similar cost-effectiveness of the ombitasvir/paritaprevir/ritonavir regimen in genotype 1 Japanese population.[42] In contrast, initial reports from less developed countries were, generally, less favorable toward the immediate use of the second-generation DAAs at their current price levels.[43–47] Nevertheless, national strategies in some countries have led to price negotiations for the new anti-HCV regimens, and this will likely allow making these regimens affordable and cost-effective in the future.[46,48] This example also highlights the importance of having a national strategy to deal with HCV on a country-by-country basis, because solutions suitable for developed countries may be not directly applicable to countries with fewer resources.

In addition to cost-effectiveness as seen from patient's and/or payer's perspective, it is also essential to consider the economic value of curing the chronic communicable disease for society. Even in developed countries, the ultimate aim of eliminating HCV infection requires adopting a long-term, societal perspective-based strategy, and substantial initial investments will be inevitable. However, in recent studies from the United States, it was estimated that overall long-term savings might exceed $60 to $170 billion solely owing to reduction in morbidity and mortality in the most prevalent HCV genotype 1 carriers even without accounting for less palpable benefits of the cure, such as prevention or resolution of EHMs of HCV, improved quality of life, and increased labor force participation and/or work productivity.[5,29,49]

Despite the generally favorable pharmacoeconomic profile described, substantial barriers for access to treatment remain. In the United States, coverage of DAA-based HCV treatment is not included or limited by some payers,[3,50,51] and the rate of any insurance coverage among generally more socially disadvantaged HCV population remains relatively low.[52] At the same time, recent studies have shown that treating the infection sooner rather than later might by the most efficient in the long run, thus challenging the present budget-saving rationing policies.[27,29,53] Alas, the budgetary cost of these regimens presents an obstacle to the ultimate goal of immediate treatment of all viremic patients with highly effective and safe DAAs.[54] In contrast, a rational national policy coupled with more price competitive treatment options for HCV around the world[46,48,55,56] could make the state-of-the-art treatment of chronic hepatitis C more accessible.

THE COST OF HEPATITIS C VIRUS-RELATED LIVER DISEASE

In the context of the cost of HCV treatment, it might be useful to understand what exactly HCV-associated economic burden is and what contributes to it. Because HCV in the leading cause of advanced liver disease worldwide, it is reasonable to conclude that its burden is enormous. Nevertheless, it remains important to relate its value to the costs of other diseases, with the aim to refer to that value in resource allocation and health care policy discussions.

A study from early 2000s suggested that in the United States, one-third of the total burden of HCV could be attributable to direct medical care, and two-thirds were indirect or productivity costs.[57] Twenty years ago, the total burden of HCV was estimated to be $5.5 billion per year (in 1997 dollars), which would project into nearly $10 billion in US dollars of 2017, assuming that the distribution of expenses remained the same. The direct costs included medical expenses such as inpatient hospital admissions, outpatient hospital and doctors' office visits, emergency room fees, other payments to medical providers and vendors, prescription drugs and medical device costs, and other health care–related expenses such as rehabilitation centers and nursing homes. These direct costs did not include impaired work productivity, lost wages and benefits, or expenses patients and families incurred owing to impaired daily functioning of a patient with HCV-related liver disease, the value of family care, or the socioeconomic consequences of the patient's premature death. Also, these costs did not include the cost of the EHMs of the virus. Even so, the total national annual burden of chronic HCV was reported to be close to that of asthma and rheumatoid arthritis, but was the only one projected to increase.[57,58]

Of more recent studies, in 2011, the total direct economic burden of HCV-related liver disease in the United States was estimated to be $6.5 billion ($4.3 to $8.2) annually.[59] Therefore, an increase in direct medical expenses was indeed nearly 2-fold from the late 1990s. Out of that, approximately $2.7 billion was covered by Medicare alone.[60] The most expensive state of health associated with HCV was the first year after liver transplantation, with different reports suggesting an average annual per-patient per-year (PPPY) expenses exceeding $140,000 in late 2000s.[61,62] Within the remainder of the spectrum of HCV-related liver disease, as reported from a large US health care management organization study, asymptomatic patients with HCV incurred approximately $6000 PPPY in incremental costs (in 2009 US dollars). That amount expectedly increased with the severity of liver disease but, when multiplied by the number of affected patients, the greatest share of the total direct medical burden (33% of all payer's expenses) was still accounted for by monitoring and managing HCV patients without liver disease, although closely followed by the share taken by patients with decompensated cirrhosis (25%).[61] In contrast, in the Medicare population, the greatest share of expenditures (64%) was owing to decompensated cirrhosis.[60] Among the sequelae of advanced liver disease caused by HCV, hepatocellular carcinoma, variceal hemorrhage, and refractory ascites were the most expensive, each exceeding $25,000 PPPY (2010 US dollars),[63] followed by hepatic encephalopathy ($17,800 per inpatient admission in 2009).[64]

These studies of the total HCV burden cited were conducted before the era of DAAs, which could have potentially shifted the trajectory of both the costs and consequences of HCV infection. In this context, there are a few studies estimating the dynamics in clinical burden of HCV caused by the use of DAAs.[65,66] In 1 study from the United States, the authors projected a decrease in the infection prevalence of nearly 50% by 2020 in comparison with 2015, and of 70% by 2030; notably, the projected remaining prevalence would be primarily owing to people being unaware of their infection and, thus, the cost-effectiveness of universal screening will probably have to be revisited.[67,68] The decrease in adverse outcomes is expected to follow at a slower pace, with a 20% to 35% reduction by 2020 in the numbers of liver-related deaths, new cases of decompensated cirrhosis, hepatocellular carcinoma and HCV-associated liver transplantations[66]; the disparity in the changes of the prevalence of the infection and of its adverse sequelae might be explained by a disproportionally higher prevalence of HCV positivity in older patients at present.[69] Given that, the direct economic burden of HCV infection is also expected to decrease proportionally. In the nearest years, however, it will be largely driven by treatment capacity, which is changing rapidly.[66]

Similar studies from Europe and Asia have confirmed the tremendous economic burden of chronic HCV infection. A report from Italy suggested the total nationwide burden of approximately €1 billion annually (as of 2013), with less than 40% of it being allocated for direct medical expenses.[70] Additionally, €100 million has been reported for HCV infection in Belgium (2014).[71] A similar estimate from Switzerland suggested that the direct annual burden of HCV was €74 million excluding any antiviral treatment costs.[72] The projected burden for the entire European region was €17 billion per year (2010) with approximately 25% of that burden being accounted for by direct medical expenditures.[73] In another study from Canada, only direct medical costs were estimated to be $161 million per year (as of 2013), despite a relatively low prevalence of HCV in that country (<1%).[74] Similarly low prevalence still resulted in more than $1 billion per year of HCV-associated burden in Iran.[75] From Egypt, and annual US$4 billion (2015) has been reported, with only 20% being attributed to direct medical expenses.[76] Finally, an estimate from Australia suggested direct medical expenses of $220 million annually (2013 US dollars),[77] and another estimate from Japan reported up to $3.2 billion per year (2005 US dollars).[78] Furthermore, because more than one-half of the worldwide HCV-infected population lives in South and East Asia,[79] the estimates are likely a fraction of the global economic burden of HCV infection. However, none of the cited estimates of the national economic burden of HCV included the cost of treatment with the most recent DAAs, so these numbers will certainly change in the near future, but most likely not monotonically over time owing to the initial costs of treatment which, in the long term, are supposed to be compensated by the savings from prevented morbidity and mortality.

ECONOMIC BURDEN OF THE EXTRAHEPATIC MANIFESTATIONS OF HEPATITIS C VIRUS

EHMs of HCV, although being less frequently emphasized historically, have become increasingly recognized. Nevertheless, in all the studies presented, the total direct economic burden of HCV infection had been calculated without accounting for EHMs and associated expenses. In this context, there are challenges in estimating the true epidemiologic burden of EHMs of HCV in different countries. Additionally, there may be substantial confounders which could interfere with the present way of calculating the prevalence and incidence of EHMs as an excessive prevalence (incidence) of the condition in infected population in comparison with the general population. For illustration, the high prevalence of depression in HCV patients might be caused by the neurologic effects of the virus.[80] At the same time, both having depression and having acquired HCV infection in the first place might be consequences of a common cause, such as a history of drug use. Additional research beyond sheer subtraction of the prevalence rates is needed to factor out the true contribution of HCV to the excessive prevalence of what is believed to be an EHM of HCV. This makes estimating the total economic burden of HCV's EHMs challenging because it is highly sensitive to the prevalence rates and, thus, the impact of different confounders.

Nevertheless, there has been an attempt to estimate the cost of EHMs in the United States. The study suggested that the total direct annual burden of EHMs for the United States could be as high as $1.5 billion (2014 US dollars).[81] In PPPY expenses, the most expensive EHM was suggested to be end-stage renal disease, and the overall contribution to the national EHM burden was estimated to be the greatest for HCV-induced type 2 diabetes and depression (both accounting for approximately 30% of all direct medical expenses). In addition, excessive prevalence of cardiovascular diseases and mixed cryoglobulinemia in patients with HCV were estimated to cost more than $100 million per year each. However, in that study, the cost calculations were based on the respective Medicare fees and, thus, might have underestimated the average cost of illness by not accounting for generally higher costs incurred by patients covered by private insurers. Another recent study from France estimated the same burden of EHMs of HCV to be €256 million per year (2015).[82] It is important to note that the prevalence of EHMs in this study were high in comparison with other similar reports (eg, the prevalence of mixed cryoglobulinemia in HCV was 51% with the rate of hospitalization for it of 26%, which well exceeds other similar estimates[81,83,84]) and, thus, the reported national cost of the EHMs substantially exceeded the cost of all HCV-related inpatient hospital stays in the country, including those for liver transplantation.[85] A number of reports on the prevalence rates of EHMs of HCV in other countries suggested notably high rates of up to 75%,[86–89] but so far have not been accompanied by the cost of illness analyses.

Although still preliminary and in need of validation, the studies of the economic burden of EHMs for HCV suggest a substantial contribution of these conditions to the total economic burden of the disease. From the estimates published so far, that burden seems to be comparable with or exceed that of all the liver transplants in HCV patients and, thus, should not be omitted in pharmacoeconomic analyses of hepatitis C. In addition to improving patient management strategies for providers and payers, accounting for the EHMs of HCV may also point out a window of opportunity for gaining additional benefits of HCV cure. However, the rate of resolution of EHMs in patients who cleared their virus is currently, for the most part, unknown.

ECONOMIC BURDEN OWING TO WORK PRODUCTIVITY LOSSES IN HEPATITIS C VIRUS–INFECTED SUBJECTS

In addition to the economic burden of HCV incurred from direct medical costs presented, a few studies suggested that the loss in productivity and other nonmedical consequences of the chronic disease might be even more costly.[57,70,73,76] Indeed, despite a higher prevalence of HCV in older people in the United States, the vast majority of HCV-infected Americans are still of working age.[52] Outside developed countries with both higher prevalence rates and more new infections, the HCV-infected population is even younger.[90,91] This makes decreased work productivity in the HCV population an important potential concern for societies.

The burden of HCV infection on work productivity is largely driven by limited labor force participation among patients with HCV, which results in lost wages and benefits; indeed, low employment rate in patients with HCV (54% vs 62% national) has been confirmed in a recent report from the United States,[92] supported by similar reports from other countries.[73,93–95] Another contributor to that burden is impaired work productivity in patients who are employed; it includes both lost hours of work (absenteeism) and decreased productivity while working (presenteeism).[96] Physical fatigue and cognitive and emotional impairment have been shown to be the major drivers of lower work productivity in patients with HCV.[97,98]

Substantial absenteeism, which includes an increase in the number of sick days and time spent on short- and long-term disability leave, has been reported in multiple studies.[73,93,99–101] From the study by Baran and colleagues,[99] it can be projected that employed people with HCV incur, on average, approximately $1200 per year (in 2013 US dollars) in absenteeism-related losses. That, when multiplied by the number of chronically infected individuals in the United States (2.7 million[102]) and by the employment rate of approximately 50% cited, suggests the national annual burden of absenteeism caused by HCV of approximately $1.65 billion. The same European burden projected from the estimates reported by Vietri and colleagues[73] (9 million infected in the region, approximately €800 PPPY in absenteeism-relates losses, 48% employed) would result in the total annual burden of €3.5 billion.

The impact of presenteeism was studied less, although it has been reported that it accounts for approximately 75% of work productivity losses in patients with HCV when estimated using the standard Work Productivity and Activity Impairment Questionnaire: Specific Health Problem (WPAI:SHP) instrument.[73,103] Given that, when spread over the entire US population living with HCV (calculated for HCV genotype 1 only which is the most prevalent in the United States), the total productivity-related burden of HCV has been reported to exceed $7 billion.[104] A similar projection of the European estimates[73] would result in €3000 PPPY, or €13.0 billion for the entire region. Another study reported that productivity burden to be €2.6 billion per year for 5 European countries (Germany, the UK, France, Italy, and Spain) in genotype 1 patients only[105]; this is, in fact, consistent with the former estimate if multiplied by the proportion of European HCV population living in these countries (approximately 25%, with 60%–70% having HCV genotype 1[106]). Furthermore, preliminary estimates from Asian countries suggested similarly enormous productivity losses: $349 million per year in Taiwan, $146 million in South Korea, $17 million in Singapore, and $11 million in Hong Kong (in 2014 US dollars).[107]

In contrast, as the studies suggested, curing HCV infection in HCV genotype 1 carriers in the United States only could save up to $2.7 billion over a 1-year time horizon solely owing to an increase in work productivity,[104] and from €340 to €435 million in the 5 European countries cited.[105] Additionally, in Asian countries, treatment with all-oral interferon-free regimens would presumably result in the productivity gains of $138 million, $58.7 million, $6.8 million, and $4.5 million in Taiwan, Korea, Singapore, and Hong Kong, respectively.[107] Notably, in those studies, the savings were projected to come from improved presenteeism only, because the short-term data available to the authors did not suggest any improvement in absenteeism; thus, those estimates might increase with longer follow-up of cured patients. It is, however, important to note that calculated work productivity used self-reports collected by the WPAI:SHP instrument, so the true gain in employers' and society benefits might differ if measured by more objective algorithms. These estimates also do not include any future productivity burden incurred by pediatric patients with HCV who are not yet in labor force, but will also generate substantial productivity losses if left untreated.[108,109]

Finally, in addition to the impact on workers' productivity in terms of lost hours, wages, and other work-related outcomes, chronic HCV infection may also impair activities other than work, such as study, housework, and child care, all of which add to the total disease burden. This can result in additional monetary expenses, and in the loss of productivity by unpaid caregivers (families or friends). Although the latter aspect of the disease is rarely considered, 1 report suggested that it could be sometimes comparable with the productivity burden experienced by the patients themselves[93] and, thus, should be accounted for by future pharmacoeconomic studies of the disease.

OTHER ASPECTS OF HEPATITIS C VIRUS ECONOMICS

There are other economic aspects related to chronic HCV from the public health point of view that have not been included in this review. Some examples are the impact of HCV infection on the families and caregivers, the economic burden of HCV related to its associated stigma, and also the economics of HCV transmission and prevention. Because there is no vaccine for HCV, it is only prevention of blood-to-blood contacts that is effective. In developed countries, implementation of standard universal precautions, such as the use of safe injections and safe components of shared equipment that have contact with blood, mass testing of donors' blood, and, potentially, behavioral interventions, have resulted in a relatively low rate of new infections and, as a result, a decreasing prevalence even before the era of DAAs.[66,110,111] In the rest of the world, however, expanding access to treatment must be accompanied by complex prevention strategies so that limited resources allocated for treatment do not end up being poured into a bottomless pit.

Another economic aspect of hepatitis C is the cost of HCV screening. In the United States, universal screening is recommended only for individuals born in 1945 to 1965 owing to known high prevalence[69]; the screening of asymptomatic average-risk people has been shown to be not cost-effective in Western countries.[67,112,113] However, prior screening cost-effectiveness studies presumed relatively low treatment uptake by diagnosed patients, which was typical for interferon-based regimens. At the same time, recent epidemiologic studies suggest that, even with the current management practices, the majority of people diagnosed with chronic HCV infection in the United States will have been treated within the next decade or so[66]; therefore, the majority of remaining viremic individuals will be unaware of their infection, which is, in fact, the only predictor of not receiving treatment.[114] In that context, it is possible that identifying that population may become cost-effective in the future[68] and, thus, a universal screening policy may be needed, similar to that for human immunodeficiency virus.[115] Furthermore, similar policies may also be potentially useful in other countries, especially those with a high prevalence of viremia at present.[47] However, unlike prevention-aimed policies, cost-effectiveness of screening is sensitive to the treatment uptake rate and, therefore, expanding screening needs to follow rather than precede improving access to effective treatment.

SUMMARY

Being a multifaceted disease, chronic HCV infection does cause a multifaceted economic burden worldwide. That burden, in addition to direct medical expenses and drug costs, morbidity, and mortality, includes indirect outcomes such as higher unemployment in infected patients, lower wages, and impairment in work productivity and nonwork activities. Universal access to highly effective curing medications will decrease that burden if not eliminate the disease completely, but it also requires investments that are currently unaffordable in most of the world. Thus, cost-effective rationing strategies are currently being developed in many countries, with the aim to get the most benefit for the least expenditure. In that context, multiple studies have consistently demonstrated that earlier treatment results in greater long-term savings owing to prevented morbidity and saved years of productive life. Because it is unlikely that any individual payer may carry such an expense, the implementation of national and potentially global initiatives and campaigns is of immediate importance and will most likely pay us all back in the long run.

REFERENCES

1. Suhrcke M, Nugent RA, Stuckler D, et al. Chronic disease: an economic perspective. London: Oxford Health Alliance; 2006.

2. El Khoury AC, Wallace C, Klimack WK, et al. Economic burden of hepatitis C-associated diseases: Europe, Asia Pacific, and the Americas. J Med Econ 2012;15(5):887–96.

3. Trooskin SB, Reynolds H, Kostman JR. Access to costly new hepatitis C drugs: medicine, money, and Advocacy. Clin Infect Dis 2015;61(12):1825–30.

4. San Miguel R, Gimeno-Ballester V, Mar J. Cost-effectiveness of protease inhibitor based regimens for chronic hepatitis C: a systematic review of published literature. Expert Rev Pharmacoecon Outcomes Res 2014;14(3):387–402.

5. Younossi ZM, Park H, Dieterich D, et al. The value of cure associated with treating treatment-naïve chronic hepatitis C genotype 1: are the new all-oral regimens good value to society? Liver Int 2016. http://dx.doi.org/10.1111/liv.13298.

6. Luhnen M, Waffenschmidt S, Gerber-Grote A, et al. Health economic evaluations of sofosbuvir for treatment of chronic hepatitis C: a systematic review. Appl Health Econ Health Policy 2016;14(5):527–43.

7. Chhatwal J, Kanwal F, Roberts MS, et al. Cost-effectiveness and budget impact of hepatitis C virus treatment with sofosbuvir and ledipasvir in the United States. Ann Intern Med 2015;162(6):397–406.

8. Cure S, Guerra I, Cammà C, et al. Cost-effectiveness of sofosbuvir plus ribavirin with or without pegylated interferon for the treatment of chronic hepatitis C in Italy. J Med Econ 2015;18(9):678–90.

9. Cure S, Guerra I, Dusheiko G. Cost-effectiveness of sofosbuvir for the treatment of chronic hepatitis C-infected patients. J Viral Hepat 2015;22(11):882–9.

10. Gissel C, Götz G, Mahlich J, et al. Cost-effectiveness of Interferon-free therapy for Hepatitis C in Germany–an application of the efficiency frontier approach. BMC Infect Dis 2015;15:297.

11. Liu S, Watcha D, Holodniy M, et al. Sofosbuvir-based treatment regimens for chronic, genotype 1 hepatitis C virus infection in U.S. incarcerated populations: a cost-effectiveness analysis. Ann Intern Med 2014;161(8):546–53.

12. Pfeil AM, Reich O, Guerra IM, et al. Cost-effectiveness analysis of sofosbuvir compared to current standard treatment in Swiss patients with chronic hepatitis C. PLoS One 2015;10(5):e0126984.

13. Tapper EB, Hughes MS, Buti M, et al. The optimal timing of hepatitis C therapy in transplant eligible patients with Child B and C cirrhosis: a cost-effectiveness analysis. Transplantation 2016. [Epub ahead of print].

14. Saab S, Virabhak S, Parisé H, et al. Cost-effectiveness of genotype 1 chronic hepatitis C virus treatments in patients coinfected with human immunodeficiency virus in the United States. Adv Ther 2016;33(8):1316–30.

15. Levin HM, McEwan PJ. Cost-effectiveness analysis: methods and applications. 2nd edition. London: Sage; 2000.

16. Younossi ZM, Birerdinc A, Henry L. Hepatitis C infection: a multi-faceted systemic disease with clinical, patient reported and economic consequences. J Hepatol 2016;65(1 Suppl):S109–19.

17. Grosse SD. Assessing cost-effectiveness in healthcare: history of the $50,000 per QALY threshold. Expert Rev Pharmacoecon Outcomes Res 2008;8(2):165–78.

18. Raftery JP. NICE's cost-effectiveness range: should it be lowered? Pharmacoeconomics 2014;32(7):613–5.

19. Donaldson C, Baker R, Mason H, et al. European value of a quality adjusted life year. Final Publishable Report. Available at: http://research.ncl.ac.uk/eurovaq/EuroVaQ_Final_Publishable_Report_and_Appendices.pdf. Accessed January 1, 2017.

20. Neumann PJ, Cohen JT, Weinstein MC. Updating cost-effectiveness–the curious resilience of the $50,000-per-QALY threshold. N Engl J Med 2014;371(9):796–7.

21. Braithwaite RS, Meltzer DO, King JT Jr, et al. What does the value of modern medicine say about the $50,000 per quality-adjusted life-year decision rule? Med Care 2008;46(4):349–56.

22. Marseille E, Larson B, Kazi DS, et al. Thresholds for the cost–effectiveness of interventions: alternative approaches. Bull World Health Organ 2015;93:118–24.

23. Vaidya A, Perry CM. Simeprevir: first global approval. Drugs 2013;73(18): 2093–106.

24. Lawitz E, Mangia A, Wyles D, et al. Sofosbuvir for previously untreated chronic hepatitis C infection. N Engl J Med 2013;368(20):1878–87.

25. Henry L, Younossi Z. Patient-reported and economic outcomes related to sofosbuvir and ledipasvir treatment for chronic hepatitis C. Expert Rev Pharmacoecon Outcomes Res 2016;16(6):659–65.

26. Hagan LM, Yang Z, Ehteshami M, et al. All-oral, interferon-free treatment for chronic hepatitis C: cost-effectiveness analyses. J Viral Hepat 2013;20(12): 847–57.

27. Younossi ZM, Park H, Saab S, et al. Cost-effectiveness of all-oral ledipasvir/sofosbuvir regimens in patients with chronic hepatitis C virus genotype 1 infection. Aliment Pharmacol Ther 2015;41(6):544–63.

28. Younossi ZM, Park H, Dieterich D, et al. Assessment of cost of innovation versus the value of health gains associated with treatment of chronic hepatitis C in the United States: the quality-adjusted cost of care. Medicine (Baltimore) 2016; 95(41):e5048.

29. Chahal HS, Marseille EA, Tice JA, et al. Cost-effectiveness of early treatment of hepatitis C virus genotype 1 by stage of liver fibrosis in a us treatment-naive population. JAMA Intern Med 2016;176(1):65–73.

30. Saab S, Parisé H, Virabhak S, et al. Cost-effectiveness of currently recommended direct-acting antiviral treatments in patients infected with genotypes 1 or 4 hepatitis C virus in the US. J Med Econ 2016;19(8):795–805.

31. Poonsapaya JM, Einodshofer M, Kirkham HS, et al. New all oral therapy for chronic hepatitis C virus (HCV): a novel long-term cost comparison. Cost Eff Resour Alloc 2015;13:17.

32. Linas BP, Barter DM, Morgan JR, et al. The cost-effectiveness of sofosbuvir-based regimens for treatment of hepatitis C virus genotype 2 or 3 infection. Ann Intern Med 2015;162(9):619–29.

33. Njei B, McCarty TR, Fortune BE, et al. Optimal timing for hepatitis C therapy in US patients eligible for liver transplantation: a cost-effectiveness analysis. Aliment Pharmacol Ther 2016;44(10):1090–101.

34. van Santen DK, de Vos AS, Matser A, et al. Cost-effectiveness of hepatitis C treatment for people who inject drugs and the impact of the type of epidemic; extrapolating from Amsterdam, The Netherlands. PLoS One 2016;11(10): e0163488.

35. Tapper EB, Bacon BR, Curry MP, et al. Real-world effectiveness for 12 weeks of ledipasvir-sofosbuvir for genotype 1 hepatitis C: the Trio Health study. J Viral Hepat 2016;24(1):22–7.

36. Younossi ZM, Park H, Gordon SC, et al. Real-world outcomes of ledipasvir/sofosbuvir in treatment-naive patients with hepatitis C. Am J Manag Care 2016; 22(6 Spec No):SP205–11.

37. Thokala P, Simpson EL, Tappenden P, et al. Ledipasvir-sofosbuvir for treating chronic hepatitis C: a NICE single technology Appraisal-an evidence review group perspective. Pharmacoeconomics 2016;34(8):741–50.

38. Borgia SM, Rowaiye A. Increased eligibility for treatment of chronic hepatitis C infection with shortened duration of therapy: implications for access to care and elimination strategies in Canada. Can J Gastroenterol Hepatol 2015;29(3): 125–9.

39. Gimeno-Ballester V, Mar J, O'Leary A, et al. Cost-effectiveness analysis of therapeutic options for chronic hepatitis C genotype 3 infected patients. Expert Rev Gastroenterol Hepatol 2017;11(1):85–93.

40. Igarashi A, Tang W, Guerra I, et al. Cost-utility analysis of ledipasvir/sofosbuvir for the treatment of genotype 1 chronic hepatitis C in Japan. Curr Med Res Opin 2017;33(1):11–21.

41. Igarashi A, Tang W, Cure S, et al. Cost-utility analysis of sofosbuvir for the treatment of genotype 2 chronic hepatitis C in Japan. Curr Med Res Opin 2017; 33(1):1–10.

42. Virabhak S, Yasui K, Yamazaki K, et al. Cost-effectiveness of direct-acting antiviral regimen ombitasvir/paritaprevir/ritonavir in treatment-naïve and treatment-experienced patients infected with chronic hepatitis C virus genotype 1b in Japan. J Med Econ 2016;19(12):1144–56.

43. Chen GF, Wei L, Chen J, et al. Will sofosbuvir/ledipasvir (Harvoni) be cost-effective and affordable for Chinese patients infected with hepatitis C virus? An economic analysis using real-world data. PLoS One 2016;11(6):e0155934.

44. Fraser I, Burger J, Lubbe M, et al. Cost-effectiveness modelling of sofosbuvir-containing regimens for chronic genotype 5 hepatitis C virus infection in South Africa. Pharmacoeconomics 2016;34(4):403–17.

45. Pantiri K, Westerhout KY, Obando CA. Cost-effectiveness analysis of simeprevir and sofosbuvir combination therapy for the treatment of genotype 1 HCV patients in the Dominican Republic. Value Health 2015;18(7):A872.

46. Puri P, Anand AC, Saraswat VA, et al. Indian national association for study of the liver (INASL) guidance for antiviral therapy against HCV infection in 2015. J Clin Exp Hepatol 2015;5(3):221–38.

47. Kim DD, Hutton DW, Raouf AA, et al. Cost-effectiveness model for hepatitis C screening and treatment: implications for Egypt and other countries with high prevalence. Glob Public Health 2015;10(3):296–317.

48. Andrieux-Meyer I, Cohn J, de Araújo ES, et al. Disparity in market prices for hepatitis C virus direct-acting drugs. Lancet Glob Health 2015;3(11):e676–7.

49. Younossi ZM, Tanaka A, Eguchi Y, et al. The impact of hepatitis C virus outside the liver: evidence from Asia. Liver Int 2016;37(2):159–72.

50. Barua S, Greenwald R, Grebely J, et al. Restrictions for Medicaid reimbursement of sofosbuvir for the treatment of hepatitis C virus infection in the United States. Ann Intern Med 2015;163(3):215–23.

51. Younossi ZM, Bacon BR, Dieterich DT, et al. Disparate access to treatment regimens in chronic hepatitis C patients: data from the TRIO network. J Viral Hepat 2016;23(6):447–54.

52. Stepanova M, Younossi ZM. Interferon-free regimens for chronic hepatitis C: barriers due to treatment candidacy and insurance coverage. Dig Dis Sci 2015;60(11):3248–51.

53. Faria R, Woods B, Griffin S, et al. Prevention of progression to cirrhosis in hepatitis C with fibrosis: effectiveness and cost effectiveness of sequential therapy with new direct-acting anti-virals. Aliment Pharmacol Ther 2016;44(8):866–76.

54. Iyengar S, Tay-Teo K, Vogler S, et al. Prices, costs, and affordability of new medicines for hepatitis C in 30 countries: an economic analysis. PLoS Med 2016; 13(5):e1002032.

55. Zoulim F, Liang TJ, Gerbes AL, et al. Hepatitis C virus treatment in the real world: optimising treatment and access to therapies. Gut 2015;64(11):1824–33.

56. Hill A, Simmons B, Gotham D, et al. Rapid reductions in prices for generic sofosbuvir and daclatasvir to treat hepatitis C. J Virus Erad 2016;2(1):28–31.

57. Leigh JP, Bowlus CL, Leistikow BN, et al. Costs of hepatitis C. Arch Intern Med 2001;161(18):2231–7.
58. Shah BB, Wong JB. The economics of hepatitis C virus. Clin Liver Dis 2006; 10(4):717–34.
59. Razavi H, Elkhoury AC, Elbasha E, et al. Chronic hepatitis C virus (HCV) disease burden and cost in the United States. Hepatology 2013;57(6):2164–70.
60. Rein DB, Borton J, Liffmann DK, et al. The burden of hepatitis C to the United States Medicare system in 2009: descriptive and economic characteristics. Hepatology 2016;63(4):1135–44.
61. McAdam-Marx C, McGarry LJ, Hane CA, et al. All-cause and incremental per patient per year cost associated with chronic hepatitis C virus and associated liver complications in the United States: a managed care perspective. J Manag Care Pharm 2011;17(7):531–46.
62. Wai H, Stepanova M, Saab S, et al. Inpatient economic and mortality assessment for liver transplantation: a nationwide study of the United States data from 2005 to 2009. Transplantation 2014;97(1):98–103.
63. El Khoury AC, Klimack WK, Wallace C, et al. Economic burden of hepatitis C-associated diseases in the United States. J Viral Hepat 2012;19(3):153–60.
64. Stepanova M, Mishra A, Venkatesan C, et al. In-hospital mortality and economic burden associated with hepatic encephalopathy in the United States from 2005 to 2009. Clin Gastroenterol Hepatol 2012;10(9):1034–41.e1.
65. Holmberg SD, Spradling PR, Moorman AC, et al. Hepatitis C in the United States. N Engl J Med 2013;368(20):1859–61.
66. Chhatwal J, Wang X, Ayer T, et al. Hepatitis C Disease Burden in the United States in the era of oral direct-acting antivirals. Hepatology 2016;64(5):1442–50.
67. Singer ME, Younossi ZM. Cost effectiveness of screening for hepatitis C virus in asymptomatic, average-risk adults. Am J Med 2001;111(8):614–21.
68. Younossi ZM, Blissett D, Blissett R, et al. In the era of highly effective direct acting anti-viral Agents, screening the entire United States population for hepatitis C is cost effective. Hepatology 2016;64(1 Suppl):369A.
69. Younossi ZM, LaLuna LL, Santoro JJ, et al. Implementation of baby boomer hepatitis C screening and linking to care in gastroenterology practices: a multicenter pilot study. BMC Gastroenterol 2016;16:45.
70. Marcellusi A, Viti R, Capone A, et al. The economic burden of HCV-induced diseases in Italy. A probabilistic cost of illness model. Eur Rev Med Pharmacol Sci 2015;19(9):1610–20.
71. Vandijck D, Moreno C, Stärkel P, et al. Current and future health and economic impact of hepatitis C in Belgium. Acta Gastroenterol Belg 2014;77(2):285–90.
72. Müllhaupt B, Bruggmann P, Bihl F, et al. Modeling the health and economic burden of hepatitis C virus in Switzerland. PLoS One 2015;10(6):e0125214.
73. Vietri J, Prajapati G, El Khoury AC. The burden of hepatitis C in Europe from the patients' perspective: a survey in 5 countries. BMC Gastroenterol 2013;13:16.
74. Myers RP, Krajden M, Bilodeau M, et al. Burden of disease and cost of chronic hepatitis C infection in Canada. Can J Gastroenterol Hepatol 2014;28(5): 243–50.
75. Zare F, Fattahi MR, Sepehrimanesh M, et al. Economic burden of hepatitis C virus infection in different stages of disease: a report from southern Iran. Hepat Mon 2016;16(4):e32654.
76. Estes C, Abdel-Kareem M, Abdel-Razek W, et al. Economic burden of hepatitis C in Egypt: the future impact of highly effective therapies. Aliment Pharmacol Ther 2015;42(6):696–706.

77. Sievert W, Razavi H, Estes C, et al. Enhanced antiviral treatment efficacy and uptake in preventing the rising burden of hepatitis C-related liver disease and costs in Australia. J Gastroenterol Hepatol 2014;29(Suppl 1):1–9.

78. Liu GG, DiBonaventura MD, Yuan Y, et al. The burden of illness for patients with viral hepatitis C: evidence from a national survey in Japan. Value Health 2012; 15(1 Suppl):S65–71.

79. Messina JP, Humphreys I, Flaxman A, et al. Global distribution and prevalence of hepatitis C virus genotypes. Hepatology 2015;61(1):77–87.

80. Féray C. Is HCV infection a neurologic disorder? Gastroenterology 2012;142(3): 428–31.

81. Younossi Z, Park H, Henry L, et al. Extrahepatic manifestations of hepatitis C: a meta-analysis of prevalence, quality of life, and economic burden. Gastroenterology 2016;150(7):1599–608.

82. Cacoub P, Vautier M, Desbois AC, et al. Direct medical costs associated with the extrahepatic manifestations of hepatitis C infection in France. Hepatology 2016; 64(1 Suppl):376A–7A.

83. Jacobson IM, Cacoub P, Dal Maso L, et al. Manifestations of chronic hepatitis C virus infection beyond the liver. Clin Gastroenterol Hepatol 2010;8(12):1017–29.

84. Ferri C, Ramos-Casals M, Zignego AL, et al. International diagnostic guidelines for patients with HCV-related extrahepatic manifestations. A multidisciplinary expert statement. Autoimmun Rev 2016;15(12):1145–60.

85. Rotily M, Vainchtock A, Jouaneton B, et al. How did chronic hepatitis C impact costs related to hospital health care in France in 2009? Clin Res Hepatol Gastroenterol 2013;37(4):365–72.

86. Nagao Y, Tanaka J, Nakanishi T, et al. High incidence of extrahepatic manifestations in an HCV hyperendemic area. Hepatol Res 2002;22(1):27–36.

87. Nuño Solinís R, Arratibel Ugarte P, Rojo A, et al. Value of treating all stages of chronic hepatitis C: a comprehensive review of clinical and economic evidence. Infect Dis Ther 2016;5(4):491–508.

88. Younossi ZM, Stepanova M, Henry L, et al. The prevalence and costs associated with clinically overt extrahepatic manifestations of hepatitis C virus infection in Japan. In Proc. of the 26th Conference of the Asian Pacific Association for the Study of the Liver (APASL'2017), Shanghai, China, February 15–19, 2017.

89. Cacoub P, Gragnani L, Comarmond C, et al. Extrahepatic manifestations of chronic hepatitis C virus infection. Dig Liver Dis 2014;46(Suppl 5):S165–73.

90. Sievert W, Altraif I, Razavi HA, et al. A systematic review of hepatitis C virus epidemiology in Asia, Australia and Egypt. Liver Int 2011;31(Suppl 2):61–80.

91. Bruggmann P, Berg T, Øvrehus AL, et al. SJ. Historical epidemiology of hepatitis C virus (HCV) in selected countries. J Viral Hepat 2014;21(Suppl 1):5–33.

92. Stepanova M, De Avila L, Afendy M, et al. Direct and indirect economic burden of chronic liver disease in the United States. Clin Gastroenterol Hepatol 2016. http://dx.doi.org/10.1016/j.cgh.2016.07.020.

93. Scalone L, Fagiuoli S, Ciampichini R, et al. The societal burden of chronic liver diseases: results from the COME study. BMJ Open Gastroenterol 2015;2(1): e000025.

94. John-Baptiste AA, Tomlinson G, Hsu PC, et al. Sustained responders have better quality of life and productivity compared with treatment failures long after antiviral therapy for hepatitis C. Am J Gastroenterol 2009;104(10):2439–48.

95. Mauss S, Petersen J, Witthoeft T, et al. Sustained responders have lower rates of liver-related events and a better quality of life and productivity compared with

non-responders/relapsers after antiviral treatment of chronic hepatitis C. Hepatology 2012;56(4 Suppl):582A–3A.

96. Gosselin E, Lemyre L, Corneil W. Presenteeism and absenteeism: differentiated understanding of related phenomena. J Occup Health Psychol 2013;18(1): 75–86.

97. Younossi I, Weinstein A, Stepanova M, et al. Mental and emotional impairment in patients with hepatitis C is related to lower work productivity. Psychosomatics 2016;57(1):82–8.

98. Younossi ZM, Stepanova M, Henry L, et al. Association of work productivity with clinical and patient-reported factors in patients infected with hepatitis C virus. J Viral Hepat 2016;23(8):623–30.

99. Baran RW, Samp JC, Walker DR, et al. Costs and absence of HCV-infected employees by disease stage. J Med Econ 2015;18(9):691–703.

100. Su J, Brook RA, Kleinman NL, et al. The impact of hepatitis C virus infection on work absence, productivity, and healthcare benefit costs. Hepatology 2010; 52(2):436–42.

101. DiBonaventura MD, Wagner JS, Yuan Y, et al. The impact of hepatitis C on labor force participation, absenteeism, presenteeism and non-work activities. J Med Econ 2011;14(2):253–61.

102. Zalesak M, Francis K, Gedeon A, et al. Current and future disease progression of the chronic HCV population in the United States. PLoS One 2013;8(5): e63959.

103. Younossi ZM, Stepanova M, Henry L, et al. An in-depth analysis of patient-reported outcomes in patients with chronic hepatitis C treated with different anti-viral regimens. Am J Gastroenterol 2016;111(6):808–16.

104. Younossi ZM, Jiang Y, Smith NJ, et al. Ledipasvir/sofosbuvir regimens for chronic hepatitis C infection: insights from a work productivity economic model from the United States. Hepatology 2015;61(5):1471–8.

105. Younossi Z, Brown A, Buti M, et al. Impact of eradicating hepatitis C virus on the work productivity of chronic hepatitis C (CH-C) patients: an economic model from five European countries. J Viral Hepat 2016;23(3):217–26.

106. Gower E, Estes C, Blach S, et al. Global epidemiology and genotype distribution of the hepatitis C virus infection. J Hepatol 2014;61(1 Suppl):S45–57.

107. Younossi ZM, Chan HLY, Dan YY, et al. Impact of ledipasvir/sofosbuvir on the work productivity of chronic hepatitis C patients in Asia. In Proc. of the Annual Meeting of the Asian Pacific Association for the Study of the Liver (APASL'2016), Tokyo, Japan, February 20-24, 2017.

108. El-Shabrawi MH, Kamal NM. Burden of pediatric hepatitis C. World J Gastroenterol 2013;19(44):7880–8.

109. Younossi ZM, Stepanova M, Balistreri W, et al. High efficacy and significant improvement of quality of life (QoL) in adolescent patients with hepatitis C genotype 1 (GT1) treated with sofosbuvir (SOF) and ledipasvir (LDV). Hepatology 2016;64(1 Suppl):351A–2A.

110. Chen SL, Morgan TR. The natural history of hepatitis C virus (HCV) infection. Int J Med Sci 2006;3(2):47–52.

111. Younossi ZM, Stepanova M, Afendy M, et al. Changes in the prevalence of the most common causes of chronic liver diseases in the United States from 1988 to 2008. Clin Gastroenterol Hepatol 2011;9(6):524–30.e1.

112. Bruggmann P, Negro F, Bihl F, et al. Birth cohort distribution and screening for viraemic hepatitis C virus infections in Switzerland. Swiss Med Wkly 2015;145: w14221.

113. Coward S, Leggett L, Kaplan GG, et al. Cost-effectiveness of screening for hepatitis C virus: a systematic review of economic evaluations. BMJ Open 2016; 6(9):e011821.

114. Younossi ZM, Stepanova M, Afendy M, et al. Knowledge about infection is the only predictor of treatment in patients with chronic hepatitis C. J Viral Hepat 2013;20(8):550-5.

115. Branson BM, Handsfield HH, Lampe MA, et al. Revised recommendations for HIV testing of adults, adolescents, and pregnant women in health-care settings. MMWR Recomm Rep 2006;55(RR14):1-17.

Extrahepatic Manifestations of Hepatitis C Virus After Liver Transplantation

Robert J. Wong, MD, MS[a],*, Sammy Saab, MD, MPH[b,c],
Aijaz Ahmed, MD[d]

KEYWORDS

- Diabetes mellitus • Lymphoproliferative disorders • Health-related quality of life
- Chronic kidney disease • Liver transplantation

KEY POINTS

- Extrahepatic manifestations of chronic hepatitis C virus (HCV) infection in the posttransplant setting are equally important than those seen in the absence of liver transplantation.
- Increased risks of metabolic abnormalities, especially diabetes mellitus, are compounded in the posttransplant setting.
- Although chronic HCV infection increases risk of lymphoproliferative disorders, these risks can be exacerbated by the increased risk of posttransplant Epstein–Barr virus–associated lymphoproliferative disorders.
- Understanding and addressing health-related quality of life impairments associated with chronic HCV is particularly important in the posttransplant setting.

INTRODUCTION

Chronic hepatitis C virus (HCV) infection remains a leading cause of chronic liver disease and is one of the leading causes of cirrhosis and hepatocellular carcinoma

Disclosure: Dr. S Saab is a consultant and is on the speaker's bureau for Gilead and Bristol Myers Squibb; Dr. A Ahmed is a consultant, is on the advisory board, and receives research grants from Gilead. Dr. R Wong is a consultant, is on the advisory board, speaker's bureau and receives research grants from Gilead.
[a] Division of Gastroenterology and Hepatology, Alameda Health System – Highland Hospital, 1411 East 31st Street, Highland Hospital – Highland Care Pavilion 5th Floor, Oakland, CA 94602, USA; [b] Department of Medicine, David Geffen School of Medicine, University of California at Los Angeles, 200 UCLA Medical Plaza, Suite 214, Los Angeles, CA 90095, USA; [c] Department of Surgery, David Geffen School of Medicine, University of California at Los Angeles, 200 UCLA Medical Plaza, Suite 214, Los Angeles, CA 90095, USA; [d] Division of Gastroenterology and Hepatology, Stanford University School of Medicine, 750 Welch Road, Suite # 210, Palo Alto, CA 94304, USA
* Corresponding author.
E-mail address: Rowong@alamedahealthsystem.org

requiring liver transplantation.[1-3] Although the emergence of highly effective antiviral therapies for the treatment of chronic HCV has revolutionized the treatment approach, leading to successful cure rates of greater than 90% to 95% associated with current available treatment regimens, there remains a large cohort of patients with HCV cirrhosis that will still progress to need for liver transplantation.[1,4] In addition, although highly effective therapies are available, barriers in access to these therapies will continue to contribute to HCV disease progression to cirrhosis and hepatocellular carcinoma.[5,6]

Several studies have reported on the beneficial effects of HCV cure, not only in terms of the benefits and improvements in hepatic disease, but improvements in extrahepatic and systemic manifestations of chronic HCV are also well-studied.[6,7] In particular, several recent studies have demonstrated significant improvements in patient-reported outcomes achieved with successful HCV treatment.[7-10] Despite these successes, disease progression to need for liver transplantation is not averted in all patients, and few studies have specifically evaluated extrahepatic manifestations of chronic HCV after liver transplantation. There is much debate on the optimal timing of HCV treatment among those awaiting liver transplantation. However, treatment of chronic HCV after liver transplantation is no longer a significant hurdle and the vast armamentarium of treatment options with short duration and high efficacy have made it much easier to achieve HCV cure in this population.[11-13]

The extrahepatic manifestations of chronic HCV in the posttransplant setting are similar to the manifestations exhibited in the pretransplant setting.[7,14-18] However, the overall milieu of the posttransplant state may interact with HCV such that certain extrahepatic manifestations become more relevant clinically and may impact the patient to a greater extent. As such, the current review focuses on the extrahepatic manifestations of chronic HCV that may be exacerbated in the posttransplant milieu (**Table 1**).

METABOLIC ABNORMALITIES

Significant metabolic abnormalities associated with chronic HCV infection are well-reported, with insulin resistance in the form of impaired glucose tolerance or diabetes mellitus having the greatest impact.[14,15,19-21] A recent metaanalysis evaluating the prevalence and burden of extrahepatic manifestations of chronic HCV included 31 studies evaluating the association of diabetes mellitus and chronic HCV.[15] Among these studies, which included 61,843 chronic HCV patients, the pooled prevalence of diabetes mellitus was 15% (95% confidence interval, 13–18) among chronic HCV patients compared with 10% (95% confidence interval, 6–15) among non-HCV controls. Furthermore, the authors calculated a pooled odds ratio of 1.58 (95% confidence interval, 1.30–1.86) for the association of DM in chronic HCV patients.[6] Despite being the second most common extrahepatic manifestation of chronic HCV, concurrent diabetes mellitus carries a much greater clinical burden given that it also increases risk of cardiovascular disease and chronic renal disease.[16,17,22,23] The prevalence of concurrent diabetes mellitus may also contribute to a higher risk of concurrent nonalcoholic fatty liver disease, which in the setting of chronic HCV contributes to more aggressive disease progression to cirrhosis and hepatocellular carcinoma. For example, 2 recent systematic reviews evaluated the impact of concurrent diabetes on the risk of disease progression and risk of hepatocellular carcinoma among chronic HCV patients.[24,25] Among a total of 20 observation studies included in the final analyses, the authors observed that concurrent obesity (odds ratio, 1.08–7.69), the presence of significant steatosis (odds ratio, 1.80–14.3), and concurrent diabetes mellitus (odds ratio,

Table 1
Extrahepatic manifestations of chronic HCV that are exacerbated in the post-liver transplant setting

Extrahepatic Manifestations	Features of the Posttransplant Environment that Increase the Risk and Severity
Insulin resistance	Glucocorticoid-related insulin resistance Direct pancreatic islet cell injury by calcineurin inhibitors and cyclosporine have been reported
Cardiovascular events	Immunosuppression regimens may increase risk of cardiovascular risk factors, including hypertension and dyslipidemia Increased risk of insulin resistance may further affect cardiovascular risk Increased risk of posttransplant steatosis from immunosuppression regimens may increase cardiovascular disease risk
Lymphoproliferative diseases	Posttransplant immunosuppression may allow dysregulated lymphoproliferation Specifically, Epstein–Barr virus–associated lymphoproliferative disorders is propagated by immunosuppression
Renal diseases	Potential nephrotoxicity of posttransplant immunosuppression regimen, including calcineurin inhibitors Appropriate selection of direct acting antivirals for treatment of chronic HCV in the posttransplant setting must take into account presence of advanced renal dysfunction
Mixed cryoglobulinemia	Nephrotoxic risks in the posttransplant setting, including those related to HCV and immunosuppression may further exacerbate cryoglobulinemia associated renal dysfunction
Health-related quality of life	Postoperative complications and prolonged hospitalization can contribute to psychosocial impairments including depression

Abbreviation: HCV, hepatitis C virus.

2.25–9.24) were all associated with an increased risk of advanced fibrosis among chronic HCV patients.[25] In a subsequent analysis, the same group evaluated the impact of concurrent metabolic abnormalities on the risk of developing hepatocellular carcinoma among chronic HCV patients and only observed a significantly increased risk associated with concurrent diabetes mellitus.[24] Thus, the combined effects of metabolic derangements associated with chronic HCV are far reaching. Furthermore, the presence of metabolic abnormalities, whether coexisting or directly caused by chronic HCV infection, also affects posttransplant mortality.[26,27] Using the 2003 to 2013 United Network for Organ Sharing Organ Procurement and Transplant Network registry data, Aguilar and colleagues[26] demonstrated that concurrent diabetes mellitus was associated with a 22% higher posttransplant mortality when compared with patients without diabetes mellitus. In light of the multitude of negative effects associated with diabetes mellitus, the estimated economic burden of diabetes among chronic HCV patients is in excess of $440 million annually.[15]

Although it is clear that concurrent diabetes among chronic HCV patients contributes to increased morbidity and mortality, the risk of concurrent diabetes and the consequences of diabetes are perhaps even more significant in the posttransplant state.[26,28,29] Previous studies have reported on the increased risk of de novo diabetes mellitus and steatosis after liver transplantation.[19,30–32] The prevalence of posttransplant new-onset diabetes mellitus ranged from 13% to 28%.[19,32–34] Although there are several risk factors for de novo diabetes mellitus in the posttransplant setting, the immunosuppression regimen can contribute to significant metabolic derangements, including diabetes mellitus.[34–36] It has been observed that calcineurin inhibitors may promote de novo development of diabetes mellitus through direct injury to the pancreatic islet cells. In addition, both tacrolimus and cyclosporine have been implicated in potential islet cell injury that may promote insulin resistance in the post-transplant setting.[35,36] The increased risk of concurrent diabetes associated with posttransplant risk factors is compounded further with the potential diabetogenic risks of chronic HCV infection in the posttransplant setting.[32,37]

The increased risk of diabetes associated with chronic HCV and the posttransplant setting also contribute to increased risks of cardiovascular disease.[22,23] This is particularly important given that chronic HCV infection itself has been shown to increase the risk of cardiovascular disease and stroke.[6,23] Although several studies have evaluated this association, a recent metaanalysis demonstrated a 20% increased odds of cardiovascular disease associated with chronic HCV infection and a 35% increased odds of developing stroke.[15] This extrahepatic manifestation of chronic HCV is especially relevant in the posttransplant setting, because many additional factors contribute to an environment that increases the risks of cardiovascular events. The increased risks of metabolic derangements in the posttransplant setting including hypertension, dyslipidemia, and diabetes mellitus further compound the risk of cardiovascular events.[19,38–40] Furthermore, there is an increased risk of concurrent nonalcoholic fatty liver disease in posttransplant patients, even when the initial etiology of chronic liver disease was not related to nonalcoholic fatty liver disease.[41–44] This further complicates the clinical scenario given that nonalcoholic fatty liver disease itself is well-correlated with an increased risk of cardiovascular disease, such that one of the leading causes of morbidity and mortality among nonalcoholic fatty liver disease patients is cardiovascular related.[45–49] A recent metaanalysis by Targher and colleagues[49] included a total of 16 observational studies evaluating the association of nonalcoholic fatty liver disease with the incidence cardiovascular disease. Over a mean period of 6.9 years in the pooled analysis, patients with nonalcoholic fatty liver disease had a 64% increased risk of fatal and/or nonfatal cardiovascular disease. Thus, the risk of cardiovascular disease is affected by multiple factors, and the convergence of these factors among chronic HCV patients in the posttransplant setting highlights the importance of better understanding disease prevalence and risk factors.

Although the increased cardiovascular disease risk in the posttransplant setting is likely multifactorial, reflecting the combined effects of immunosuppression-related effects on hypertension, dyslipidemia, and insulin resistance, the etiology of the increased risk of cardiovascular disease associated with chronic HCV is not well-defined.[14,23] Previous studies have suggested that HCV itself may have proatherogenic effects.[50–52] Specifically, prior observational studies report an increased risk of carotid atherosclerosis associated with chronic HCV infection, and this increased risk persisted even after correcting for the potential confounding effect of hepatic steatosis.[53] However, other studies suggest that HCV promotes cardiovascular risk through proinflammatory pathways, such that increased systemic inflammatory cascade contributes to increased atherosclerosis development.[53,54] Nevertheless, regardless of the mechanism of action, the increased risk of cardiovascular disease among chronic HCV patients is real, and this may be especially significant in the posttransplant setting.

LYMPHOPROLIFERATIVE DISORDERS

The risks of lymphoproliferative disorders among chronic HCV patients have been well-reported. Several studies in various cohorts have demonstrated an increased risk of non-Hodgkin lymphoma among patients chronically infected with HCV.[55–58]

Most recently, the results of a large metaanalysis identified 16 studies that investigated the association between chronic HCV and lymphoproliferative disorders.[6] Among these pooled studies, the risk of lymphoma was 60% higher among patients with chronic HCV when compared with non-HCV controls. Although the exact mechanism of this increased risk is poorly understood, several hypotheses have been raised. One thought purports that chronic stimulation of lymphocytes via persistent untreated HCV over time leads to dysregulated proliferation that contributes to a pathogenic lymphoproliferative state.[59–61] Another theory suggests that viral replication of HCV within B cells may have a direct oncogenic effect such that it also contributes to a dysregulated growth and replication leading to uncontrolled proliferation.[62,63]

The increased risk of lymphoproliferative disorders associated with chronic HCV is particularly important in the posttransplant setting, given that the certain immunosuppression regimens in the posttransplant setting may also contribute to increased risk of lymphoproliferative disorders.[64] The overall prevalence of posttransplant lymphoproliferative disorders is as high as 20% in some studies.[64,65] However, the risk is relatively lower among post-liver transplant patients compared with patients who receive lung and heart transplants. However, despite the relative lower risk of posttransplant lymphoproliferative disorders in renal and liver transplant recipients, given that the majority of solid organ transplants in the United States are those involving kidney and liver, the overall burden of posttransplant lymphoproliferative disorders among post-liver transplant patients is much greater. The overall incidence of posttransplant lymphoproliferative disorders among liver transplant recipients has ranged from 0.8% to 3.6% in some studies.[64,65] Lymphoproliferative disorders in the posttransplant setting are thought to be propagated through Epstein–Barr virus (EBV) infection.[66] The immunosuppressed state in the posttransplant patient allows uncontrolled EBV-associated promotion of lymphoproliferation. Although difficult to manage in the posttransplant setting, with the need to balance the importance of immunosuppression for the prevention of solid organ rejection and the need to balance pulling back on immunosuppression to better control the EBV-associated consequences, the concurrence of chronic HCV infection can pose an even more difficult dilemma. As such, the combined risk of lymphoproliferative disorders in the posttransplant setting is an important extrahepatic manifestation of chronic HCV to be particularly cognizant of.

RENAL DISORDERS

The risk of kidney injury associated with chronic HCV infection is a particularly complex extrahepatic manifestation, given that HCV contributes to renal dysfunction through a variety of mechanisms.[67] One of the more prevalent extrahepatic manifestations of chronic HCV, mixed cryoglobulinemia, is a vasculitis that contributes directly to renal dysfunction.[7,16,17] The presence of mixed cryoglobulinemia further exacerbates the risk of HCV-related renal disease. Even in the absence of cryoglobulinemia, HCV-associated glomerulonephritis has been well-documented. Furthermore, as previously mentioned, HCV contributes to increased risk of diabetes mellitus, and the negative impact of chronic insulin resistance on the development of chronic renal dysfunction is also well-established.[20,37] In a recent metaanalysis that included 14 studies specifically evaluating the association of chronic HCV infection with development of chronic renal disease, the authors demonstrated a 26% increased risk of having renal disease progression among chronic HCV patients compared with non-HCV controls.[6] A multicenter study using data from the Multinational Observational Study in Transplantation (MOST) evaluated predictors of post-liver transplantation renal dysfunction. On multivariate analysis, positivity for chronic HCV was an independent predictor of posttransplant renal dysfunction even after correcting for baseline serum creatinine levels before liver transplantation.[68] The increased risk of chronic kidney disease associated with HCV is particularly important in the posttransplant setting given that immunosuppression with calcineurin inhibitors have also been reported to contribute to nephrotoxicity. Other immunosuppressive regimens including cyclosporine also need to be monitored closely in the setting of renal dysfunction.

Although renal disease is an important extrahepatic manifestation of chronic HCV, an equally important consideration is the management of chronic HCV in the post-kidney transplant setting. The significant burden of chronic HCV in the kidney transplant setting is demonstrated in a recent systematic review reporting up to a 10% chronic HCV prevalence among kidney transplant recipients.[69] Furthermore, the presence of concurrent chronic HCV in kidney transplant recipients is also associated with increased graft loss and overall posttransplant mortality.[70,71] Thus, the need for safe and effective therapies for eradicating HCV after kidney transplant are paramount to improve long-term outcomes. Before the availability of current direct-acting antiviral therapies, treatment of chronic HCV in the post-kidney transplant setting presented a dilemma given the high risk, including allograft rejection and loss together with the low effectiveness of antiviral therapies.[72,73] However, the current era of interferon-free and ribavirin-free regimens have demonstrated high efficacy and an acceptable safety profile in treating chronic HCV in the post-kidney transplant setting.[74–76]

MIXED CRYOGLOBULINEMIA

Another common extrahepatic manifestation of chronic HCV, mixed cryoglobulinemia has a reported prevalence ranging from 10% to nearly 50% among chronic HCV patients.[58] In addition to renal disease in the form of membranoproliferative glomerulonephritis, the clinical manifestations of mixed cryoglobulinemia reflect the systemic nature of this disease, ranging from mild symptoms of palpable purpura, weakness, and arthralgias to severe manifestations, such as pulmonary hemorrhage and central nervous system involvement.[16,18,58,77] Most commonly, though, skin, joints, and renal involvement are the primary manifestations of cryoglobulinemia. A recent metaanalysis that included 21 studies reported a pooled prevalence of 30.1% among chronic HCV patients compared with 1.9% among non-HCV populations.[15] However, this high prevalence of mixed cryoglobulinemia included both symptomatic and asymptomatic patients. The prevalence of symptomatic cryoglobulinemia is much lower at approximately 5% of chronic HCV patients.[15,58] Although the exact pathogenesis is not well-described, it has been hypothesized that chronic antigenic stimulation by the HCV contributes to risk of cryoglobulinemia in the same manner as the increased risk of HCV-related autoimmune and lymphoproliferative disorders.[58] In the post-liver transplant setting, the prevalence of mixed cryoglobulinemia is also similarly high, with some studies reporting prevalence of nearly 50%, with 20% of those patients reporting symptomatic cryoglobulinemia.[77–79] Furthermore, concurrent cryoglobulinemia in the posttransplant setting can further complicate the risk of acute kidney injury associated with HCV itself and concurrent immunosuppression therapies. However, the current era of highly effective direct acting antivirals have demonstrated success in treatment HCV-associated mixed cryoglobulinemia, thus emphasizing the importance of early recognition of this extrahepatic manifestation to that timely therapy can be initiated.[80]

HEALTH-RELATED QUALITY OF LIFE

The importance of health-related quality of life assessment among patients with chronic HCV is becoming more important as we realize the encompassing negative impact of untreated HCV infection.[6,7,81] The emphasis on health-related quality of life assessment reflects the perceived impact on patients' overall well-being, including both physical and mental health.

Understanding and addressing the impact of disease processes on health-related quality of life is not only important to consider the holistic approach to improving patient outcomes, but also that impairments in health-related quality of life has been demonstrated to contribute to significant economic deficits resulting from decreased productivity or increased use of health care resources.[6,81–83] A recent metaanalysis evaluating the impact of HCV on health-related quality of life demonstrated that, among the physical health domains, the lowest scores were seen among the general health categories.[6] Among the mental health domains, HCV patients scored the lowest in those categories assessing social functioning. Overall scores were lower in HCV patients when compared with their non-HCV counterparts.[6] Furthermore, fatigue, also an important factor that affects health-related quality of life, was found to be significantly more prominent among HCV patients compared with healthy controls.[81,82,84] The prevalence of concurrent depression as a potential manifestation of chronic HCV has also been evaluated, and the pooled risk assessment observed that chronic HCV patients were more than twice as likely as non-HCV controls to have significant depression.[6] Assessment of health-related quality of life is equally important in the posttransplant setting and the interplay between impaired quality of life associated with chronic HCV can be compounded by the quality of life impairments seen after liver transplantation.[85–89] The concurrence of chronic HCV in this posttransplant setting may further contribute to decreased quality of life.

The economic burden of extrahepatic manifestations is particularly significant in the post-liver transplant setting. Among all chronic HCV patients, the total direct medical costs associated with management of extrahepatic manifestations of chronic HCV was estimated at \$1.5 billion in 2014, with HCV-associated diabetes mellitus (\$443.4 million) and HCV-related depression (\$430.7 million) account for the leading comorbidities in terms of direct medical costs.[15] The negative impact of extrahepatic manifestations in posttransplant patients can further exacerbate this economic burden, leading to prolonged hospitalization, increased use of outpatient resources, and overall worse posttransplant outcomes.

SUMMARY

It has become more apparent that the detrimental effects of untreated chronic HCV infection extend beyond the hepatic manifestations and extrahepatic manifestations impart significant health consequences for patients. These extrahepatic manifestations in the posttransplant setting are particularly important given that the posttransplant setting itself contributes to and potentially compounds the detrimental effects. Furthermore, the highly immunosuppressed environment of the posttransplant setting not only contributes to increased metabolic abnormalities, but increases the risk for EBV-associated lymphoproliferative disorders. Chronic kidney disease and mixed-type cryoglobulinemia is also important to consider in the posttransplant setting, given the multitude of factors contributing to renal dysfunction, both HCV related and non–HCV related. This is particularly important in its effect on appropriate adjustments to immunosuppressive regimens. Finally, the impact of chronic HCV infection on health-related quality of life is particularly important in the posttransplant setting given the tenuous physical and mental health affected by the stressors of undergoing successful liver transplantation.

REFERENCES

1. Hajarizadeh B, Grebely J, Dore GJ. Epidemiology and natural history of HCV infection. Nature reviews. Gastroenterol Hepatol 2013;10(9):553–62.
2. Wong RJ, Aguilar M, Cheung R, et al. Nonalcoholic steatohepatitis is the second leading etiology of liver disease among adults awaiting liver transplantation in the United States. Gastroenterology 2015;148(3):547–55.
3. Wong RJ, Cheung R, Ahmed A. Nonalcoholic steatohepatitis is the most rapidly growing indication for liver transplantation in patients with hepatocellular carcinoma in the U.S. Hepatology 2014;59(6):2188–95.
4. Thrift AP, El-Serag HB, Kanwal F. Global epidemiology and burden of HCV infection and HCV-related disease. Nat Rev Gastroenterol Hepatol 2016;14(2):122–32.
5. Saab S, Jimenez M, Fong T, et al. Accessibility to oral antiviral therapy for patients with chronic hepatitis C in the United States. J Clin Translational Hepatol 2016; 4(2):76–82.
6. Younossi ZM, Bacon BR, Dieterich DT, et al. Disparate access to treatment regimens in chronic hepatitis C patients: data from the TRIO network. J Viral Hepat 2016;23(6):447–54.
7. van der Meer AJ, Berenguer M. Reversion of disease manifestations after HCV eradication. J Hepatol 2016;65(1 Suppl):S95–108.
8. Younossi ZM, Stepanova M, Feld J, et al. Sofosbuvir/velpatasvir improves patient-reported outcomes in HCV patients: results from ASTRAL-1 placebo-controlled trial. J Hepatol 2016;65(1):33–9.
9. Younossi ZM, Stepanova M, Sulkowski M, et al. Sofosbuvir and ribavirin for treatment of chronic hepatitis C in patients coinfected with hepatitis C virus and HIV: the impact on patient-reported outcomes. J Infect Dis 2015;212(3):367–77.
10. Younossi ZM, Stepanova M, Chan HL, et al. Patient-reported outcomes in Asian patients with chronic hepatitis C treated with ledipasvir and sofosbuvir. Medicine 2016;95(9):e2702.
11. Chhatwal J, Samur S, Kues B, et al. Optimal timing of hepatitis C treatment for patients on the liver transplant waiting list. Hepatology 2016;65(3):777–88.
12. Kwok RM, Ahn J, Schiano TD, et al. Sofosbuvir plus ledispasvir for recurrent hepatitis C in liver transplant recipients. Liver Transpl 2016;22(11):1536–43.
13. Elfeki M, Abou Mrad R, Modaresi Esfeh J, et al. Sofosbuvir/Ledipasvir without ribavirin achieved high sustained virologic response for hepatitis C recurrence after liver transplantation: two-center experience. Transplantation 2016. [Epub ahead of print].
14. Wong RJ, Gish RG. Metabolic manifestations and complications associated with chronic hepatitis C virus infection. Gastroenterol Hepatol 2016;12(5):293–9.
15. Younossi Z, Park H, Henry L, et al. Extrahepatic manifestations of hepatitis C: a meta-analysis of prevalence, quality of life, and economic burden. Gastroenterology 2016;150(7):1599–608.
16. Vigano M, Colombo M. Extrahepatic manifestations of hepatitis C virus. Gastroenterol Clin North Am 2015;44(4):775–91.
17. Negro F, Forton D, Craxi A, et al. Extrahepatic morbidity and mortality of chronic hepatitis C. Gastroenterology 2015;149(6):1345–60.

18. Ferri C, Ramos-Casals M, Zignego AL, et al. International diagnostic guidelines for patients with HCV-related extrahepatic manifestations. A multidisciplinary expert statement. Autoimmun Rev 2016;15(12):1145–60.
19. Barnard A, Konyn P, Saab S. Medical management of metabolic complications of liver transplant recipients. Gastroenterol Hepatol 2016;12(10):601–8.
20. Kralj D, Virovic Jukic L, Stojsavljevic S, et al. Hepatitis C virus, insulin resistance, and steatosis. J Clin Translational Hepatol 2016;4(1):66–75.
21. Garcia-Compean D, Gonzalez-Gonzalez JA, Lavalle-Gonzalez FJ, et al. Current concepts in diabetes mellitus and chronic liver disease: clinical outcomes, hepatitis C virus association, and therapy. Dig Dis Sci 2016;61(2):371–80.
22. Wong RJ, Kanwal F, Younossi ZM, et al. Hepatitis C virus infection and coronary artery disease risk: a systematic review of the literature. Dig Dis Sci 2014;59(7):1586–93.
23. Petta S, Maida M, Macaluso FS, et al. Hepatitis C virus infection is associated with increased cardiovascular mortality: a meta-analysis of observational studies. Gastroenterology 2016;150(1):145–55.e4 [quiz: e115–6].
24. Dyal HK, Aguilar M, Bartos G, et al. Diabetes mellitus increases risk of hepatocellular carcinoma in chronic hepatitis C virus patients: a systematic review. Dig Dis Sci 2016;61(2):636–45.
25. Dyal HK, Aguilar M, Bhuket T, et al. Concurrent obesity, diabetes, and steatosis increase risk of advanced fibrosis among HCV patients: a systematic review. Dig Dis Sci 2015;60(9):2813–24.
26. Aguilar M, Liu B, Holt EW, et al. Impact of obesity and diabetes on waitlist survival, probability of liver transplantation and post-transplant survival among chronic hepatitis C virus patients. Liver Int 2016;36(8):1167–75.
27. Huang TS, Lin CL, Shyu YC, et al. Diabetes, hepatocellular carcinoma, and mortality in hepatitis C-infected patients: a population-based cohort study. J Gastroenterol Hepatol 2016. [Epub ahead of print].
28. Gane EJ. Diabetes mellitus following liver transplantation in patients with hepatitis C virus: risks and consequences. Am J Transplant 2012;12(3):531–8.
29. Younossi ZM, Stepanova M, Saab S, et al. The impact of type 2 diabetes and obesity on the long-term outcomes of more than 85 000 liver transplant recipients in the US. Aliment Pharmacol Ther 2014;40(6):686–94.
30. Garcia-Pajares F, Penas-Herrero I, Sanchez-Ocana R, et al. Metabolic syndrome after liver transplantation: five-year prevalence and risk factors. Transplant Proc 2016;48(9):3010–2.
31. Saab S, Shpaner A, Zhao Y, et al. Prevalence and risk factors for diabetes mellitus in moderate term survivors of liver transplantation. Am J Transplant 2006;6(8):1890–5.
32. Baid S, Cosimi AB, Farrell ML, et al. Posttransplant diabetes mellitus in liver transplant recipients: risk factors, temporal relationship with hepatitis C virus allograft hepatitis, and impact on mortality. Transplantation 2001;72(6):1066–72.
33. Nair S, Verma S, Thuluvath PJ. Obesity and its effect on survival in patients undergoing orthotopic liver transplantation in the United States. Hepatology 2002;35(1):105–9.
34. Bianchi G, Marchesini G, Marzocchi R, et al. Metabolic syndrome in liver transplantation: relation to etiology and immunosuppression. Liver Transpl 2008;14(11):1648–54.
35. Drachenberg CB, Klassen DK, Weir MR, et al. Islet cell damage associated with tacrolimus and cyclosporine: morphological features in pancreas allograft biopsies and clinical correlation. Transplantation 1999;68(3):396–402.

36. Hjelmesaeth J, Hartmann A, Kofstad J, et al. Glucose intolerance after renal transplantation depends upon prednisolone dose and recipient age. Transplantation 1997;64(7):979–83.

37. Delgado-Borrego A, Casson D, Schoenfeld D, et al. Hepatitis C virus is independently associated with increased insulin resistance after liver transplantation. Transplantation 2004;77(5):703–10.

38. Fussner LA, Heimbach JK, Fan C, et al. Cardiovascular disease after liver transplantation: when, what, and who is at risk. Liver Transpl 2015;21(7):889–96.

39. Rabkin JM, Corless CL, Rosen HR, et al. Immunosuppression impact on long-term cardiovascular complications after liver transplantation. Am J Surg 2002; 183(5):595–9.

40. Desai S, Hong JC, Saab S. Cardiovascular risk factors following orthotopic liver transplantation: predisposing factors, incidence and management. Liver Int 2010;30(7):948–57.

41. Hejlova I, Honsova E, Sticova E, et al. Prevalence and risk factors of steatosis after liver transplantation and patient outcomes. Liver Transpl 2016;22(5):644–55.

42. Dumortier J, Giostra E, Belbouab S, et al. Non-alcoholic fatty liver disease in liver transplant recipients: another story of "seed and soil". Am J Gastroenterol 2010; 105(3):613–20.

43. Contos MJ, Cales W, Sterling RK, et al. Development of nonalcoholic fatty liver disease after orthotopic liver transplantation for cryptogenic cirrhosis. Liver Transpl 2001;7(4):363–73.

44. Kim H, Lee K, Lee KW, et al. Histologically proven non-alcoholic fatty liver disease and clinically related factors in recipients after liver transplantation. Clin Transplant 2014;28(5):521–9.

45. Ma J, Hwang SJ, Pedley A, et al. Bi-directional analysis between fatty liver and cardiovascular disease risk factors. J Hepatol 2016;66:390–7.

46. Targher G. Non-alcoholic fatty liver disease as driving force in coronary heart disease? Gut 2016;66(2):213–4.

47. Wu S, Wu F, Ding Y, et al. Association of non-alcoholic fatty liver disease with major adverse cardiovascular events: a systematic review and meta-analysis. Scientific Rep 2016;6:33386.

48. Chimakurthi CR, Rowe IA. Establishing the independence and clinical importance of non-alcoholic fatty liver disease as a risk factor for cardiovascular disease. J Hepatol 2016;65(6):1265–6.

49. Targher G, Byrne CD, Lonardo A, et al. Non-alcoholic fatty liver disease and risk of incident cardiovascular disease: a meta-analysis. J Hepatol 2016;65(3): 589–600.

50. Miyajima I, Kawaguchi T, Fukami A, et al. Chronic HCV infection was associated with severe insulin resistance and mild atherosclerosis: a population-based study in an HCV hyperendemic area. J Gastroenterol 2013;48(1):93–100.

51. Fukui M, Kitagawa Y, Nakamura N, et al. Hepatitis C virus and atherosclerosis in patients with type 2 diabetes. JAMA 2003;289(10):1245–6.

52. Maruyama S, Koda M, Oyake N, et al. Myocardial injury in patients with chronic hepatitis C infection. J Hepatol 2013;58(1):11–5.

53. Adinolfi LE, Restivo L, Zampino R, et al. Chronic HCV infection is a risk of atherosclerosis. Role of HCV and HCV-related steatosis. Atherosclerosis 2012;221(2): 496–502.

54. Oliveira CP, Kappel CR, Siqueira ER, et al. Effects of hepatitis C virus on cardiovascular risk in infected patients: a comparative study. Int J Cardiol 2013;164(2): 221–6.

55. Gisbert JP, Garcia-Buey L, Pajares JM, et al. Prevalence of hepatitis C virus infection in B-cell non-Hodgkin's lymphoma: systematic review and meta-analysis. Gastroenterology 2003;125(6):1723–32.
56. de Sanjose S, Benavente Y, Vajdic CM, et al. Hepatitis C and non-Hodgkin lymphoma among 4784 cases and 6269 controls from the International Lymphoma Epidemiology Consortium. Clin Gastroenterol Hepatol 2008;6(4):451–8.
57. Matsuo K, Kusano A, Sugumar A, et al. Effect of hepatitis C virus infection on the risk of non-Hodgkin's lymphoma: a meta-analysis of epidemiological studies. Cancer Sci 2004;95(9):745–52.
58. Martyak LA, Yeganeh M, Saab S. Hepatitis C and lymphoproliferative disorders: from mixed cryoglobulinemia to non-Hodgkin's lymphoma. Clin Gastroenterol Hepatol 2009;7(8):900–5.
59. Cacoub P, Gragnani L, Comarmond C, et al. Extrahepatic manifestations of chronic hepatitis C virus infection. Dig Liver Dis 2014;46(Suppl 5):S165–73.
60. Rasul I, Shepherd FA, Kamel-Reid S, et al. Detection of occult low-grade B-cell non-Hodgkin's lymphoma in patients with chronic hepatitis C infection and mixed cryoglobulinemia. Hepatology 1999;29(2):543–7.
61. Peveling-Oberhag J, Arcaini L, Hansmann ML, et al. Hepatitis C-associated B-cell non-Hodgkin lymphomas. Epidemiology, molecular signature and clinical management. J Hepatol 2013;59(1):169–77.
62. Zignego AL, Giannelli F, Marrocchi ME, et al. T(14;18) translocation in chronic hepatitis C virus infection. Hepatology 2000;31(2):474–9.
63. Ellis M, Rathaus M, Amiel A, et al. Monoclonal lymphocyte proliferation and bcl-2 rearrangement in essential mixed cryoglobulinaemia. Eur J Clin Invest 1995; 25(11):833–7.
64. Petrara MR, Giunco S, Serraino D, et al. Post-transplant lymphoproliferative disorders: from epidemiology to pathogenesis-driven treatment. Cancer Lett 2015; 369(1):37–44.
65. Morscio J, Dierickx D, Tousseyn T. Molecular pathogenesis of B-cell posttransplant lymphoproliferative disorder: what do we know so far? Clin Dev Immunol 2013;2013:150835.
66. Izadi M, Taheri S. Features, predictors and prognosis of lymphoproliferative disorders post-liver transplantation regarding disease presentation time: report from the PTLD.Int. survey. Ann Transplant 2011;16(1):39–47.
67. Park H, Adeyemi A, Henry L, et al. A meta-analytic assessment of the risk of chronic kidney disease in patients with chronic hepatitis C virus infection. J Viral Hepat 2015;22(11):897–905.
68. Burra P, Senzolo M, Masier A, et al. Factors influencing renal function after liver transplantation. Results from the MOST, an international observational study. Dig Liver Dis 2009;41(5):350–6.
69. Fabrizi F, Martin P, Dixit V, et al. Hepatitis C virus antibody status and survival after renal transplantation: meta-analysis of observational studies. Am J Transplant 2005;5(6):1452–61.
70. Mahmoud IM, Elhabashi AF, Elsawy E, et al. The impact of hepatitis C virus viremia on renal graft and patient survival: a 9-year prospective study. Am J Kidney Dis 2004;43(1):131–9.
71. Carpio R, Pamugas GE, Danguilan R, et al. Outcomes of renal allograft recipients with hepatitis C. Transplant Proc 2016;48(3):836–9.
72. Scott DR, Wong JK, Spicer TS, et al. Adverse impact of hepatitis C virus infection on renal replacement therapy and renal transplant patients in Australia and New Zealand. Transplantation 2010;90(11):1165–71.

73. Wei F, Liu J, Liu F, et al. Interferon-based anti-viral therapy for hepatitis C virus infection after renal transplantation: an updated meta-analysis. PLoS One 2014; 9(4):e90611.

74. Fernandez I, Munoz-Gomez R, Pascasio JM, et al. Efficacy and tolerability of interferon-free antiviral therapy in kidney transplant recipients with chronic hepatitis c. J Hepatol 2016;66(4):718–23.

75. Colombo M, Aghemo A, Liu H, et al. Treatment with ledipasvir-sofosbuvir for 12 or 24 Weeks in kidney transplant recipients with chronic hepatitis C virus genotype 1 or 4 infection: a randomized trial. Ann Intern Med 2017;166(2):109–17.

76. Lin MV, Sise ME, Pavlakis M, et al. Efficacy and safety of direct acting antivirals in kidney transplant recipients with chronic hepatitis C virus infection. PLoS One 2016;11(7):e0158431.

77. Abrahamian GA, Cosimi AB, Farrell ML, et al. Prevalence of hepatitis C virus-associated mixed cryoglobulinemia after liver transplantation. Liver Transpl 2000;6(2):185–90.

78. Duvoux C, Tran Ngoc A, Intrator L, et al. Hepatitis C virus (HCV)-related cryoglobulinemia after liver transplantation for HCV cirrhosis. Transpl Int 2002;15(1):3–9.

79. Garrouste C, Kamar N, Boulestin A, et al. Prevalence of cryoglobulinemia and autoimmune markers in liver transplant patients. Exp Clin Transplant 2008;6(3): 184–9.

80. Gragnani L, Visentini M, Fognani E, et al. Prospective study of guideline-tailored therapy with direct-acting antivirals for hepatitis C virus-associated mixed cryoglobulinemia. Hepatology 2016;64(5):1473–82.

81. Younossi ZM, Stepanova M, Henry L, et al. Association of work productivity with clinical and patient-reported factors in patients infected with hepatitis C virus. J Viral Hepat 2016;23(8):623–30.

82. Younossi ZM, Stepanova M, Nader F, et al. Patient-reported outcomes in chronic hepatitis C patients with cirrhosis treated with sofosbuvir-containing regimens. Hepatology 2014;59(6):2161–9.

83. Manne V, Sassi K, Allen R, et al. Hepatitis C and work impairment: a review of current literature. J Clin Gastroenterol 2014;48(7):595–9.

84. Younossi ZM, Stepanova M, Sulkowski M, et al. Sofosbuvir and ledipasvir improve patient-reported outcomes in patients co-infected with hepatitis C and human immunodeficiency virus. J Viral Hepat 2016;23(11):857–65.

85. Tanikella R, Kawut SM, Brown RS Jr, et al. Health-related quality of life and survival in liver transplant candidates. Liver Transpl 2010;16(2):238–45.

86. Sullivan KM, Radosevich DM, Lake JR. Health-related quality of life: two decades after liver transplantation. Liver Transpl 2014;20(6):649–54.

87. Duffy JP, Kao K, Ko CY, et al. Long-term patient outcome and quality of life after liver transplantation: analysis of 20-year survivors. Ann Surg 2010;252(4):652–61.

88. Volk ML, Hagan M. Organ quality and quality of life after liver transplantation. Liver Transpl 2011;17(12):1443–7.

89. Saab S, Ng V, Landaverde C, et al. Development of a disease-specific questionnaire to measure health-related quality of life in liver transplant recipients. Liver Transpl 2011;17(5):567–79.

Other Extrahepatic Manifestations of Hepatitis C Virus Infection (Pulmonary, Idiopathic Thrombocytopenic Purpura, Nondiabetes Endocrine Disorders)

Daniel Segna, MD[a,b], Jean-François Dufour, MD[b,*]

KEYWORDS

- Hepatitis C • Extrahepatic manifestations • Pulmonary • Endocrine
- Idiopathic thrombocytopenic purpura

KEY POINTS

- Hepatitis C Virus (HCV) infection may increase the risk for obstructive, interstitial, and vascular lung disease, lung cancer, and mortality in HCV-infected lung transplant recipients.
- HCV infection may increase the risk of idiopathic thrombocytopenic purpura, nonresponse to corticosteroids during the treatment, and higher rates of splenectomy.
- HCV infection may increase the risk of autoimmune thyroiditis, infertility, growth hormone and adrenal deficiency, osteoporosis, and low-trauma fractures.
- Targeted prospective cohorts may confirm these results mostly obtained from small case-control studies with different study populations and low level of evidence.

INTRODUCTION

Hepatitis C virus (HCV) is a widespread infection with an estimated prevalence of at least 1.8% in the American population and is a leading cause of liver-related morbidity and mortality worldwide.[1] In addition to hepatocytes, it also infects, and replicates in, extrahepatic tissues and peripheral mononuclear blood cells.[2,3] Therefore, it is not surprising that HCV infection is also associated with extrahepatic manifestations evolving

Disclosure Statement: The authors have nothing to disclose.
[a] Department of General Internal Medicine, Inselspital - Bern University Hospital, Freiburgstrasse 4, Bern 3010, Switzerland; [b] Division of Hepatology, Department of Visceral Surgery and Medicine, Inselspital- Bern University Hospital, Freiburgstrasse 4, Bern 3010, Switzerland
* Corresponding author.
E-mail address: jean-francois.dufour@dkf.unibe.ch

simultaneously with, or independent from, viral hepatitis, cirrhosis, portal hypertension, or hepatocellular cancer. The prevalence of extrahepatic manifestations in HCV infection largely depends on the definition of this condition, but seems to concern up to 0.9% to 1.4% of 16,761 HCV-infected patients identified in various high-risk groups in Lazio, Italy.[4]

In this review, we summarize the current evidence for potential pulmonary and non-diabetic endocrine extrahepatic manifestations of HCV.

Pulmonary Manifestations of Hepatitis C Virus Infection

There is accumulating evidence on a potential interaction between HCV virus infection and pulmonary extrahepatic manifestations (**Table 1**). These range from potentially increased rates of obstructive and restrictive pneumopathies, as well as malignant and autoimmune manifestations. In addition to HCV-induced cirrhosis and/or portal hypertension, lung health seems to be influenced directly by HCV through changes to immune response by an alteration in T lymphocytes, eosinophilic granulocytes, and inflammatory cytokines, which may account for interstitial or alveolar inflammation and a higher rate of obstructive lung disease and lung fibrosis.[5–7]

Lung function and obstructive lung diseases

There are controversial data on the relationship between HCV infection and lung function. Cross-sectional analyses from the Third National Health and Nutrition Examination Survey among 9159 patients suggest an increase in forced expiratory volume in 1 second (FEV_1) and full vital capacity in anti-HCV antibody–positive versus –negative subjects; however, these associations were no longer significant after additional adjustment for cocaine and marijuana use as well as poverty income ratio.[8] Another cross-sectional study on the prevalence of HCV infection among patients with chronic obstructive pulmonary disease found a notably increased prevalence of HCV infection (7.5%; 95% confidence interval [CI], 6.52–8.48) in comparison with blood donors as a control group (0.41%; 95% CI, 0.40–0.42). In contrast with the aforementioned study, HCV-positive patients showed a significantly lower FEV_1 than HCV-negative patients (34.7 ± 8.6% vs 42.7 ± 16.5%).[9] However, these results may be due to a generally more advanced chronic obstructive pulmonary disease stage, leading to a significant selection bias. A small prospective cohort study among 59 patients assessed the decline in FEV_1 and diffusing capacity of the lung for carbon monoxide in current smokers and ex-smokers, which were significantly higher in HCV-positive patients than in HCV-negative patients.[10] The same study group interestingly detected an increased impaired reversibility with salbutamol among asthmatic HCV patients with no response to interferon therapy.[11]

Nevertheless, these results could not be confirmed in a cross-sectional analysis among 1068 human immunodeficiency virus (HIV)-infected individuals with no evidence of an independent association between markers of HCV exposure, chronicity, viremia, or HCV-associated end-organ damage with obstructive lung disease.[12] Whether HCV infection leads to a faster decline in lung function and to a potentially higher prevalence of obstructive lung disease still needs to be verified in large, prospective cohort studies in the general population.

Pulmonary hypertension

The role of HCV in the development, progression and improvement of pulmonary hypertension (PH), independent from or simultaneously with liver cirrhosis and portal hypertension, is not well-understood.

Table 1
Pulmonary manifestations of HCV infection

Authors	Design	Study Population	Results/Conclusion
Lung function/obstructive lung diseases			
Fischer et al,[12] 2014	Cross-sectional study	1068 participants with intravenous drug use from the Acquired Immunodeficiency Syndrome Linked to the Intravenous Experience Study	No independent association between markers of HCV exposure, chronicity, viremia, or HCV-associated end-organ damage with obstructive lung disease.
Kanazawa & Yoshikawa,[11] 2004	Prospective cohort study	55 HCV-positive patients with asthma undergoing IFN treatment vs HCV-negative patients (matched for age, sex, and baseline pulmonary function)	Nonresponders to IFN therapy with chronic HCV infection showed a significantly accelerated decline in lung function and impaired reversibility with salbutamol compared with IFN responders and HCV-negative controls.
Kanazawa et al,[10] 2003	Prospective cohort study	59 COPD patients	Chronic HCV infection might accelerate decline in lung function (FEV_1, DLCO) in patients with preexisting COPD.
Goh et al,[8] 2014	Cross-sectional study	9159 participants from a population-based cohort (NHANES III)	Exposure to HCV was significantly associated with an increase in FEV_1 and functional vital capacity. These associations were no longer significant after additionally adjusting for cocaine and marijuana use as well as poverty income ratio.
Silva et al,[9] 2010	Cross-sectional study	184 patients with COPD vs 16,138 blood donors	COPD patients showed a significantly higher prevalence of HCV infection than blood donors (OR, 29.2; 95% CI, 17.3–49.2; $P<.01$). HCV-positive patients had a significantly lower FEV_1 than the control group ($P = .01$).
Kubo et al,[6] 1996	Case-control study	13 patients with chronic HCV vs 13 healthy controls	Lavage lymphocyte and eosinophil numbers were increased in patients with HCV, but not total cell count. Surface marker analysis of the lymphocyte populations showed increases in CD2, CD3, CD4, and HLA-DR, but no difference in CD4/CD8 ratio.

(continued on next page)

Table 1
(*continued*)

Authors	Design	Study Population	Results/Conclusion
PH			
Chen et al,[13] 2013	Cross-sectional study	100 cirrhotic patients	Cirrhotic patients with PPH had more frequently a history of HCV infection (20.0 vs 1.1%, $P = .03$) than those without PPH. However, HCV infection was not significantly associated with PPH in backward stepwise regression models.
Demir & Demir,[15] 2014	Case-control study	50 HCV-infected patients vs 50 healthy controls (prevalence of cirrhosis not reported)	HCV infection was significantly associated with right ventricular systolic dysfunction and PH (higher systolic pulmonary artery pressure and pulmonary vascular resistance, all $P<.01$) compared with healthy controls.
Sangal et al,[14] 2014	Cross-sectional study within a retrospective cohort	68 noncirrhotic patients with HIV–HCV coinfection	The prevalence of echocardiographic PH was higher (26%) in HIV–HCV coinfected individuals than the previously reported prevalence in HIV monoinfection (0.5%). IFN-based HCV treatment and time since HCV diagnosis were associated with the development of PH as assessed by echocardiography.
Renard et al,[16] 2016	Case series	3 cirrhotic patients (2 with HIV coinfection, 1 with PH)	Three cases of newly diagnosed or exacerbated pulmonary arterial hypertension in patients treated with sofosbuvir.
Lung transplantation			
Koenig et al,[17] 2016	Retrospective cohort study	17,762 lung transplant recipients from the Scientific Registry of Transplant Recipients (1994–2011) in the United States	In multivariate survival analysis, HCV infection was associated with higher mortality in lung transplant recipients (aHR, 1.24; 95% CI, 1.04–1.46; $P = .01$), whereas there was no association of HCV infection with time to graft loss.
Doucette et al,[18] 2016	Retrospective cohort study	14 HCV-positive vs 456 HCV-negative lung transplant recipients from the University of Alberta Lung Transplant Program (1986–2011)	1-, 3-, and 5-y survival rates were similar in HCV-positive and HCV-negative recipients.

Englum et al,[19] 2016	Retrospective cohort study	16,604 lung recipients from the United Network for Organ Sharing database (1994–2011)	Overall survival was shorter in the HCV-positive compared with HCV-negative donor group (median 1.3 vs 5.1 y; P<.01). Results were confirmed in adjusted analyses.
Lung cancer			
Allison et al,[20] 2015	Retrospective analysis of different cohorts/ registries	12,126 chronic HCV-infected persons from the Chronic Hepatitis Cohort Study vs 133,795,010 records from 13 cancer registries	HCV infection was associated with an increased for lung cancer compared with noninfected peers (standardized relative risk, 1.6; 95% CI, 1.3–1.9).
PE			
Ambrosino et al,[21] 2016	Systematic review and metaanalysis of case-control and retrospective cohort studies	VTE analysis: 100,364 HCV-infected patients vs 8,470,176 controls; PE analysis: 100,254 HCV-infected patients vs 8,470,055 controls	HCV-infected subjects may exhibit an increased risk of VTE (OR, 1.88; 95% CI, 1.33–2.65, P<.01) with a nonsignificant trend toward an increased risk of PE compared with healthy controls (OR, 1.81; 95% CI, 0.90–3.66; P = .09).
Pulmonary fibrosis			
Ueda et al,[23] 1992	Case-control study	66 IPF patients vs 9464 age-matched controls	Prevalence of HCV infection was significantly higher in IPF patients than in healthy controls (28.8% vs 3.7%, P<.05).
Arase et al,[25] 2008	Case-control study	6150 HCV-infected patients vs 2050 HBV-infected patients (age and sex-matched)	Cumulative incidence rate of IPF after 20 y was significantly higher in HCV- than in HBV-infected patients (0.9% vs 0.0%, P = .02).
Irving et al,[24] 1993	Cross-sectional study	62 IPF patients	None of 62 IFP patients suffered from HCV infection; therefore. no increased prevalence of HCV infection compared with the general population.
Pulmonary sarcoidosis			
Goldberg et al,[26] 2006	Case reports, systematic literature review	667 HCV-infected patients treated with recombinant alpha-IFN vs 3862 IFN-naive HCV patients	3 cases of biopsy-proven sarcoidosis in recombinant alpha-IFN recipients vs none in therapy- naive patients (incidence rate 0.4% vs 0.0%, P<.01).

(continued on next page)

Table 1
(continued)

Authors	Design	Study Population	Results/Conclusion
Ramos-Casals et al,[27] 2005	Case reports, systematic literature review	68 HCV-infected patients with incident sarcoidosis (20 treated with alpha-IFN monotherapy, 30 treated with alpha-IFN and ribavirin, 18 therapy-naïve patients)	In HCV infection, sarcoidosis may either be triggered by antiviral therapy (in 75% of cases) or occur spontaneously. Of 18 treatment-naïve HCV patients with sarcoidosis, 14 (87%) suffered from pulmonary involvement.
Faurie et al,[28] 2010	Case series from retrospective cohort study	11 patients with chronic HCV infection and sarcoidosis, partly obtained from a retrospective cohort of 3194 patients with chronic HCV infection	Sarcoidosis triggered by antiviral therapy was more frequent after completion of therapy and presented a benign outcome. In treatment-naïve HCV patients, systemic corticosteroids had to be used more often and outcome was less favorable.
Tuberculosis			
Wu et al,[31] 2015	Case-cohort analysis from a prospective population-based cohort	5454 HCV-infected vs 54,274 noninfected Taiwanese patients	HCV infection was significantly associated with active tuberculosis disease in multivariate Cox regression (aHR, 3.20; 95% CI, 1.85–5.53; $P<.01$) and competing death risk event analysis (aHR, 2.11; 95% CI, 1.39–3.20; $P<.01$).
Richards et al,[32] 2006	Cross-sectional study	272 hospitalized patients with tuberculosis in Georgia	Of 272 patients with tuberculosis, 61 (22.4%) were seropositive for HCV infection.
El-Serag et al,[33] 2003	Case-control study	34,204 HCV-infected patients vs 136,816 uninfected controls	HCV-infected patients showed a significantly higher prevalence of tuberculosis vs controls (3.3% vs 1.3%; $P<.01$), with similar results after exclusion of immunocompromised patients.

Lomtadze et al,[34] 2013	Prospective cohort study	326 patients with culture-confirmed tuberculosis and serial ALAT/ASAT measurements	In multivariable analysis, HCV coinfection was found to be an independent risk factor for incident antituberculosis drug-induced hepatotoxicity (aHR, 3.2; 95% CI, 1.6–6.5; $P<.01$).
Liu et al,[35] 2014	Retrospective cohort study	553 patients with active tuberculosis	Incidence of transient liver function impairment was significantly increased in patients with HCV than in controls (12% [20/161] vs 2% [9/392]; $P<.01$). However, mean onset times of drug-induced hepatotoxicity were not significantly different.

Abbreviations: aHR, adjusted hazard ratio; ALAT, alanine aminotransaminase; anti-Hbc, antibody against hepatitis B core protein; ASAT, aspartate aminotransaminase; CI, confidence interval; COPD, chronic obstructive pulmonary disease; DLCO, diffusing capacity of the lung for carbon monoxide; FEV_1, forced expiratory volume in 1 second; HCV, hepatitis C virus; HIV, human immunodeficiency virus; HR, hazard ratio; IFN, interferon; IPF, idiopathic pulmonary fibrosis; NHANES III, Third National Health and Nutrition Examination Survey; OR, odds ratio; PE, pulmonary embolism; PH, pulmonary hypertension; PPH, portopulmonary hypertension; VTE, venous thromboembolism.

Portopulmonary hypertension (PPH), a pulmonary vasoconstriction and vascular remodeling after chronic portal hypertension, is a rare condition. Chen and colleagues[13] conducted a small, cross-sectional study among 100 hospitalized cirrhotic patients. Ten patients presented with PPH, 8 with a viral etiology of their cirrhosis. The results showed a significantly higher rate of HCV infection compared with the control group without PPH (20.0% vs 1.1%, respectively; $P = .03$). However, HCV was not shown to be an independent risk factor for PPH.[13] Interestingly, another cross-sectional analysis among 68 noncirrhotic HIV–HCV coinfected patients reported a comparable high prevalence of PH/right heart dysfunction of 26%, as determined by transthoracic echocardiography. Despite the missing control group, the authors compared it with a generally lower frequency of 0.5% among HIV-monoinfected patients from other studies. Moreover, treatment with interferon, but not ribavirin, was significantly associated with PH (odds ratio [OR], 5.65; 95% CI, 1.07–29.93; $P = .04$).[14]

Another case-control study among 50 HCV-infected versus noninfected patients detected a significantly increased rate of right heart dysfunction and PH based on different hemodynamic markers measured by transthoracic echocardiography[15]; however, there was no information on concomitant portal hypertension and cirrhosis.

Curiously, a case series of 3 cirrhotic HCV-infected patients treated with sofosbuvir and ribavirin showed a newly diagnosed pulmonary arterial hypertension in 2 cases after completion of antiviral therapy with sustained virologic response, and a worsening of a preexisting pulmonary arterial hypertension in 1 patient about 2 months after start of treatment. The authors hypothesized that a decrease in vasodilatory inflammatory mediators after or during antiviral therapy may result in a clinical progression of pulmonary arterial hypertension.[16] However, 2 of those patients had HIV coinfection, whereas 1 suffered from portal hypertension, which may be potential confounders.

The role of HCV infection as an independent risk factor for PH merits further investigation. Similarly, PH as a potential adverse event of current antiviral therapy strategies may be studied further on.

Lung transplantation

In the field of lung transplantation, there are rather heterogeneous data on the role of HCV infection in mortality and transplant survival among both recipients and donors. A large prospective cohort study of 17,762 lung transplant recipients from the American Scientific Registry of Transplant Recipients found a significant association between HCV infection and greater overall mortality with an adjusted hazard ratio of 1.24 (95% CI, 1.04–1.46; $P = .01$). This was especially true for long-term mortality 3 years after transplantation, whereas the first 2 years did not show different death rates in HCV-positive versus HCV-negative individuals.[17] On the basis of these data, treatment of HCV infection in lung transplant recipients may result in a longer posttransplant survival. Another small case-control study, however, found no different 1-, 3-, and 5-year survival rates between HCV-positive versus HCV-negative recipients.[18] Changing the perspective, transplantation of HCV-positive donor lungs was shown to be associated with a poorer survival (median, 1.3 vs 5.1 years; $P<.01$) in their recipients compared with HCV-negative donor organs. Conversely, HCV infection in recipients did not significantly impact survival.[19]

Lung cancer

HCV infection has been hypothesized to be associated with a higher incidence rate of extrahepatic cancer. Among 12,126 chronic HCV-infected persons in the Chronic Hepatitis Cohort Study,[20] the risk of developing lung cancer was significantly increased with a standardized rate ratio of 1.6 (95% CI, 1.3–1.9). Further studies may verify these results and investigate the potential mechanisms linking these 2 conditions.

Pulmonary embolism

The relationship between HCV infection and the risk of pulmonary embolism remains debatable. Recently, Ambrosino and colleagues[21] conducted a systematic literature search and meta-analysis of retrospective cohort, case-control and cross-sectional studies identifying an increased risk of deep vein thrombosis (6 studies, OR: 1.92; 95% CI, 1.35–2.72; $P<.01$); however, this was not confirmed in pulmonary embolism, with a trend toward an increased risk in this population (4 studies: OR, 1.81; 95% CI, 0.90–3.66). Because the number of participants was considerably high for the latter analysis, a power issue is rather improbable. However, because the studies were cross-sectional or retrospective and considerably varied in study design, an association between HCV can neither be reliably confirmed nor discarded.

Pulmonary fibrosis

There is some, however contradictive, literature on a possible association between HCV infection and idiopathic pulmonary fibrosis (IPF). A systematic literature review by Aliannejad and Ghanei[22] suggested that a higher frequency of HCV markers in IPF patients,[23] an increase in lymphocyte and neutrophil numbers in bronchoalveolar lavage of chronic HCV patients, and the development of IPF in interferon-treated HCV patients may predispose for pulmonary fibrosis. Whereas a small Japanese case-control study found a significantly increased prevalence of HCV seropositivity among 66 IPF patients compared with 9464 age-matched controls (28.8% vs 3.7%, respectively; $P<.05$),[23] these results could not be confirmed in a subsequent analysis of IPF patients in the United Kingdom.[24]

Conversely, HCV infection was significantly associated with incident IPF in a retrospective analysis of 6150 HCV-infected versus 2050 HBV-infected Japanese patients,[25] which may indicate an HCV-specific role in the development of lung fibrosis.

Pulmonary sarcoidosis

The role of HCV infection in extrahepatic sarcoidosis is not completely understood. In a case-control study, Goldberg and colleagues[26] reported 3 cases of histologically proven sarcoidosis with pulmonary involvement among HCV-infected patients treated with recombinant interferon-alpha, whereas no event was recorded in the interferon-naïve control group. However, there was also evidence of sarcoidosis in therapy-naïve HCV patients in a systematic review and retrospective case series,[27] including patients with HCV infections with 87% of pulmonary involvement. Interestingly, a different degree of aggressiveness of disease and steroid requirement was discussed for these 2 groups. For instance, a series of 11 cases with chronic HCV infection and histologically confirmed sarcoidosis from a retrospective French cohort study indicated systemic corticosteroids had to be used more often and outcome was less favorable in treatment-naïve patients[28] compared with those receiving interferon.

In a case report of a patient with chronic therapy-naïve HCV infection,[29] treatment with pegylated interferon-alpha and ribavirin for 48 weeks led to a complete clinical and histologic remission of symptoms, which corroborates the hypothesis of a direct virologic effect on the development and clinical course of this disease. As in other autoimmune and hematooncologic extrahepatic manifestations of HCV, a dysregulation of the cytokine/chemokine network may predispose for granulomatous diseases.[30] In light of the revolutionary changes in HCV therapy, examining the effect of new antiviral agents in the reversibility of sarcoidosis may warrant further investigation.

Tuberculosis

As shown in previous studies, HCV infection and tuberculosis share the comparable high-risk population with a high rate of HIV coinfection and socially difficult circumstances, such as homelessness and imprisonment.[31] Richards and colleagues[32] found a surprisingly high prevalence of 22.4% HCV coinfection among hospitalized patients with tuberculosis in Georgia. Conversely, in a case-control study among American veterans, there was an increased prevalence of tuberculosis coinfection in HCV-infected cases compared with noninfected controls,[33] however, to a lesser extent. These data were drawn from selected study samples, which may not represent the general population. However, a population-based, nationwide case-cohort study in Taiwan recently found a significantly increased risk of developing active tuberculosis in HCV-infected patients compared with age- and sex-matched peers the general population in Taiwan.[31] This strengthens the hypothesis of a shared cooccurrence owing to currently unknown mechanisms. However, a direct alteration of immune response to HCV seropositivity may exert a certain impact on the vulnerability to developing tuberculosis.

Despite a considerable hepatotoxicity of most antituberculosis drugs, little is known about the implication of HCV coinfection. In a prospective cohort study from Georgia including 326 patients with culture-confirmed tuberculosis, HCV coinfection resulted to be an independent risk factor for incident antituberculosis drug-induced hepatotoxicity as determined by monthly measured alanine aminotransferase levels during follow-up with an almost 3-fold risk increase compared with monoinfected peers and a faster development of liver injury after onset of antituberculosis therapy.[34] Likewise, a retrospective cohort study among 553 Taiwanese patients with active tuberculosis showed a higher rate of transient liver function impairment during antituberculosis treatment among HCV-infected patients.[35]

Once the controversy on the effect of HCV coinfection will be solved, it may be worthwhile to investigate the interactions of current antiviral and antituberculosis therapy in case of simultaneous occurrence.

Idiopathic Thrombocytopenic Purpura in Hepatitis C Virus–Infected Patients

Idiopathic thrombocytopenic purpura (ITP) is characterized by the destruction of thrombocytes in the spleen with the appearance of cutaneous and mucosal petechiae, epistaxis, menorrhagia, eventually causing major bleedings such as intracerebral hemorrhages (**Table 2**). Although the pathogenetic mechanisms are not completely understood, an alteration of immune response with formation of autoantibodies or cytotoxic T-lymphocytes directed against thrombocytic surface proteins as well as a suppressed platelet production may play a major role.[36] As potential triggering factors, especially viral infections,[37,38] lymphoproliferative and autoimmune diseases are discussed.[39,40] HCV may enhance autoimmune responses leading to thrombocytopenia by means of molecular mimicry[41] of platelet surface proteins and production of correspondent antibodies. Aref and colleagues investigated the most likely surface antigens in 50 HCV-infected patients (30 with thrombocytopenia) by flow cytometry and quantitative monoclonal immobilization of platelet antibodies. The most frequent platelet membrane glycoproteins (GP) were GP IIb/IIIa, GP IIIa, GP IIb, GP Ib, and GP Ia.[41,42] Moreover, HCV infection was associated with a significant elevation of platelet-associated immunoglobulin G compared with HBV-infected or healthy controls in a cross-sectional study among 421 patients with chronic hepatitis.[43]

In the 1990s, a cross-sectional study among 300 patients with lymphoproliferative or autoimmune diseases found a statistically significant correlation between HCV prevalence and number of autoimmune alterations in both conditions, suggesting

Table 2
ITP in HCV-infected patients

Authors	Design	Study Population	Results/Conclusion
Chiao et al,[37] 2009	Retrospective case-cohort study	120,908 American veterans with HCV	HCV was associated with elevated risk for ITP (HR, 1.8; 95% CI, 1.4–2.3) and overall incidence rates of ITP were higher compared with HCV-negative participants (30.2 vs 18.5 per 100,000 person-years). ITP incidence was increased among both untreated and treated HCV-infected persons.
Pivetti et al,[40] 1996	Cross-sectional study	300 patients with autoimmune disorders, thereof 33 patients with ITP and 167 with lymphoid malignancies	Statistically significant correlation between HCV prevalence and number of autoimmune alterations in both lymphoproliferative and connective tissue disorders, which was not found for anti-HBc positive patients. HCV may skew the immune system toward the production of autoantibodies.
Pockros et al,[44] 2002	Retrospective chart review	7 cases of ITP in 3440 patients with chronic HCV infection	ITP occurs more commonly in patients with chronic HCV infection than expected by chance.
Rajan et al,[45] 2005	Retrospective cohort study	250 patients with chronic thrombocytopenia	HCV patients (30%) had less severe thrombocytopenia. Symptoms and signs of thrombocytopenia were less frequent in HCV patients, but major bleeding was more frequent (25% vs 10%; $P<.01$).
Aref et al,[42] 2009	Cross-sectional study	50 patients with HCV	Platelet-specific antibodies in 86.7% of HCV patients. Target antigens for platelets antibodies: GP IIb/IIIa (30%), GP IIIa (20.5%), GP IIb (13.3%), GP Ib (13.3%), GP Ia (10%). Platelets count was inversely correlated with the levels of platelet GP-specific antibodies ($r = -0.42$, $P = .02$), and significantly parallel to spleen size ($P = .02$).
Sakuraya et al,[46] 2002	Prospective cohort study	79 patients with chronic ITP	HCV-infected patients with ITP required more often prednisolone treatment and splenectomy, but response rate to prednisolone treatment was significantly lower, as compared with noninfected controls (all $P<.01$).

Abbreviations: anti-Hbc, antibody against hepatitis B core protein; CI, confidence interval; GP, glycoprotein; HBV, hepatitis B virus; HCV, hepatitis C virus; HR, hazard ratio; ITP, idiopathic thrombocytopenic purpura.

that ITP may be potentially linked with HCV infection.[40] In a cohort of 3440 newly diagnosed HCV-infected patients, 7 developed ITP with 6 of 7 positive for anti-GP IIb/IIIA antibodies. Furthermore, the occurrence of ITP was significantly increased compared with data from the general population, which corroborated the hypothesis of an increased risk of ITP in HCV patients.[44]

In a large, retrospective analysis of HCV-infected US veterans compared with HCV-negative individuals matched by age, gender, visit date, and outpatient/inpatient consultation, HCV-infection was associated with an increased risk for ITP (HR, 1.8%; 95% CI, 1.4–2.3), which was true for both untreated and treated patients.[37] In a retrospective cohort study among 250 patients with chronic thrombocytopenia, those with exclusively noncirrhotic HCV infection exhibited fewer symptoms of thrombocytopenia, such as bruising, petechiae, and mucosal bleeding, but higher rates of major bleeding compared with HCV-seronegative peers,[45] so that the authors discuss HCV-mediated idiopathic thrombocytopenia as a different entity from other etiologies.

Whereas an association between HCV infection and ITP is probable, there is little evidence investigating its impact on ITP treatment. Sakuraya and colleagues[46] found a significantly higher rate of prednisolone therapy and splenectomy, and lower response rate to corticosteroids in HCV-infected patients compared with seronegative controls. Conversely, ITP as a potential serious adverse event during or even after interferon treatment in HCV patients has been described in some case reports.[47–49] With the arrival of interferon-free regimens, it is still unknown whether they are associated with a change in the rate of ITP during therapy and after a sustained virologic response.

Nondiabetic Endocrine Manifestations of Hepatitis C Virus Infection

HCV infection may lead to various endocrine extrahepatic manifestations in addition to diabetes mellitus type 2 (**Table 3**). In the following sections, we aim to give an overview of current literature on frequent as well as rare endocrine diseases with a potential association with HCV. Notwithstanding, the great majority of evidence is based on small, case-control studies that may be subject to selection biases and selective reporting. In many cases, information on the degree of resulting cirrhosis is lacking; therefore, the effect of HCV infection in noncirrhotic patients may not be accurately measurable.

Thyroid disease

Autoimmune thyroiditis Autoimmune thyroiditis has largely been recognized as a common extrahepatic endocrine manifestation of HCV with the first case reports in the early 1990s.[50] Additionally, Tran and colleagues[51] detected a significant association between HCV seropositivity and Hashimoto's thyroiditis when compared with hepatitis B surface antigen–positive controls, which may indicate an HCV-specific effect on the thyroid gland. Thyroid antibodies are very frequent in HCV infection and reach a prevalence of up to 42% in this population.[52] Conversely, HCV antibodies were significantly increased in 112 patients with autoimmune thyroiditis, as compared with 88 controls with nontoxic goiter (11.6% vs 2.3%; $P<.05$).[53] Another cross-sectional study among randomly selected patients with Hashimoto's thyroiditis found a highly significantly increased prevalence of HCV seropositivity compared with patients with either nontoxic goiter, myxedema, or Grave's disease.[54] In a case-control study, patients with untreated HCV infection without hepatocellular carcinoma or cirrhosis (n = 630) were more likely to present with hypothyroidism and positive antithyroglobulin, and antithyroid peroxidase antibodies than healthy controls from both iodine-sufficient (n = 268) and -deficient areas (n = 389) and HBV-infected patients.[55] In the past, several indirect mechanisms were discussed as potential links

Table 3
Nondiabetic endocrine manifestations of HCV infection

Authors	Design	Study Population	Results/Conclusion
Autoimmune thyroiditis			
Tran et al,[51] 1993	Cross-sectional study	72 chronic HCV patients before IFN therapy vs 60 chronic HBsAg-positive patients	Significant association between chronic HCV infection and prevalent thyroid autoantibodies ($P = .02$), whereas only one HbsAg-positive man had thyroid microsome autoantibodies.
Testa et al,[53] 2006	Case-control study	112 patients with autoimmune thyroid disease vs 88 patients with nontoxic goiter	Significant association between positive HCV antibodies and autoimmune thyroid disease, compared with HbsAg/anti-Hbs positive controls (11.6% vs 2.3%; $P<.05$).
Duclos-Vallée et al,[54] 1994	Cross-sectional study	200 patients with thyroid disease (50 with simple goiter, 50 with Graves' disease, 50 with Hashimoto's thyroiditis, 50 with myxedema)	12 of 50 patients with Hashimoto's thyroiditis had a positive ELISA for HCV RNA, whereas only 3 of 100 patients with other thyroid diseases were seropositive ($P<.01$). Comparable results from recombinant immunoblot assay ($P = .01$).
Nair Kesavachandran et al,[61] 2013	Systematic review	HCV patients receiving IFN treatment (both single and combination treatment)	Other risk factors than IFN treatment may account for the association between HCV infection and thyroid-related disorders. Validity of pooled risk estimates limited (high variability, variation in IFN criteria, dosage, and treatment.
Thyroid cancer			
Fiorino et al,[67] 2015	Systematic review	Studies on the association between HCV infection and different cancer types	No definitive and univocal conclusion for the association between HCV and thyroid cancer.
Amin et al,[65] 2006	Retrospective data-linkage study	75,834 HCV vs 39,109 HBV vs 2604 HBV/HCV coinfected patients	Lower incidence rate of thyroid cancer in HCV monoinfected patients, as compared with incidence from the New South Wales Central Cancer Registry (SIR = 0.3; 95% CI, 0.2–0.7; $P<.05$).
Giordano et al,[66] 2007	Retrospective data-linkage study	146,394 HCV-infected patients vs 572,293 seronegative patients	No association between HCV infection and thyroid cancer (adjusted HR, 0.72; 95% CI, 0.52–0.99; $P = .04$).

(continued on next page)

Table 3
(continued)

Authors	Design	Study Population	Results/Conclusion
Montella et al,[63] 2001	Case-control study	495 patients with different cancer types (130 with thyroid cancer) vs 226 healthy controls	Significant association between HCV and thyroid cancer (OR, 2.8; 95% CI, 1.2–6.3; $P = .01$).
Antonelli et al,[62] 1999	Case-control study	139 patients with HCV infection vs 835 individuals from a population-based study in an iodine-deficient area in Italy	Significantly higher prevalence of papillary thyroid cancer among patients with HCV infection compared with controls (no exact figures, Fisher's exact test $P<.01$).
Male infertility			
Yang et al,[76] 2015	Case-control study	Couples undergoing in-vitro fertilization: 90 HCV-infected women only vs 78 HCV-infected men only vs 1256 noninfected controls	Similar sperm parameters, ovarian stimulation, fertilization, and pregnancy results across subgroups. HCV infection may have no effect on IVF treatment outcomes.
El-Serafi et al,[70] 2016	Case-control study	55 male patients with HCV infection vs 21 healthy controls	Increased androstenedione, prolactin, and testosterone, but decreased dehydroepiandrosterone sulfate levels in HCV-infected men vs controls (all $P<.01$).
Durazzo et al,[71] 2006	Case-control study	10 HCV-infected men before and during treatment with IFN and ribavirin at 6 and 12 months vs 16 healthy controls	Lower nemaspermic motility and morphology, lower testosterone and inhibin B levels in HCV-infected men vs controls (all $P<.01$). Treatment improved spermatic function and increased testosterone and inhibin B levels.
Menopause			
Calvet et al,[73] 2015	Prospective cohort study	667 HIV-infected women	HCV coinfection was an additional risk factor for menopause earlier than 45 y of age compared with HIV-monoinfected women (HR, 6.26; 95% CI, 2.12–18.52; $P<.01$).
Cieloszyk et al,[72] 2009	Cross-sectional study	559 middle-aged, impoverished women	Women infected with HCV were more likely to be postmenopausal than were uninfected women (age-adjusted OR, 1.68; 95% CI, 1.02–2.77; $P = .04$).

IVF			
Yang et al,[76] 2015	Case-control study	90 couples undergoing IVF: 90 HCV-infected women only vs 78 HCV-infected men only vs 1256 noninfected controls	Similar sperm parameters, ovarian stimulation, fertilization, and pregnancy results. HCV infection may have no affection on IVF treatment outcomes.
Englert et al,[77] 2007	Case-control study	42 HCV-seropositive women vs 84 healthy controls undergoing IVF	HCV-seropositive women display a decreased ovarian response to IVF.
Pregnancy			
Pergam et al,[75] 2008	Retrospective cohort study	506 HCV-positive vs 2022 HCV-negative vs 1439 drug-using HCV-negative mothers	HCV-positive pregnant women seem to be at risk for adverse neonatal and maternal outcomes.
GH axis			
Plöckinger et al,[80] 2007	Cross-sectional study	21 HCV-infected patients before and during antiviral therapy	High rate (81%) of GH insufficiency in chronic HCV infection. Treatment leads to improvement of GH levels, while IGF-1 levels remain low.
Helaly & El-Afandy,[79] 2009	Case-control study	25 HCV-infected patients vs 15 healthy controls	IGF-1 levels were significantly lower in HCV-infected patients than in controls. Negative correlation between HCV viral load and GH levels ($P<.05$).
Adrenal insufficiency			
Ben-Shlomo et al,[78] 2014	Retrospective cohort study	4668 inpatients with random morning cortisol levels ≤15 μg/dL	Biochemical adrenal-cortisol insufficiency in hospitalized patients is associated with HCV infection ($P = .01$).
Bone health			
Hansen et al,[83] 2014	Comparison of 2 prospective cohort studies	12,013 HCV-infected patients vs age- and sex-matched 60,065 individuals from the general population	HCV-infected patients had increased risk of all fracture types (aIRR, 2.15; 95% CI, 2.03-2.28). In contrast, overall risk of fracture did not differ between patients with chronic vs cleared HCV infection.
Orsini et al,[84] 2013	Case-control study	60 noncirrhotic untreated men with chronic HCV infection vs 59 healthy controls (matched for age, sex, weight, AND smoking status)	Noncirrhotic untreated HCV patients have lower BMD at the femur as compared with healthy men ($P = .04$).

(continued on next page)

Table 3
(continued)

Authors	Design	Study Population	Results/Conclusion
Lin et al,[85] 2012	Case-control study	69 chronic HCV-infected patients vs 275 age- and sex-matched controls	In chronic HCV infection, mean BMD, Z score, and T score at the lumbar spine were significantly lower (P<.01), whereas the rate of osteoporosis in patients aged 45–54 y was significantly higher (P = .01) than among healthy controls.
Lange et al,[86] 2011	Case-control study	468 HCV-infected, treatment-naïve patients vs 6000 healthy controls	Chronic HCV infection is associated with a higher prevalence of vitamin D deficiency compared with healthy controls (25% vs 12%, P<.01).
Arteh et al,[87] 2010	Cross-sectional study	118 consecutive patients with chronic liver disease.	In cirrhotic HCV patients, 16.3% had mild, 48.8% had moderate, and 30.2% had severe vitamin D deficiency. In HCV patients without cirrhosis, 22.8% had mild, 52.6% had moderate, and 14% had severe vitamin D deficiency. In the non–HCV-related cirrhosis group, 38.9% had mild, 27.8% had moderate, and 27.8% had severe vitamin D deficiency.
Marek et al,[82] 2015	Case-control study	80 noncirrhotic patients with HBV or HCV infection vs 40 healthy controls	In patients with chronic HBV or HCV infection, daily secretion of calcidiol was lower (P<.01), diurnal concentration of intact parathyroid hormone higher (P<.01) compared with the control group.

Abbreviations: aIRR, adjusted incidence rate ratio; anti-Hbs, antibody against hepatitis B surface protein; BMD, bone mineral density; CI, confidence interval; GH, growth hormone; GP, glycoprotein; HbsAg, hepatitis B surface antigen; HBV, hepatitis B virus; HCV, hepatitis C virus; HIV, human immunodeficiency virus; HR, hazard ratio; IFN, interferon; IGF-1, insulin-like growth factor 1; IVF, in vitro fertilization; OR, odds ratio; SIR, standardized incidence ratio.

between these 2 conditions, especially the interference with self-recognition in the interaction between immune system and thyrocytes,[56,57] including molecular mimicry or cross-reactivity of HCV with thyroid antigens,[57,58] formation of heat shock proteins, and changes in major histocompatibility complex II antigens on thyrocytes.[59] Interestingly, new evidence suggests that HCV can directly infect human thyroid cell lines, potentially contributing to the persistence of viral infection and to the development of thyroid autoimmunity through additional inflammatory mechanisms.[60]

At present, interferon-based HCV treatment still plays a major role in the development in autoimmune thyroiditis, also called interferon-induced thyroiditis.[61] In the light of recent dramatic improvements in the treatment of HCV infections with a shift to interferon-free regimens based on direct-acting antiviral and host-targeted agents, their role in thyroid disease still needs to be verified.

Thyroid cancer Overall, the literature on the relationship between HCV infection and thyroid cancer is controversial. Several case-control studies identified a possible association between HCV infection and thyroid cancer. In a study by Antonelli and colleagues,[62] the prevalence of histologically confirmed papillary thyroid cancer was significantly increased in patients with HCV infection compared with healthy controls (2.2% vs 0.0%; $P<.01$). Similar evidence comes from a case-control study from South Italy with an increased risk of thyroid cancer with an OR of 2.8 for thyroid cancers among HCV-infected patients compared with seronegative peers.[63] However, these data could not be confirmed in another case-control study[64] and 2 large retrospective record-linkage studies.[65,66] In a recent systematic review from 2015, Fiorino and colleagues[67] concluded from the existing literature that previously positive results from case-control studies were not confirmed in large, prospective cohort studies, which may be owing to the different and unspecific study designs of these 2 retrospective cohort studies for thyroid cancer. Therefore, targeted prospective cohort studies on this relationship may be useful to solve this divergence.

Interaction with sexual hormones: Infertility, reproduction, menopause, and pregnancy Current data suggest that HCV infection may interact with sexual function and reproduction in male and female patients, as well as in the development of menopause in women. However, there were mostly case-control studies increasing the chance of a selection bias.

A systematic review by Garolla and colleagues[68] concluded that HCV sperm infection worsens parameters such as motility and abnormal morphology with some data suggesting an improvement in semen quality after antiviral therapy. However, sperm infection may not be the sole pathway to male infertility in this population. A case-control study including 57 patients with persistent HCV monoinfection and maintained hepatic function additionally showed significantly lower testosterone (1.43 vs 3.51 ng/mL), but higher estradiol (18.24 vs 8.6 ng/mL) and prolactin (10.0 vs 6.7 ng/mL) levels compared with healthy controls.[69] Another case-control study also indicated either a reduced sperm quality or potentially altered androgen, increased prolactin and estrogen levels.[70,71] However, a small case-control study among noncirrhotic patients with chronic hepatitis B and C found a comparable response to gonadoliberin testing in comparison with healthy controls.

Some data suggest that menopause may occur earlier in HCV-infected women than in controls[72,73] and HCV infection was found to be an additional risk factor for younger age at menopause in HIV-infected Brazilian women.[73] Overall, data for the role of HCV in conception, pregnancy, and birth are somewhat contradicting, as also described in the systematic review by Floreani.[74] Although the author concluded that there is no unfavorable effect of HCV infection in pregnancy, other studies suggest the opposite, with low birth weight, need for assisted ventilation of the fetus, and admission to a neonatal intensive care unit.[75] Yet, future research may focus on this topic and clarify potential interactions of HCV virus with sexual hormones during this dynamic episode in women.

In reproductive medicine, a case-control study including 1424 couples undergoing in vitro fertilization with either HCV-infected men or women did not show significant alterations in sperm parameters, ovarian stimulation, fertilization, and pregnancy results.[76] In contrast, Englert and colleagues[77] showed significantly lower ovarian response to stimulation in 42 HCV-seropositive women undergoing in vitro fertilization compared with 84 healthy controls.

Overall, HCV infection may negatively impact both male and female sexual function through direct infectious mechanisms or interaction with the hormonal axis of sexual hormones. Notwithstanding, data are scarce and partly contradicting; therefore, this field still deserves future research.

Adrenal insufficiency There is evidence that HCV can infect a plethora of tissues of our body, also the adrenal gland.[3] In a cross-sectional analysis by Ben-Shlomo and colleagues,[78] patients with adrenal insufficiency showed a higher prevalence of liver disease, especially HCV infection. However, there was no information on the degree of infection. Further studies may examine the prevalence and incidence of adrenal insufficiency in larger cohort studies.

Growth hormone and insulin-like growth factor There are some data suggesting a possible affection of the growth hormone (GH) axis by HCV infection, which could also serve as a potential link to HCV-associated hyperglycemic status.[79] In a case series of 21 patients with HCV, 17 (81%) presented with severe GH insufficiency and with 9 of these having decreased insulin-like growth factor (IGF) levels. After treatment with pegylated interferon-alpha plus either ribavirin or levovirin and sustained virologic response in most of the patients, severe GH insufficiency persisted only in 4 of these. However, IGF-1 levels remained low, indicating persistent GH resistance in hepatocytes.[80] In an Egyptian case-control study of 25 chronic HCV patients, IGF-1 and GH levels were significantly lower compared with 15 controls. Moreover, there was a significantly negative correlation between HCV viral load and GH levels ($P<.05$) with a nonsignificant trend for IGF-1 levels.[79] Nevertheless, there was no clear information on the degree of cirrhosis in HCV infection, which may be a potent confounder in these associations.[81] A recent case-control study from Poland[82] investigated the GH–IGF-1 axis as well as calciotropic hormones in noncirrhotic HCV- and HBV-infected patients. Although GH concentrations were increased in these patients, IGF-1 levels were decreased in comparison with healthy controls. Considering the limitations of these studies, there may be an induction of GH resistance in the liver, which may affect IGF-1 levels and increase the chance of diabetes mellitus type 2, a condition that is discussed elsewhere.

Bone health The impact of HCV infection on bone metabolism is not well-understood.

In a cohort study including 12,013 HCV-exposed patients compared with 60,065 age- and sex-matched individuals from the general population, those with HCV had a 2-fold increased risk for all fractures and low-energy fractures.[83] Although there was no difference between cleared and chronic HCV infection, one may speculate that HCV exerts a certain influence on the endocrine regulation of bone turnover. Additionally, a small case-control study among noncirrhotic HCV-infected men showed a lower femoral bone mineral density ($P = .04$) and higher rate of osteoporosis ($P = .01$)

compared with healthy peers. However, lower levels of activity and greater immobilization were also more common in HCV-infected patients, which may be possible confounders in this association.[84] Comparable results were found for a decreased lumbar spine bone mineral density and prevalence of osteoporosis in 69 HCV-infected patients compared with 275 age- and sex-matched controls in Taiwan.[85]

Whether HCV infection directly deteriorates bone health through endocrine pathways remains controversial. A possible endocrine reason for these findings could be the comparably high prevalence of vitamin D deficiency in HCV-infected patients with and, interestingly, without cirrhosis as well.[86,87] Additionally, a Polish case-cohort study found increased levels of intact parathyroid hormone in patients with either HBV or HCV infection,[82] but this could not be confirmed in a small study among exclusively HCV-infected individuals. Overall, the role of HCV infection in the endocrine regulation of bone metabolism deserves further investigation.

SUMMARY

There is accumulating evidence of an association between HCV infection and pulmonary, endocrine extrahepatic, and hematologic manifestations. Potential mechanisms of interaction are direct infection or alteration of immune response, which may result in an increased risk for obstructive and interstitial lung disease, ITP, autoimmune thyroiditis, infertility, and potentially lung and thyroid cancers. However, findings are mostly obtained from small case-control studies. Generalizability and external validity may be highly compromised owing to different study designs and populations, residual confounding, and low statistical power. This may be the reason for divergent or inconclusive results. Future efforts are needed to study the strength of association and the linking mechanisms in this population.

REFERENCES

1. NIH Consensus Statement on Management of Hepatitis C: 2002. NIH Consens State Sci Statements 2002;19(3):1–46.
2. Blackard JT, Kemmer N, Sherman KE. Extrahepatic replication of HCV: insights into clinical manifestations and biological consequences. Hepatology 2006; 44(1):15–22.
3. Yan FM, Chen AS, Hao F, et al. Hepatitis C virus may infect extrahepatic tissues in patients with hepatitis C. World J Gastroenterol 2000;6(6):805–11.
4. Faustini A, Colais P, Fabrizi E, et al. Hepatic and extra-hepatic sequelae, and prevalence of viral hepatitis C infection estimated from routine data in at-risk groups. BMC Infect Dis 2010;10:97.
5. Kanazawa H. Relationship between hepatitis C virus infection and pulmonary disorders: potential mechanisms of interaction. Expert Rev Clin Immunol 2006;2(5): 801–10.
6. Kubo K, Yamaguchi S, Fujimoto K, et al. Bronchoalveolar lavage fluid findings in patients with chronic hepatitis C virus infection. Thorax 1996;51(3):312–4.
7. Moorman J, Saad M, Kosseifi S, et al. Hepatitis C virus and the lung: implications for therapy. Chest 2005;128(4):2882–92.
8. Goh LY, Card T, Fogarty AW, et al. The association of exposure to hepatitis B and C viruses with lung function and respiratory disease: a population based study from the NHANES III database. Respir Med 2014;108(12):1733–40.
9. Silva DR, Stifft J, Cheinquer H, et al. Prevalence of hepatitis C virus infection in patients with COPD. Epidemiol Infect 2010;138(2):167–73.

10. Kanazawa H, Hirata K, Yoshikawa J. Accelerated decline of lung function in COPD patients with chronic hepatitis C virus infection: a preliminary study based on small numbers of patients. Chest 2003;123(2):596–9.

11. Kanazawa H, Yoshikawa J. Accelerated decline in lung function and impaired reversibility with salbutamol in asthmatic patients with chronic hepatitis C virus infection: a 6-year follow-up study. Am J Med 2004;116(11):749–52.

12. Fischer WA 2nd, Drummond MB, Merlo CA, et al. Hepatitis C virus infection is not an independent risk factor for obstructive lung disease. COPD 2014;11(1):10–6.

13. Chen H-S, Xing S-R, Xu W-G, et al. Portopulmonary hypertension in cirrhotic patients: prevalence, clinical features and risk factors. Exp Ther Med 2013;5(3): 819–24.

14. Sangal RB, Taylor LE, Gillani F, et al. Risk of echocardiographic pulmonary hypertension in individuals with human immunodeficiency virus-hepatitis C virus coinfection. Ann Am Thorac Soc 2014;11(10):1553–9.

15. Demir C, Demir M. Effect of hepatitis C virus infection on the right ventricular functions, pulmonary artery pressure and pulmonary vascular resistance. Int J Clin Exp Med 2014;7(8):2314–8.

16. Renard S, Borentain P, Salaun E, et al. Severe pulmonary arterial hypertension in patients treated for hepatitis C with sofosbuvir. Chest 2016;149(3):e69–73.

17. Koenig A, Stepanova M, Saab S, et al. Long-term outcomes of lung transplant recipients with hepatitis C infection: a retrospective study of the U.S. transplant registry. Aliment Pharmacol Ther 2016;44(3):271–8.

18. Doucette KE, Halloran K, Kapasi A, et al. Outcomes of lung transplantation in recipients with hepatitis C virus infection. Am J Transplant 2016;16(8):2445–52.

19. Englum BR, Ganapathi AM, Speicher PJ, et al. Impact of donor and recipient hepatitis C status in lung transplantation. J Heart Lung Transplant 2016;35(2): 228–35.

20. Allison RD, Tong X, Moorman AC, et al. Increased incidence of cancer and cancer-related mortality among persons with chronic hepatitis C infection, 2006-2010. J Hepatol 2015;63(4):822–8.

21. Ambrosino P, Tarantino L, Criscuolo L, et al. The risk of venous thromboembolism in patients with hepatitis C. A systematic review and meta-analysis. Thromb Haemost 2016;116(4):958.

22. Aliannejad R, Ghanei M. Hepatitis C and pulmonary fibrosis: hepatitis C and pulmonary fibrosis. Hepat Mon 2011;11(2):71–3.

23. Ueda T, Ohta K, Suzuki N, et al. Idiopathic pulmonary fibrosis and high prevalence of serum antibodies to hepatitis C virus. Am Rev Respir Dis 1992;146(1): 266–8.

24. Irving WL, Day S, Johnston ID. Idiopathic pulmonary fibrosis and hepatitis C virus infection. Am Rev Respir Dis 1993;148(6 Pt 1):1683–4.

25. Arase Y, Suzuki F, Suzuki Y, et al. Hepatitis C virus enhances incidence of idiopathic pulmonary fibrosis. World J Gastroenterol 2008;14(38):5880–6.

26. Goldberg HJ, Fiedler D, Webb A, et al. Sarcoidosis after treatment with interferon-alpha: a case series and review of the literature. Respir Med 2006;100(11): 2063–8.

27. Ramos-Casals M, Mana J, Nardi N, et al. Sarcoidosis in patients with chronic hepatitis C virus infection: analysis of 68 cases. Medicine 2005;84(2):69–80.

28. Faurie P, Broussolle C, Zoulim F, et al. Sarcoidosis and hepatitis C: clinical description of 11 cases. Eur J Gastroenterol Hepatol 2010;22(8):967–72.

29. Brjalin V, Salupere R, Tefanova V, et al. Sarcoidosis and chronic hepatitis C: a case report. World J Gastroenterol 2012;18(40):5816–20.

30. Fallahi P, Ferri C, Ferrari SM, et al. Cytokines and HCV-related disorders. Clin Dev Immunol 2012;2012:468107.
31. Wu PH, Lin YT, Hsieh KP, et al. Hepatitis C virus infection is associated with an increased risk of active tuberculosis disease: a nationwide population-based study. Medicine 2015;94(33):e1328.
32. Richards DC, Mikiashvili T, Parris JJ, et al. High prevalence of hepatitis C virus but not HIV co-infection among patients with tuberculosis in Georgia. Int J Tuberc Lung Dis 2006;10(4):396–401.
33. El-Serag HB, Anand B, Richardson P, et al. Association between hepatitis C infection and other infectious diseases: a case for targeted screening? Am J Gastroenterol 2003;98(1):167–74.
34. Lomtadze N, Kupreishvili L, Salakaia A, et al. Hepatitis C virus co-infection increases the risk of anti-tuberculosis drug-induced hepatotoxicity among patients with pulmonary tuberculosis. PLoS One 2013;8(12):e83892.
35. Liu YM, Cheng YJ, Li YL, et al. Antituberculosis treatment and hepatotoxicity in patients with chronic viral hepatitis. Lung 2014;192(1):205–10.
36. Nugent D, McMillan R, Nichol JL, et al. Pathogenesis of chronic immune thrombocytopenia: increased platelet destruction and/or decreased platelet production. Br J Haematol 2009;146(6):585–96.
37. Chiao EY, Engels EA, Kramer JR, et al. Risk of immune thrombocytopenic purpura and autoimmune hemolytic anemia among 120 908 US veterans with hepatitis C virus infection. Arch Intern Med 2009;169(4):357–63.
38. DiMaggio D, Anderson A, Bussel JB. Cytomegalovirus can make immune thrombocytopenic purpura refractory. Br J Haematol 2009;146(1):104–12.
39. Cines DB, Bussel JB, Liebman HA, et al. The ITP syndrome: pathogenic and clinical diversity. Blood 2009;113(26):6511–21.
40. Pivetti S, Novarino A, Merico F, et al. High prevalence of autoimmune phenomena in hepatitis C virus antibody positive patients with lymphoproliferative and connective tissue disorders. Br J Haematol 1996;95(1):204–11.
41. Zhang W, Nardi MA, Borkowsky W, et al. Role of molecular mimicry of hepatitis C virus protein with platelet GPIIIa in hepatitis C-related immunologic thrombocytopenia. Blood 2009;113(17):4086–93.
42. Aref S, Sleem T, El Menshawy N, et al. Antiplatelet antibodies contribute to thrombocytopenia associated with chronic hepatitis C virus infection. Hematology 2009;14(5):277–81.
43. Nagamine T, Ohtuka T, Takehara K, et al. Thrombocytopenia associated with hepatitis C viral infection. J Hepatol 1996;24(2):135–40.
44. Pockros PJ, Duchini A, McMillan R, et al. Immune thrombocytopenic purpura in patients with chronic hepatitis C virus infection. Am J Gastroenterol 2002;97(8):2040–5.
45. Rajan SK, Espina BM, Liebman HA. Hepatitis C virus-related thrombocytopenia: clinical and laboratory characteristics compared with chronic immune thrombocytopenic purpura. Br J Haematol 2005;129(6):818–24.
46. Sakuraya M, Murakami H, Uchiumi H, et al. Steroid-refractory chronic idiopathic thrombocytopenic purpura associated with hepatitis C virus infection. Eur J Haematol 2002;68(1):49–53.
47. Elefsiniotis IS, Pantazis KD, Fotos NV, et al. Late onset autoimmune thrombocytopenia associated with pegylated interferon-alpha-2b plus ribavirin treatment for chronic hepatitis C. J Gastroenterol Hepatol 2006;21(3):622–3.
48. Hsiao CH, Tseng KC, Tseng CW, et al. Late-onset immune thrombocytopenic purpura after withdrawal of interferon treatment for chronic hepatitis C infection: a case report. Medicine 2015;94(34):e1296.

49. Fujii H, Kitada T, Yamada T, et al. Life-threatening severe immune thrombocyto-penia during alpha-interferon therapy for chronic hepatitis C. Hepatogastroenter-ology 2003;50(51):841–2.

50. Tran A, Quaranta JF, Beusnel C, et al. Hepatitis C virus and Hashimoto's thyroid-itis. Eur J Med 1992;1(2):116–8.

51. Tran A, Quaranta JF, Benzaken S, et al. High prevalence of thyroid autoantibodies in a prospective series of patients with chronic hepatitis C before interferon ther-apy. Hepatology 1993;18(2):253–7.

52. Tomer Y, Villanueva R. Hepatitis C and thyroid autoimmunity: is there a link? Am J Med 2004;117(1):60–1.

53. Testa A, Castaldi P, Fant V, et al. Prevalence of HCV antibodies in autoimmune thyroid disease. Eur Rev Med Pharmacol Sci 2006;10(4):183–6.

54. Duclos-Vallée JC, Johanet C, Trinchet JC, et al. High prevalence of serum anti-bodies to hepatitis C virus in patients with Hashimoto's thyroiditis. BMJ 1994;309(6958):846–7.

55. Antonelli A, Ferri C, Pampana A, et al. Thyroid disorders in chronic hepatitis C. Am J Med 2004;117(1):10–3.

56. Lunel F. Hepatitis C virus and autoimmunity: fortuitous association or reality? Gastroenterology 1994;107(5):1550–5.

57. Pastore F, Martocchia A, Stefanelli M, et al. Hepatitis C virus infection and thyroid autoimmune disorders: a model of interactions between the host and the environ-ment. World J Hepatol 2016;8(2):83–91.

58. Martocchia A, Falaschi P. Amino acid sequence homologies between HCV poly-protein and thyroid antigens. Intern Emerg Med 2007;2(1):65–7.

59. Tomer Y, Davies TF. Infection, thyroid disease, and autoimmunity. Endocr Rev 1993;14(1):107–20.

60. Blackard JT, Kong L, Huber AK, et al. Hepatitis C virus infection of a thyroid cell line: implications for pathogenesis of hepatitis C virus and thyroiditis. Thyroid 2013;23(7):863–70.

61. Nair Kesavachandran C, Haamann F, Nienhaus A. Frequency of thyroid dysfunc-tions during interferon alpha treatment of single and combination therapy in hep-atitis C virus-infected patients: a systematic review based analysis. PLoS One 2013;8(2):e55364.

62. Antonelli A, Ferri C, Fallahi P. Thyroid cancer in patients with hepatitis c infection. JAMA 1999;281(17):1588.

63. Montella M, Crispo A, de Bellis G, et al. HCV and cancer: a case-control study in a high-endemic area. Liver 2001;21(5):335–41.

64. Malaguarnera M, Gargante MP, Risino C, et al. Hepatitis C virus in elderly cancer patients. Eur J Intern Med 2006;17(5):325–9.

65. Amin J, Dore GJ, O'Connell DL, et al. Cancer incidence in people with hepatitis B or C infection: a large community-based linkage study. J Hepatol 2006;45(2):197–203.

66. Giordano TP, Henderson L, Landgren O, et al. Risk of non-Hodgkin lymphoma and lymphoproliferative precursor diseases in US veterans with hepatitis C virus. JAMA 2007;297(18):2010–7.

67. Fiorino S, Bacchi-Reggiani L, de Biase D, et al. Possible association between hepatitis C virus and malignancies different from hepatocellular carcinoma: a sys-tematic review. World J Gastroenterol 2015;21(45):12896–953.

68. Garolla A, Pizzol D, Bertoldo A, et al. Sperm viral infection and male infertility: focus on HBV, HCV, HIV, HPV, HSV, HCMV, and AAV. J Reprod Immunol 2013;100(1):20–9.

69. Hofny ER, Ali ME, Taha EA, et al. Semen and hormonal parameters in men with chronic hepatitis C infection. Fertil Steril 2011;95(8):2557–9.
70. El-Serafi AT, Osama S, El-Zalat H, et al. Dysregulation of male sex hormones in chronic hepatitis C patients. Andrologia 2016;48(1):82–6.
71. Durazzo M, Premoli A, Di Bisceglie C, et al. Alterations of seminal and hormonal parameters: an extrahepatic manifestation of HCV infection? World J Gastroenterol 2006;12(19):3073–6.
72. Cieloszyk K, Hartel D, Moskaleva G, et al. Effects of hepatitis C virus infection on menopause status and symptoms. Menopause 2009;16(2):401–6.
73. Calvet GA, Grinsztejn BG, Quintana Mde S, et al. Predictors of early menopause in HIV-infected women: a prospective cohort study. Am J Obstet Gynecol 2015; 212(6):765.e1–13.
74. Floreani A. Hepatitis C and pregnancy. World J Gastroenterol 2013;19(40): 6714–20.
75. Pergam SA, Wang CC, Gardella CM, et al. Pregnancy complications associated with hepatitis C: data from a 2003-2005 Washington state birth cohort. Am J Obstet Gynecol 2008;199(1):38.e1-9.
76. Yang L, Zhao R, Zheng Y, et al. Effect of hepatitis C virus infection on the outcomes of in vitro fertilization. Int J Clin Exp Med 2015;8(4):6230–5.
77. Englert Y, Moens E, Vannin AS, et al. Impaired ovarian stimulation during in vitro fertilization in women who are seropositive for hepatitis C virus and seronegative for human immunodeficiency virus. Fertil Steril 2007;88(3):607–11.
78. Ben-Shlomo A, Mirocha J, Gwin SM, et al. Clinical factors associated with biochemical adrenal-cortisol insufficiency in hospitalized patients. Am J Med 2014;127(8):754–62.
79. Helaly GF, El-Afandy NM. Influence of HCV infection on insulin-like growth factor 1 and proinflammatory cytokines: association with risk for growth hormone resistance development. Egypt J Immunol 2009;16(2):115–24.
80. Plöckinger U, Kruger D, Bergk A, et al. Hepatitis-C patients have reduced growth hormone (GH) secretion which improves during long-term therapy with pegylated interferon-alpha. Am J Gastroenterol 2007;102(12):2724–31.
81. Caufriez A, Reding P, Urbain D, et al. Insulin-like growth factor I: a good indicator of functional hepatocellular capacity in alcoholic liver cirrhosis. J Endocrinol Invest 1991;14(4):317–21.
82. Marek B, Kajdaniuk D, Niedziolka D, et al. Growth hormone/insulin-like growth factor-1 axis, calciotropic hormones and bone mineral density in young patients with chronic viral hepatitis. Endokrynol Pol 2015;66(1):22–9.
83. Hansen AB, Omland LH, Krarup H, et al. Fracture risk in hepatitis C virus infected persons: results from the DANVIR cohort study. J Hepatol 2014;61(1):15–21.
84. Orsini LG, Pinheiro MM, Castro CH, et al. Bone mineral density measurements, bone markers and serum vitamin D concentrations in men with chronic noncirrhotic untreated hepatitis C. PLoS One 2013;8(11):e81652.
85. Lin JC, Hsieh TY, Wu CC, et al. Association between chronic hepatitis C virus infection and bone mineral density. Calcif Tissue Int 2012;91(6):423–9.
86. Lange CM, Bojunga J, Ramos-Lopez E, et al. Vitamin D deficiency and a CYP27B1-1260 promoter polymorphism are associated with chronic hepatitis C and poor response to interferon-alfa based therapy. J Hepatol 2011;54(5):887–93.
87. Arteh J, Narra S, Nair S. Prevalence of vitamin D deficiency in chronic liver disease. Dig Dis Sci 2010;55(9):2624–8.

Treatment of Extrahepatic Manifestations of Hepatitis C Virus

Elisabetta Degasperi, MD[a], Alessio Aghemo, MD, PhD[a],
Massimo Colombo, MD[b],*

KEYWORDS

- Direct-acting antivirals • Sofosbuvir • IFN-free regimens • Cryoglobulinemia
- Lymphoma • HCV • Chronic kidney disease • Lichen planus

KEY POINTS

- Antiviral treatment has been shown to prevent many non-liver-related complications and reduce all-cause mortality in patients infected with HCV, because anti-HCV therapy improves virus-related extrahepatic manifestations (EHMs).
- Antiviral treatment of patients suffering from mixed cryoglobulinemia syndrome (MCS) and non-Hodgkin lymphoma (NHL) is able to achieve clinical response of vasculitis-related manifestations and hematologic disease remission, so it should be considered a first-line treatment option in these patients.
- Extrahepatic benefits of antiviral therapy include improvement of HCV-related chronic kidney disease (CKD) and cutaneous manifestations, prevention of type 2 diabetes development and cardiovascular risks, together with improved quality of life and neurocognitive functions.
- Development of IFN-free regimens allows large-scale treatment of patients suffering from EHMs, by providing safe and efficacious options for patients previously IFN contraindicated.

Financial Disclosure and Conflict of Interest: Dr E. Degasperi has nothing to disclose. Dr M. Colombo has received grant and research support from BMS and Gilead Science; he serves on advisory committees for Merck, Roche, Novartis, Bayer, BMS, Gilead Science, Tibotec, Vertex, Janssen Cilag, Achillion, Lundbeck, GSK, GenSpera, AbbVie, AlfaWasserman, and Jennerex; he performs speaking and teaching at Tibotec, Roche, Novartis, Bayer, BMS, Gilead Science, Vertex, Merck, Janssen, Sanofi, and AbbVie. Dr A. Aghemo serves on the advisory board for AbbVie, Gilead Sciences, Janssen, Merck, and BMS; he is on the speaker bureau at AbbVie, Gilead Sciences, Janssen, Merck, and BMS; and has a research grant from Gilead Sciences.
[a] A.M. and A. Migliavacca Center for Liver Disease, Division of Gastroenterology and Hepatology, Fondazione IRCCS CA' Granda Ospedale Maggiore Policlinico, Università degli Studi di Milano, Via Francesco Sforza 35, Milan 20122, Italy; [b] Humanitas Clinical and Research Center, Via Alessandro Manzoni 56, Rozzano 20089, Italy
* Corresponding author.
E-mail address: massimo.colombo@unimi.it

INTRODUCTION

Chronic infection with hepatitis C virus (HCV) is now considered a systemic disease, because HCV-related extrahepatic manifestations (EHMs) have been shown to affect whole-organ functioning through multiple disorders. Better knowledge of HCV-associated diseases has led to understand that antiviral treatment represents a true etiologic therapy for some EHMs and, most of all, is able to prevent development of several non-liver-related complications. Recently, many studies have demonstrated that HCV clearance is associated with improved survival independently from liver-related outcomes: indeed the achievement of a sustained virologic response (SVR) to antiviral treatment has been associated with reduction of all-cause mortality in many large population studies.[1,2] Moreover, a Taiwanese study, including 12,384 patients with HCV receiving antiviral therapy matched with 24,768 untreated control subjects, showed that HCV treatment is associated with improved extrahepatic outcomes, such as lower incidence of end-stage renal disease, acute coronary syndrome, and ischemic stroke.[3]

Consequently, SVR is now regarded as a relevant survival end point also in patients with HCV with milder liver disease. Although anti-HCV treatment of patients suffering from EHMs was not systematically pursued in the past, because of reduced efficacy and high rates of adverse events typical of interferon (IFN)-based regimens, availability of potent and safe direct-acting antivirals (DAAs) has paved the way to large-scale treatment also in these patients. This article summarizes current data concerning antiviral therapy of common HCV-related EHMs.

MIXED CRYOGLOBULINEMIA

Since the demonstration that HCV infection is responsible for immune complexes formation in mixed cryoglobulinemia (MC), antiviral treatment has become one of the mainstays for treating MC-related vasculitis. Reports about successful MC treatment date back to the IFN-based therapy, which was shown to improve vasculitic manifestations in most patients. Several studies consistently demonstrated the strong link between virologic response, serologic response (decrease in serum cryocrit, rheumatoid factor negativization, normalization of C4 complement fraction levels), and clinical response (improvement in MC-related vasculitic manifestations): indeed nearly all patients achieving the SVR also showed improved biochemical profile and clinical symptoms, and conversely, virologic relapse with onset of viral replication resulted in MC recurrence.[4–8] However, SVR rates were still suboptimal (48%–60%) because of low efficacy of pegylated (Peg) IFN plus ribavirin (Rbv) therapy, and most studies were retrospective or lacked adequate follow-up.

An Italian study tried to prospectively evaluate long-term outcomes of viral eradication in MC, by comparing 121 patients with HCV with symptomatic MC (MC syndrome [MCS]), 132 asymptomatic patients with MC, and 158 patients with HCV without cryoglobulins treated with PegIFN plus Rbv, with a mean follow-up of 92.5 months. SVR was achieved by 52% of patients in the MCS group, and was associated with a persistent clinical and serologic response in all but two patients. On the contrary, non-SVR patients were also clinical nonresponders, although transient improvement of MCS was observed concomitantly to viremia decreasing on-therapy. Surprisingly, patients from MC and MCS groups showed lower SVR rates compared with the HCV group without MC (49% vs 61%; $P = .01$), despite similar viral kinetics on-treatment.[9] Reduced SVR in patients with MC could not be linked to higher treatment discontinuation rates for adverse events, although patients with MCS experienced more side effects than the HCV control group, mostly anemia and neutropenia. It has been hypothesized that persistent HCV replication in peripheral blood mononuclear cells from patients with MC could be a viral reservoir explaining higher treatment failure rates, although this has not been convincingly demonstrated.[10]

Lower SVR in patients with MC has been reported also in 33 patients receiving PegIFN plus Rbv and first-generation protease inhibitors (PIs),[11] but not confirmed by other authors: in a prospective study including 30 patients with MC vasculitis receiving PegIFN plus Rbv and telaprevir or boceprevir, SVR was achieved by 67% of patients, consistent with expected SVR to triple therapy. Antiviral treatment improved clinical manifestations of MC, such as purpura, arthralgia, neuropathy, and kidney impairment; cryoglobulin clearance was observed in 54% of patients at SVR24. All SVR patients displayed complete or partial clinical response, although also 8 of 10 non-SVR patients achieved a temporary response. As expected with PIs, more adverse events compared with dual treatment were reported, mainly anemia (74%), neutropenia (78%), and infections (48%).[12]

IFN-free regimens are expected to increase SVR and provide a safe treatment course to previously IFN-contraindicated patients. Reports concerning DAA-based treatment of patients with MC account for approximately 100 patients, with optimal virologic response rates.[13–16] Sise and colleagues[15] reported 83% SVR in 12 patients with MCS receiving sofosbuvir (SOF)-based combinations: of note, the only two patients failing antiviral treatment received suboptimal combinations according to current international guidelines. An Italian prospective study of 44 patients with MC treated with SOF-based combinations reported 100% SVR rates; considering MC outcomes at the SVR24 time point, 36% of patients achieved a complete clinical response (regression of all baseline vasculitis symptoms), 41% improved all MC symptoms, and 23% achieved at least a 50% reduction in MC manifestations. By comparing SVR12 and SVR24 time points, purpura, kidney disease, and skin ulcers improved faster than fatigue, sicca syndrome, and neuropathy, meaning that different features of MC vasculitis are more or less responsive to HCV eradication. Cryocrit disappeared in 40% of patients at SVR24, and decreased significantly in all others; interestingly, it did not correlate with clinical response, because some responder patients still exhibited detectable cryoglobulins.[16] Persistence of cryoglobulins has been described also in other case series[14,17]: more studies and extended follow-up are needed to prospectively evaluate long-term outcomes of MC in patients achieving viral clearance with IFN-free regimens, especially concerning risk of late MC relapse.

IFN-free regimens are expected to open new perspectives also in patients with severe MC: although antiviral therapy has always represented the first-line treatment of mild-moderate MCS, management of patients with life-threatening symptoms instead required first-line intensive immunosuppressive treatment. Administration of anti-CD20 monoclonal antibody rituximab (RTX) is now widely applied, because of the selective inhibition of B-cell compartment responsible for MCS. However, immunosuppression represents only a "symptomatic" approach, aiming at disease control but not affecting the HCV-driven stimulus to immune complex generation, so that MC relapse can occur. Combined or sequential immunosuppressive and "etiologic" antiviral therapy has been attempted in the past with PegIFN plus Rbv, showing good rates of vasculitis remission. RTX administration followed by PegIFN plus Rbv achieved 73% clinical response at 6 months in a study including 38 patients with MCS: of note, RTX combined with antiviral treatment was able to achieve faster MCS remission when compared with 55 patients receiving only anti-HCV therapy. Overall SVR rates did not differ in the two patient groups (60% vs 58%, respectively).[6] These findings have been replicated by other studies reporting combined or sequential RTX plus PegIFN and Rbv treatment of severe MCS.[18–20] However, this approach was not feasible in all patients, because neutropenia and anemia resulting from deep immunosuppression could contraindicate IFN treatment. In this field, IFN-free regimens allow for concomitant antiviral and RTX-based therapy of severe MCS, thus combining etiologic and symptomatic treatment.

Efficacy data of antiviral treatment in patients with MCS are summarized in **Fig. 1**.

HEPATITIS C VIRUS–RELATED LYMPHOPROLIFERATIVE DISORDERS

Although epidemiologic and molecular data already suggested a strong association between HCV and B-cell non-Hodgkin lymphoma (NHL), the demonstration that HCV eradication by antiviral treatment not only translated into reduced rates of NHL development, but also achieved hematologic response in many patients has changed the paradigm of NHL management. Long-lasting viral replication leading to polyclonal and eventually monoclonal B-cell proliferation is now considered the main driving force conferring the increased NHL risk in patients with HCV: indeed, a large retrospective Japanese study comparing 2708 patients with HCV receiving IFN treatment with 501 untreated patients demonstrated that SVR patients had 0% cumulative rate of incident lymphoma at 15 years compared with 2.56% of patients with persistent infection, meaning that viral clearance is responsible for the protective effect; conversely, the untreated group showed the same risk as patients not achieving viral

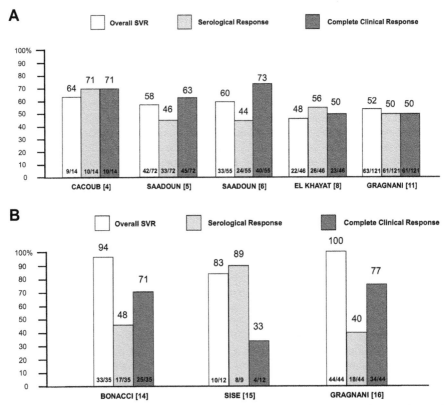

Fig. 1. Anti-HCV treatment of patients with MCS with IFN-based (A) and IFN-free (B) regimens.

eradication.[21] In the early 2000s Hermine and coworkers[22] firstly described successful IFN treatment of splenic lymphoma with villous lymphocytes (now marginal zone lymphoma [MZL]): indeed eight of nine patients displayed a partial to complete hematologic response after a median 27-month follow-up. These findings were reinforced if compared with six HCV-negative patients with the same lymphoma subtype, in which IFN administration did not achieve any hematologic response, thus strongly linking IFN efficacy to its antiviral more than antiproliferative effect.

IFN-based treatment has been shown to reverse molecular aberrations associated with clonal B-cell expansion: indeed some studies demonstrated that immunoglobulin heavy chain gene (IgH) rearrangement, t(14;18) translocation, and bcl-2 proto-oncogene overexpression, typical of hematologic malignancies, disappeared after antiviral therapy.[23,24] Other studies did not replicate these findings and found molecular aberrations to persist, probably meaning that there is a no-return point where activation of proliferative pathways becomes independent from viral stimulus.[22,25]

Antiviral treatment of indolent NHL has been largely established, because data generated with IFN/PegIFN plus Rbv in more than 200 patients have confirmed safety and efficacy of this policy, and durable benefits in terms of disease remission and survival: overall, hematologic response was achieved in more than 70% SVR patients. Data concerning IFN treatment in indolent NHL are summarized in **Table 1**.[22,25–31]

More recently, an Italian group reported a retrospective experience concerning 100 patients with indolent NHL receiving antiviral therapy as first-line treatment option (IFN/PegIFN ± Rbv): SVR was achieved in 80% of cases, consistent with 52% patients infected with the easy-to-treat HCV genotype 2. A total of 44% and 33% of patients achieved a complete or partial hematologic response, respectively, where lymphoma remission was significantly associated with HCV clearance ($P = .003$). Hematologic response rates did not differ according to lymphoma subtype, MZL accounting for most cases. The 5-year progression-free survival (PFS) and overall survival (OS) were 63% and 92%, respectively, in patients receiving antiviral therapy as first-line treatment, significantly higher if compared with 45% and 75% of untreated patients ($P = .001$ for PFS, $P = .004$ for OS, respectively).[30] Improvement in OS following antiviral treatment has been reported also in a multicenter French study enrolling 116 patients with HCV with NHL, mainly MZL (39%) but including also aggressive subtypes, such as diffuse B-cell lymphoma (DLBCL) (39%): 70 patients received antiviral treatment with PegIFN and Rbv ± first-generation PIs, and SVR was achieved in 61% of cases, reflecting a 50% to 61% prevalence of HCV-1 in patient population. Among the 14 patients receiving antiviral therapy as first-line treatment, all 11 patients achieving hematologic response were also virologic responders, thus reinforcing the strong association between viral clearance and disease remission. Antiviral treatment was confirmed the only variable significantly associated with improved OS (hazard ratio [HR], 0.18; 95% confidence interval [CI], 0.04–0.95; $P = .004$).[31]

The role of antiviral treatment in aggressive lymphomas has been less evaluated in the past, because chemotherapy (CT) was usually required as first-line option, and NHL or CT-related cytopenias often represented a contraindication to IFN administration. Nevertheless, antiviral treatment in DLBCL has been reported, either following first-line CT or by combined antiviral therapy plus CT.[32] Moreover, achievement of HCV eradication before DLBCL onset has been associated with better CT response and improved OS.[33]

The development of IFN-free regimens has dramatically changed the scenario, by providing effective and safe regimens to treat patients suffering from NHL. Successful antiviral treatment of a patient with splenic MZL by combination of the NS3 PI faldaprevir plus the nonnucleoside NS5B inhibitor deleobuvir and Rbv has been reported by

Table 1
IFN-based treatment of indolent HCV-associated NHL

Study	Patients	NHL Subtype	Treatment	SVR (%)	NHL Response (%)	CR in SVR, %
Hermine et al,[22] 2002	9 6 HCV-control subjects	SLVL	IFN ± Rbv	7 (78)	7/9 (78) CR 0%	100
Vallisa et al,[25] 2005	13	SMZL, MZL, FL, LPL	PegIFN + Rbv	6/13 (46)	7/12 (58) CR 2/12 (16) PR	100
Kelaidi et al,[26] 2004	8	SMZL, MZL	IFN/PegIFN ± Rbv	5/8 (63)	5/8 (63) CR	100
Mazzaro et al,[27] 2009	18	SLVL, FL, LPL	IFN/PegIFN + Rbv	9/18 (50)	9/18 (50) CR 4/18 (22) PR	100
Saadoun et al,[28] 2005	18	SLVL	IFN ± Rbv	14/18 (78)	16/18 (89) CR 2/18 (11) PR	100
Pellicelli et al,[29] 2011	9	SMZL, MZL, FL	PegIFN + Rbv	7/9 (78)	5/9 (56) CR 2/9 (22) PR	71
Arcaini et al,[30] 2014	100	SMZL, MZL, LPL, FL	IFN/PegIFN ± Rbv	80/100 (80)	44/100 (44) CR 33/100 (33) PR	55
Michot et al,[31] 2015	14	MZL	PegIFN + Rbv ± PI	11/14 (79)	8/14 (57) CR 3/14 (21) PR	73

Abbreviations: CR, complete response; FL, follicular lymphoma; LPL, lymphoplasmacytic lymphoma; PR, partial response; SLVL, splenic lymphoma with villous lymphocytes; SMZL, splenic marginal zone lymphoma.

Rossotti and colleagues[34]: anti-HCV therapy was able to achieve a rapid and durable hematologic response for 48 months after the end of treatment. Optimal virologic and hematologic response was confirmed in three patients with MZL and two patients with DLBCL treated with combination of SOF plus simeprevir or daclatasvir: all patients achieved the SVR and complete remission of NHL was obtained in four of five patients at 6 months. One patient with MZL with severe MC-related kidney impairment received RTX infusions during antiviral treatment to manage acute renal failure and all patients with DLBCL received CT courses before antiviral treatment without significant toxicity or drug-drug interaction (DDI) concerns, thus confirming the optimal safety profile of DAA-based therapy.[35] Data concerning 46 patients with indolent NHL (37 MZLs) from a multicenter European experience showed 90% SVR to DAA-based treatment with 67% hematologic response after 8 months. The estimated OS and PFS at 1 year were 98% and 75%, respectively. MZL displayed better response than non-MZL subtypes, with 27 of 37 (73%) versus four of nine (44%) patients achieving lymphoma remission following antiviral treatment.[36]

In conclusion, antiviral therapy of NHL is now considered a true "etiologic" treatment aimed at suppressing the proliferative hit of viral replication on B-cell population. Extended follow-up and more prospective data are required to confirm long-term outcomes of HCV-associated NHLs treated with IFN-free regimens; however, these preliminary results seem to confirm that DAAs are effective even without the IFN immunomodulatory action, thus meaning that antiviral rather than antiproliferative effect has greater importance in achieving disease remission.

HEPATITIS C VIRUS–RELATED RENAL DISEASE

The association between HCV infection and increased risk of end-stage renal disease recognizes several possible mechanisms of kidney damage, where renal involvement by MC-related vasculitis with membranoproliferative glomerulonephritis (MPGN) represents the most common type of chronic kidney disease (CKD). However, increased rates of diabetes mellitus development, together with additional cardiovascular risk demonstrated in HCV-infected patients, may contribute to renal damage. Consequently, it is not surprising that HCV treatment reduces end-stage renal disease development in a Taiwanese study including 37,152 patients with HCV (HR, 0.15; 95% CI, 0.07–0.31; $P<.001$).[3]

IFN-based antiviral treatment has been proven beneficial in MC-related MPGN, because achievement of SVR resulted in renal disease improvement together with cryocrit reduction.[4,5,37] IFN therapy, however, was associated with many side effects in patients with CKD, mostly anemia that required stimulating growth factor (erythropoietin) administration or even blood transfusion. The addition of first-generation PIs to PegIFN plus Rbv did not change the scenario, because increased SVR rates in HCV-1 patients were affected by more adverse events as counterpart.[11] Saadoun and colleagues[12] reported improvement of kidney disease in five of seven (71%) patients with MCS treated with PegIFN plus Rbv and boceprevir/telaprevir. At Week 72 (SVR24), daily proteinuria decreased significantly and hematuria disappeared in all cases. Kidney involvement was not associated with increased adverse events; however, anemia developed in 74% of the 30 patients included in the study, requiring erythropoietin administration in 93% of cases and blood transfusion in 46%.

IFN-free regimens have allowed treating patients with CKD without significant safety issues: in a retrospective series of 12 patients with MCS receiving DAAs (SOF + Rbv or SOF + simeprevir), six of seven (86%) patients with MPGN achieved the SVR and all patients showed a serologic response (cryocrit reduction) with proteinuria decrease.

Treatment was well tolerated, with no need for erythropoietin, and only two patients had hemoglobin reduction greater than 1 g/dL.[15] These good results were confirmed also in the VASCUVALDIC study, enrolling 24 patients with MC, where four of five (80%) MPGN patients treated with SOF plus Rbv showed improvement of proteinuria and hematuria.[38]

The main studies about antiviral treatment of patients with HCV-related kidney involvement are shown in **Fig. 2**.

IFN-free options for patients with HCV with CKD are still restricted, because administration of SOF-based regimens with a glomerular filtration rate (GFR) less than 30 mL/min is not recommended due to pharmacokinetic data showing accumulation of SOF metabolite GS-331007.[39] Although clinical relevance of increased exposure to GS-331007 is still debated, many data generated in real practice have reported SOF-based therapy for patients with HCV with GFR less than 30 mL/min with different treatment schedules (SOF full-dose, 400 mg/d, 200 mg/d, or 400 mg/three times a week) but optimal efficacy.[40] Concerning safety, the TARGET study demonstrated that SOF administration in patients with CKD resulted in increased side effects, mainly anemia, whereas some patients showed also renal function deterioration on-therapy.[41] As a consequence, current European guidelines suggest SOF administration in patients with advanced CKD only if treatment is considered nondeferrable for clinical urgency.[42]

The only approved regimen for patients with CKD stage 4 to 5 (GFR <30 mL/min) is the combination of paritapreivr/ombitasvir/ritonavir ± dasabuvir (3D/2D regimen), which is effective only in patients with HCV-1 and -4 and not recommended in impaired liver function (Child-Pugh score B or C). This regimen has been evaluated in 20 patients with HCV-1 CKD stage 4 to 5 receiving 3D for 12 weeks in the RUBY study, showing 90% SVR and anemia as the only side effect in patients with HCV-1a, where Rbv administration was prescribed.[43] In addition to Rbv need in HCV-1a, the 3D/2D combination has relevant DDIs because of the presence of booster ritonavir. The upcoming availability of second-generation NS3 inhibitor grazoprevir plus NS5A inhibitor elbasvir combination is expected to improve the DDI profile and to provide a Rbv-free regimen for patients with HCV-1 and -4 and CKD, because the phase 3 C-SURFER study showed 99% SVR rates in 224 patients with HCV-1 receiving grazoprevir plus elbasvir for 12 weeks, with a safety profile similar to placebo.[44] HCV 2 or 3 genotypes with advanced CKD have now limited treatment options except from off-label use of SOF-based regimens; however, the pangenotypic

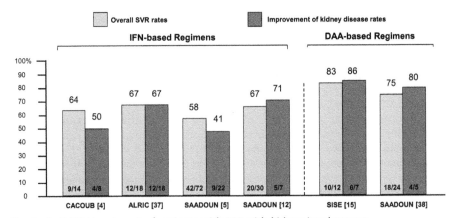

Fig. 2. Anti-HCV treatment of patients with MC with kidney involvement.

second-generation NS3 plus NS5A glecaprevir plus pibrentasvir combination, which is not renally excreted, is expected to fill the gap: indeed, recent data reported 98% SVR in patients with 104 HCV-1 to -6.[45]

IFN-free regimens have also opened the way to effective antiviral treatment after kidney transplantation, where viral eradication is of primary importance because HCV impairs graft survival, but IFN administration was contraindicated because of risk of graft rejection: a large phase 2 study evaluating SOF/ledipasvir treatment for 12 or 24 weeks in 114 kidney transplanted patients with HCV-1 or -4 with stable renal function achieved 100% SVR with optimal safety profile.[46]

In conclusion, antiviral treatment in patients with CKD is expected to dramatically change, as IFN-free options allow HCV cure in pretransplant and posttransplant phase. Decisions about optimal treatment timing could be influenced by the possibility to access the HCV-positive kidney graft pool, thus shortening the waiting list.

TYPE 2 DIABETES AND CARDIOVASCULAR OUTCOMES

HCV eradication has been associated with reduced risk of type 2 diabetes mellitus (T2DM) development. In a Spanish study including 734 patients with HCV with normal glucose values, achievement of viral clearance had a protective effect on T2DM onset, as 49 of 430 (11.4%) SVR versus 74 of 304 (24.3%) non-SVR patients developed glucose abnormalities in a 27-month follow-up. At multivariate analysis, SVR was independently associated with reduced T2DM risk (odds ratio, 0.44; 95% CI, 0.20–0.97; $P = .04$).[47] This has been confirmed also by a large retrospective Japanese study, where 143 out of 2842 patients with HCV treated with IFN developed T2DM during a mean observation period of 6.4 years: 117 out of 143 (81%) were nonresponders to antiviral treatment, and lack of SVR was independently associated with T2DM development (HR, 2.73; 95% CI, 1.77–4.20; $P<.001$).[48] The pathogenic mechanisms behind reduced T2DM incidence in SVR patients could be linked to elimination of HCV-related insulin resistance, as demonstrated by a prospective study including more than 400 HCV-infected patients, where achievement of SVR prevented insulin resistance development in patients without diabetes according to homeostasis model assessment.[49]

HCV eradication seems also to positively modify cardiovascular outcomes in patients with diabetes. A Taiwanese study on patients with T2DM compared 1411 patients with HCV treated with PegIFN plus Rbv, 1411 HCV untreated, and 5644 uninfected patients, showing that antiviral treatment was associated with a 47% risk reduction for ischemic stroke (HR, 0.53; 95% CI, 0.30–0.93) and 36% for acute coronary syndrome (HR, 0.64; 95% CI, 0.39–1.06) across an 8-year follow-up.[50] Reduced risk of acute coronary syndrome and ischemic stroke after antiviral therapy has been confirmed in patients with HCV without diabetes.[3]

QUALITY OF LIFE AND NEUROCOGNITIVE FUNCTION

In addition to fatigue, HCV has been associated with impaired neurocognitive functions and depression: antiviral treatment has demonstrated to improve health-related quality of life independently from clinically significant liver disease in patients achieving viral eradication.[51–53] Moreover, studies investigating HCV effects on central nervous system consistently demonstrated that viral eradication results in improved attention, vigilance, and working memory.[54,55] Recently, application of magnetic resonance spectroscopy in 22 patients with HCV showed improvement in cerebral inflammation markers after achievement of the SVR, meaning recovery of neuronal dysfunction following HCV cure.[56]

CUTANEOUS MANIFESTATIONS

Antiviral treatment benefits on HCV cutaneous manifestations are less defined, mainly because immune-mediated skin disorders were considered a relative contraindication to receive IFN, due to disease exacerbation risk. Moreover, Rbv and the PI telaprevir could determine drug-induced rash, so that a precise evaluation of antiviral treatment role in HCV cutaneous manifestations was complicated by many confounders. Data concerning the most characterized HCV-related skin disorder, lichen planus, are quite contradictory, because IFN treatment did not always result in lichen improvement.[57,58] IFN-free regimens allow for better outcome evaluation of HCV-related cutaneous diseases. In a Japanese report including seven patients, DAA-based treatment was shown to improve lichen planus manifestations, with complete disappearance of skin lesions in three patients 6 months after antiviral therapy.[59]

SUMMARY

It is now well demonstrated that HCV eradication following antiviral treatment positively affects not only liver-related outcomes, but also improves many disorders caused by HCV EHMs. Health gain resulting from HCV cure involves the physical and psychological spheres, with improved social and personal functioning. Consequently, achievement of the SVR is now considered a true surrogate marker of survival, as consistently demonstrated in several studies. Worldwide scaling up of DAA-based treatment toward HCV eradication will allow for real evaluation of SVR extrahepatic benefits long-term.

REFERENCES

1. van der Meer AJ, Veldt BJ, Feld JJ, et al. Association between sustained virological response and all-cause mortality among patients with chronic hepatitis C and advanced hepatic fibrosis. JAMA 2012;308:2584–93.
2. Tada T, Kumada T, Toyoda H, et al. Viral eradication reduces all-cause mortality in patients with chronic hepatitis C virus infection: a propensity score analysis. Liver Int 2016;36:817–26.
3. Hsu YC, Ho HJ, Huang YT, et al. Association between antiviral treatment and extrahepatic outcomes in patients with hepatitis C virus infection. Gut 2015;64: 495–503.
4. Cacoub P, Lidove O, Maisonobe T, et al. Interferon-alpha and ribavirin treatment in patients with hepatitis C virus-related systemic vasculitis. Arthritis Rheum 2002; 46:3317–26.
5. Saadoun D, Resche-Rigon M, Thibault V, et al. Antiviral therapy for hepatitis C virus–associated mixed cryoglobulinemia vasculitis: a long-term follow up study. Arthritis Rheum 2006;54:3696–706.
6. Saadoun D, Resche Rigon M, Sene D, et al. Rituximab plus Peg-interferon-alpha/ribavirin compared with Peg-interferon-alpha/ribavirin in hepatitis C-related mixed cryoglobulinemia. Blood 2010;116:326–34.
7. Mazzaro C, Monti G, Saccardo F, et al. Efficacy and safety of peginterferon alfa-2b plus ribavirin for HCV-positive mixed cryoglobulinemia: a multicentre open-label study. Clin Exp Rheumatol 2011;29:933–41.
8. El Khayat HR, Fouad YM, Ahmad EA, et al. Hepatitis C virus (genotype 4)-associated mixed cryoglobulinemia vasculitis: effects of antiviral treatment. Hepatol Int 2012;6:606–12.

9. Gragnani L, Fognani E, Piluso A, et al. Long-term effect of HCV eradication in patients with mixed cryoglobulinemia: a prospective, controlled, open-label, cohort study. Hepatology 2015;61:1145–53.

10. Giannini C, Petrarca A, Monti M, et al. Association between persistent lymphatic infection by hepatitis C virus after antiviral treatment and mixed cryoglobulinemia. Blood 2008;111:2943–5.

11. Gragnani L, Fabbrizzi A, Triboli E, et al. Triple antiviral therapy in hepatitis C virus infection with or without mixed cryoglobulinaemia: a prospective, controlled pilot study. Dig Liver Dis 2014;46:833–7.

12. Saadoun D, Resche Rigon M, Pol S, et al. PegIFNα/ribavirin/protease inhibitor combination in severe hepatitis C virus-associated mixed cryoglobulinemia vasculitis. J Hepatol 2015;62:24–30.

13. Makara M, Sulyok M, Csacsovszki O, et al. Successful treatment of HCV-associated cryoglobulinemia with ombitasvir/paritaprevir/ritonavir, dasabuvir and ribavirin: a case report. J Clin Virol 2015;72:66–8.

14. Bonacci M, Lens S, Londoño MC, et al. Virologic, clinical, and immune response outcomes of patients with hepatitis C virus-associated cryoglobulinemia treated with direct-acting antivirals. Clin Gastroenterol Hepatol 2017;15(4):575–83.e1.

15. Sise ME, Bloom AK, Wisocky J, et al. Treatment of hepatitis C virus-associated mixed cryoglobulinemia with direct-acting antiviral agents. Hepatology 2016; 63:408–17.

16. Gragnani L, Visentini M, Fognani E, et al. Prospective study of guideline-tailored therapy with direct-acting antivirals for hepatitis C virus-associated mixed cryoglobulinemia. Hepatology 2016;64:1473–82.

17. Cornella SL, Stine JG, Kelly V, et al. Persistence of mixed cryoglobulinemia despite cure of hepatitis C with new oral antiviral therapy including direct-acting antiviral sofosbuvir: a case series. Postgrad Med 2015;127:413–7.

18. Terrier B, Saadoun D, Sène D, et al. Efficacy and tolerability of rituximab with or without PEGylated interferon alfa-2b plus ribavirin in severe hepatitis C virus-related vasculitis: a long-term followup study of thirty-two patients. Arthritis Rheum 2009;60:2531–40.

19. Dammacco F, Tucci FA, Lauletta G, et al. Pegylated interferon-alpha, ribavirin, and rituximab combined therapy of hepatitis C virus-related mixed cryoglobulinemia: a long-term study. Blood 2010;116:343–53.

20. Urraro T, Gragnani L, Piluso A, et al. Combined treatment with antiviral therapy and rituximab in patients with mixed cryoglobulinemia: review of the literature and report of a case using direct antiviral agents-based antihepatitis C virus therapy. Case Reports Immunol 2015;2015:816424.

21. Kawamura Y, Ikeda K, Arase Y, et al. Viral elimination reduces incidence of malignant lymphoma in patients with hepatitis C. Am J Med 2007;120:1034–41.

22. Hermine O, Lefrère F, Bronowicki JP, et al. Regression of splenic lymphoma with villous lymphocytes after treatment of hepatitis C virus infection. N Engl J Med 2002;347:89–94.

23. Zuckerman E, Zuckerman T, Sahar D, et al. The effect of antiviral therapy on t(14;18) translocation and immunoglobulin gene rearrangement in patients with chronic hepatitis C virus infection. Blood 2001;97:1555–9.

24. Zignego AL, Ferri C, Giannelli F, et al. Prevalence of bcl-2 rearrangement in patients with hepatitis C virus-related mixed cryoglobulinemia with or without B-cell lymphomas. Ann Intern Med 2002;137:571–80.

25. Vallisa D, Bernuzzi P, Arcaini L, et al. Role of anti-hepatitis C virus (HCV) treatment in HCV-related, low-grade, B-cell, non-Hodgkin's lymphoma: a multicenter Italian experience. J Clin Oncol 2005;23:468–73.

26. Kelaidi C, Rollot F, Park S, et al. Response to antiviral treatment in hepatitis C virus-associated marginal zone lymphomas. Leukemia 2004;18:1711–6.

27. Mazzaro C, De Re V, Spina M, et al. Pegylated-interferon plus ribavirin for HCV-positive indolent non-Hodgkin lymphomas. Br J Haematol 2009;145:255–7.

28. Saadoun D, Suarez F, Lefrere F, et al. Splenic lymphoma with villous lymphocytes, associated with type II cryoglobulinemia and HCV infection: a new entity? Blood 2005;105:74–6.

29. Pellicelli AM, Marignani M, Zoli V, et al. Hepatitis C virus-related B cell subtypes in non Hodgkin's lymphoma. World J Hepatol 2011;3:278–84.

30. Arcaini L, Vallisa D, Rattotti S, et al. Antiviral treatment in patients with indolent B-cell lymphomas associated with HCV infection: a study of the Fondazione Italiana Linfomi. Ann Oncol 2014;25:1404–10.

31. Michot JM, Canioni D, Driss H, et al. Antiviral therapy is associated with a better survival in patients with hepatitis C virus and B-cell non-Hodgkin lymphomas, ANRS HC-13 lympho-C study. Am J Hematol 2015;90:197–203.

32. La Mura V, De Renzo A, Perna F, et al. Antiviral therapy after complete response to chemotherapy could be efficacious in HCV-positive non-Hodgkin's lymphoma. J Hepatol 2008;49:557–63.

33. Hosry J, Mahale P, Turturro F, et al. Antiviral therapy improves overall survival in hepatitis C virus infected patients who develop diffuse large B-cell lymphoma. Int J Cancer 2016;139:2519–28.

34. Rossotti R, Travi G, Pazzi A, et al. Rapid clearance of HCV-related splenic marginal zone lymphoma under an interferon-free, NS3/NS4A inhibitor-based treatment. A case report. J Hepatol 2015;62:234–7.

35. Carrier P, Jaccard A, Jacques J, et al. HCV-associated B-cell non-Hodgkin lymphomas and new direct antiviral agents. Liver Int 2015;35:2222–7.

36. Arcaini L, Besson C, Frigeni M, et al. Interferon-free antiviral treatment in B-cell lymphoproliferative disorders associated with hepatitis C virus infection. Blood 2016;128:2527–32.

37. Alric L, Plaisiser E, Thébault S, et al. Influence of antiviral therapy in hepatitis C virus-associated cryoglobulinemic MPGN. Am J Kidney Dis 2004;43:617–23.

38. Saadoun D, Thibault V, Si Ahmed SN, et al. Sofosbuvir plus ribavirin for hepatitis C virus-associated cryoglobulinaemia vasculitis: VASCUVALDIC study. Ann Rheum Dis 2016;75:1777–82.

39. Desnoyer A, Pospai D, Lê MP, et al. Pharmacokinetics, safety and efficacy of a full dose sofosbuvir-based regimen given daily in hemodialysis patients with chronic hepatitis C. J Hepatol 2016;65:40–7.

40. De Nicola S, Aghemo A. The quest for safe and effective treatments of chronic hepatitis C in patients with kidney impairment. Liver Int 2016;36:791–3.

41. Saxena V, Koraishy FM, Sise ME, et al. Safety and efficacy of sofosbuvir-containing regimens in hepatitis C-infected patients with impaired renal function. Liver Int 2016;36:807–16.

42. European Association for the Study of the Liver. EASL recommendations on treatment of hepatitis C 2016. J Hepatol 2017;66(1):153–94.

43. Pockros PJ, Reddy KR, Mantry PS, et al. Efficacy of direct-acting antiviral combination for patients with hepatitis C virus genotype 1 infection and severe renal impairment or end-stage renal disease. Gastroenterology 2016;150:1590–8.

44. Roth D, Nelson DR, Bruchfeld A, et al. Grazoprevir plus elbasvir in treatment-naive and treatment-experienced patients with hepatitis C virus genotype 1 infection and stage 4-5 chronic kidney disease (the C-SURFER study): a combination phase 3 study. Lancet 2015;386:1537–45.
45. Gane E, Lawitz E, Pugatch D, et al. EXPEDITION-4: efficacy and safety of Glecaprevir/Pibrentasvir (ABT-493/ABT-530) in patients with renal impairment and chronic hepatitis C virus genotype 1-6 infection. Abstract presented at the AASLD Liver Meeting 2016.
46. Colombo M, Aghemo A, Liu H, et al. Treatment with ledipasvir-sofosbuvir for 12 or 24 weeks in kidney transplant recipients with chronic hepatitis C virus genotype 1 or 4 infection: a randomized trial. Ann Intern Med 2017;166(2):109–17.
47. Romero-Gómez M, Fernández-Rodríguez CM, Andrade RJ, et al. Effect of sustained virological response to treatment on the incidence of abnormal glucose values in chronic hepatitis C. J Hepatol 2008;48:721–7.
48. Arase Y, Suzuki F, Suzuki Y, et al. Sustained virological response reduces incidence of onset of type 2 diabetes in chronic hepatitis C. Hepatology 2009;49: 739–44.
49. Aghemo A, Prati GM, Rumi MG, et al. Sustained virological response prevents the development of insulin resistance in patients with chronic hepatitis C. Hepatology 2012;56:1681–7.
50. Hsu YC, Lin JT, Ho HJ, et al. Antiviral treatment for hepatitis C virus infection is associated with improved renal and cardiovascular outcomes in diabetic patients. Hepatology 2014;59:1293–302.
51. Younossi Z, Park H, Henry L, et al. Extrahepatic manifestations of hepatitis C: a meta-analysis of prevalence, quality of life, and economic burden. Gastroenterology 2016;150:1599–608.
52. Sarkar S, Jiang Z, Evon DM, et al. Fatigue before, during and after antiviral therapy of chronic hepatitis C: results from the Virahep-C study. J Hepatol 2012;57: 946–52.
53. Spiegel BM, Younossi ZM, Hays RD, et al. Impact of hepatitis C on health related quality of life: a systematic review and quantitative assessment. Hepatology 2005;41:790–800.
54. Kraus MR, Schäfer A, Wissmann S, et al. Neurocognitive changes in patients with hepatitis C receiving interferon alfa-2b and ribavirin. Clin Pharmacol Ther 2005; 77:90–100.
55. Thein HH, Maruff P, Krahn MD, et al. Improved cognitive function as a consequence of hepatitis C virus treatment. HIV Med 2007;8:520–8.
56. Byrnes V, Miller A, Lowry D, et al. Effects of anti-viral therapy and HCV clearance on cerebral metabolism and cognition. J Hepatol 2012;56:549–56.
57. Nagao Y, Kawaguchi T, Ide T, et al. Exacerbation of oral erosive lichen planus by combination of interferon and ribavirin therapy for chronic hepatitis C. Int J Mol Med 2005;15:237–41.
58. Doutre MS, Beylot C, Couzigou P, et al. Lichen planus and virus C hepatitis: disappearance of the lichen under interferon alfa therapy. Dermatology 1992; 184:229.
59. Nagao Y, Kimura K, Kawahigashi Y, et al. Successful treatment of hepatitis C virus-associated oral lichen planus by interferon-free therapy with direct-acting antivirals. Clin Transl Gastroenterol 2016;7:e179.

Moving?

Make sure your subscription moves with you!

To notify us of your new address, find your **Clinics Account Number** (located on your mailing label above your name), and contact customer service at:

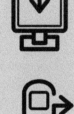

Email: **journalscustomerservice-usa@elsevier.com**

800-654-2452 (subscribers in the U.S. & Canada)
314-447-8871 (subscribers outside of the U.S. & Canada)

Fax number: **314-447-8029**

Elsevier Health Sciences Division
Subscription Customer Service
3251 Riverport Lane
Maryland Heights, MO 63043

*To ensure uninterrupted delivery of your subscription, please notify us at least 4 weeks in advance of move.

Printed and bound by CPI Group (UK) Ltd, Croydon, CR0 4YY

03/10/2024

01040495-0020